Lecture Notes in Biomathematics

Vol. 1: P. Waltman, Deterministic Threshold Models in the Theory of Epidemics. V, 101 pages. 1974.

Vol. 2: Mathematical Problems in Biology, Victoria Conference 1973. Edited by P. van den Driessche. VI, 280 pages. 1974.

Vol. 3: D. Ludwig, Stochastic Population Theories. VI, 108 pages. 1974.

Vol. 4: Physics and Mathematics of the Nervous System. Edited by M. Conrad, W. Güttinger, and M. Dal Cin. XI, 584 pages. 1974.

Vol. 5: Mathematical Analysis of Decision Problems in Ecology. Proceedings 1973. Edited by A. Charnes and W.R. Lynn. VIII, 421 pages. 1975.

Vol. 6: H.T. Banks, Modeling and Control in the Biomedical Sciences. V. 114 pages. 1975.

Vol. 7: M.C. Mackey, Ion Transport through Biological Membranes, An Integrated Theoretical Approach. IX, 240 pages. 1975.

Vol. 8: C. DeLisi, Antigen Antibody Interactions. IV, 142 pages. 1976.

Vol. 9: N. Dubin, A Stochastic Model for Immunological Feedback in Carcinogenesis: Analysis and Approximations. XIII, 163 pages. 1976.

Vol. 10: J.J. Tyson, The Belousov-Zhabotinskii Reaktion. IX, 128 pages. 1976.

Vol. 11: Mathematical Models in Medicine. Workshop 1976. Edited by J. Berger, W. Bühler, R. Repges, and P. Tautu. XII, 281 pages. 1976.

Vol. 12: A.V. Holden, Models of the Stochastic Activity of Neurones. VII, 368 pages. 1976.

Vol. 13: Mathematical Models in Biological Discovery. Edited by D.L. Solomon and C. Walter. VI, 240 pages. 1977.

Vol. 14: L.M. Ricciardi, Diffusion Processes and Related Topics in Biology. VI, 200 pages. 1977.

Vol. 15: Th. Nagylaki, Selection in One- and Two-Locus Systems. VIII, 208 pages. 1977.

Vol. 16: G. Sampath, S.K. Srinivasan, Stochastic Models for Spike Trains of Single Neurons. VIII, 188 pages. 1977.

Vol. 17: T. Maruyama, Stochastic Problems in Population Genetics. VIII, 245 pages. 1977.

Vol. 18: Mathematics and the Life Sciences. Proceedings 1975. Edited by D.E. Matthews. VII, 385 pages. 1977.

Vol. 19: Measuring Selection in Natural Populations. Edited by F.B. Christiansen and T.M. Fenchel. XXXI, 564 pages. 1977.

Vol. 20: J.M. Cushing, Integrodifferential Equations and Delay Models in Population Dynamics. VI, 196 pages. 1977.

Vol. 21: Theoretical Approaches to Complex Systems. Proceedings 1977. Edited by R. Heim and G. Palm. VI, 244 pages. 1978.

Vol. 22: F.M. Scudo and J.R. Ziegler, The Golden Age of Theoretical Ecology: 1923–1940. XII, 490 pages. 1978.

Vol. 23: Geometrical Probability and Biological Structures: Buffon's 200th Anniversary. Proceedings 1977. Edited by R.E. Miles and J. Serra. XII, 338 pages. 1978.

Vol. 24: F.L. Bookstein, The Measurement of Biological Shape and Shape Change. VIII, 191 pages. 1978.

Vol. 25: P. Yodzis, Competition for Space and the Structure of Ecological Communities. VI, 191 pages. 1978.

Vol. 26: M.B Katz, Questions of Uniqueness and Resolution in Reconstruction from Projections. IX, 175 pages. 1978.

Vol. 27: N. MacDonald, Time Lags in Biological Models. VII, 112 pages. 1978.

Vol. 28: P.C. Fife, Mathematical Aspects of Reacting and Diffusing Systems. IV, 185 pages. 1979.

Vol. 29: Kinetic Logic – A Boolean Approach to the Analysis of Complex Regulatory Systems. Proceedings, 1977. Edited by R. Thomas. XIII, 507 pages. 1979.

Vol. 30: M. Eisen, Mathematical Models in Cell Biology and Cancer Chemotherapy. IX, 431 pages. 1979.

Vol. 31: E. Akin, The Geometry of Population Genetics. IV, 205 pages. 1979.

Vol. 32: Systems Theory in Immunology. Proceedings, 1978. Edited by G. Bruni et al. XI, 273 pages. 1979.

Vol. 33: Mathematical Modelling in Biology and Ecology. Proceedings, 1979. Edited by W.M. Getz. VIII, 355 pages. 1980.

Vol. 34: R. Collins, T.J. van der Werff, Mathematical Models of the Dynamics of the Human Eye. VII, 99 pages. 1980.

Vol. 35: U. an der Heiden, Analysis of Neural Networks. X, 159 pages. 1980.

Vol. 36: A. Wörz-Busekros, Algebras in Genetics. VI, 237 pages. 1980.

Vol. 37: T. Ohta, Evolution and Variation of Multigene Families. VIII, 131 pages. 1980.

Vol. 38: Biological Growth and Spread: Mathematical Theories and Applications. Proceedings, 1979. Edited by W. Jäger, H. Rost and P. Tautu. XI, 511 pages. 1980.

Vol. 39: Vito Volterra Symposium on Mathematical Models in Biology. Proceedings, 1979. Edited by C. Barigozzi. VI, 417 pages. 1980.

Vol. 40: Renewable Resource Management. Proceedings, 1980. Edited by T. Vincent and J. Skowronski. XII, 236 pages. 1981.

Vol. 41: Modèles Mathématiques en Biologie. Proceedings, 1978. Edited by C. Chevalet and A. Micali. XIV, 219 pages. 1981.

Vol. 42: G.W. Swan, Optimization of Human Cancer Radiotherapy. VIII, 282 pages. 1981.

Vol. 43: Mathematical Modeling on the Hearing Process. Proceedings, 1980. Edited by M.H. Holmes and L.A. Rubenfeld. V, 104 pages. 1981.

Vol. 44: Recognition of Pattern and Form. Proceedings, 1979. Edited by D.G. Albrecht. III, 226 pages. 1982.

Vol. 45: Competition and Cooperation in Neutral Nets. Proceedings, 1982. Edited by S. Amari and M.A. Arbib. XIV, 441 pages. 1982.

Vol. 46: E. Walter, Identifiability of State Space Models with applications to transformation systems. VIII, 202 pages. 1982.

Vol. 47: E. Frehland, Stochastic Transport Processes in Discrete Biological Systems. VIII, 169 pages. 1982.

Vol. 48: Tracer Kinetics and Physiologic Modeling. Proceedings, 1983. Edited by R.M. Lambrecht and A. Rescigno. VIII, 509 pages. 1983.

Vol. 49: Rhythms in Biology and Other Fields of Application. Proceedings, 1981. Edited by M. Cosnard, J. Demongeot and A. Le Breton. VII, 400 pages. 1983.

Vol. 50: D.H. Anderson, Compartmental Modeling and Tracer Kinetics. VII, 302 pages. 1983.

Vol. 51: Oscillations in Mathematical Biology. Proceedings, 1982. Edited by J.P.E. Hodgson. VI, 196 pages. 1983.

Vol. 52: Population Biology. Proceedings, 1982. Edited by H.I. Freedman and C. Strobeck. XVII, 440 pages. 1983.

Vol. 53: Evolutionary Dynamics of Genetic Diversity. Proceedings, 1983. Edited by G.S. Mani. VII, 312 pages. 1984.

Vol. 54: Mathematical Ecology. Proceedings, 1982. Edited by S.A. Levin and T.G. Hallam. XII, 513 pages. 1984.

Vol. 55: Modelling of Patterns in Space and Time. Proceedings, 1983. Edited by W. Jäger and J.D. Murray. VIII, 405 pages. 1984.

Vol. 56: H.W. Hethcote, J.A. Yorke, Gonorrhea Transmission Dynamics and Control. IX, 105 pages. 1984.

Vol. 57: Mathematics in Biology and Medicine. Proceedings, 1983. Edited by V. Capasso, E. Grosso and S.L. Paveri-Fontana. XVIII, 524 pages. 1985.

ctd. on inside back cover

Lecture Notes in Biomathematics

Managing Editor: S. Levin

83

C. Castillo-Chavez (Ed.)

Mathematical and Statistical Approaches to AIDS Epidemiology

Springer-Verlag Berlin Heidelberg GmbH

Editor

Carlos Castillo-Chavez
Biometrics Unit
Cornell University
Ithaca, NY 14853, USA

Mathematics Subject Classification (1980): 92A07, 92A15

DOI 10.1007/978-3-642-93454-4

Originally published by Springer-Verlag Berlin Heidelberg New York in 1989
MyCopy version of the original edition 1989

2146/3140-543210 – Printed on acid-free paper
www.springer.com/mycopy

Dedicated to the memory of

Sir Ronald Ross

TABLE OF CONTENTS

III. Heterogeneity and HIV Transmission Dynamics

IV. Social Dynamics and AIDS

V. The Immune System and the HIV

Foreword

Human immunodeficiency virus (HIV) disease has become one of the major public health problems in both developed and developing nations. Although the virus, HIV, has existed in humans for at least three decades, it was not recognized as a significant health problem in any country until 1981. All forecasts indicate that the current grim statistics of the number ill and dead worldwide will continue to increase for years. In many areas, health care facilities already are inadequate or barely adequate to care for those with HIV disease. The effect on society is magnified because those who become ill are relatively young, at an age when they should be making their greatest contributions to society. In some areas, children infected with HIV add substantially to infant or childhood mortality.

Though recognition of AIDS is recent, and the discovery of its causative agent, HIV, even more recent, there is an unprecedented need for understanding the scope of the problem. The severity of the clinical illness, the transmissibility of the agent, and our inability to comprehend fully and quantify the behaviors that transmit HIV throughout the world's diverse populations have resulted in a need for theoretical modeling of HIV transmission and progression in various populations. Analyses of theoretical models can assist our understanding of the long (and variable) progression rate of HIV infection to frank disease and death, as well as social and biological variables affecting transmission rates in different populations. Mathematicians and statisticians, working closely with epidemiologists and clinical researchers, can develop models to assess the potential (and actual) impact of therapeutic interventions and prevention measures.

This volume reflects many of the contributions that statisticians and mathematicians have made to our understanding of HIV disease. Mathematical modelers have obtained important insights on how the spread of HIV through a population can be affected by social mixing patterns. Examples of how modeling can lead to greater understanding of the natural history of HIV disease include modeling the human immune system, estimating the infectivity of HIV for different types of sexual contact and at different times during the course of disease, and estimating the distribution of the latency period. Finally, statisticians have made useful short-term forecasts of the future numbers of AIDS cases, as an aid to public health planning; one forecasting method is described here.

Modeling efforts are useful *per se* in organizing information, in stimulating explicit statements of assumptions, and in providing guidance on what additional data are critically needed from epidemiological and behavioral studies. Modeling also is helpful in estimating and reducing the range of uncertainty concerning various aspects of the challenges posed by HIV disease. For example, good transmission models would greatly assist the theoretical evaluation of education and prevention programs. Improved procedures to predict future numbers of AIDS cases and of people with less serious HIV disease are needed to aid in health care and public health planning. Epidemiologists, medical researchers, and public health officials look forward to important contributions from statistical and mathematical modelers in understanding HIV disease and in guiding public health policy during the coming years.

James W. Curran
Director for Division of HIV-AIDS
Centers for Disease Control
Atlanta, Georgia, U.S.A.

Acknowledgements

The experience of putting together this volume has been extremely stimulating. I would like to express my gratitude to Heather Crawford and Catherine Den Tandt, my editorial assistants, for their oustanding work, and Pam Archin and Norma Phalen, for secretarial support. I am grateful for the moral and financial support of the Biometrics Unit, and particularly recognize the efforts of my chairman, C. E. McCulloch.

I owe a debt of gratitude to the expert scientists who reviewed the manuscripts included in this volume. I also acknowledge the support of the National Science Foundation and the National Institute of Allergy and Infectious Diseases.

I owe deep appreciation to my colleague, Simon A. Levin, for his comments, criticisms, and friendship. And always, above all, my deep gratitude to Debbie Castillo for her help, love, and understanding.

Carlos Castillo-Chavez
Ithaca, N. Y.

Introduction

STATISTICAL AND MATHEMATICAL APPROACHES IN HIV/AIDS MODELING: A REVIEW

Steven J. Schwager
Biometrics Unit
337 Warren Hall
Cornell University
Ithaca, NY 14853-7801
U.S.A.

Carlos Castillo-Chavez
Biometrics Unit/Center for Applied Math.
341 Warren Hall
Cornell University
Ithaca, NY 14853-7801
U.S.A.

Herbert Hethcote
Dept. of Mathematics
University of Iowa
Iowa City, Iowa 52242
U.S.A.

Abstract

This paper provides a brief introduction to the field and the literature of statistical and mathematical approaches to HIV/AIDS modeling. The emphasis is on succinct description of the methodology and on discussion of the work of some researchers who were unable to contribute to this volume. This review is not complete; however, it is complemented to a great degree by the partial reviews of the literature provided by several authors in their contributions to this volume. An additional objective of this introductory chapter is to describe to nonspecialists, in general terms, some of the main statistical and mathematical approaches currently used in problems related to AIDS epidemiology.

1. Introduction

Mathematical models are an important tool in the study of the transmission of human immunodeficiency virus (HIV), the etiological agent for acquired immune deficiency syndrome (AIDS). These models are useful in furthering our understanding of many aspects of HIV dynamics such as short- and long-term prediction of HIV (and AIDS) incidence, the effects of behavioral changes and preventive measures on its transmission dynamics, its effects on demographic parameters, and the results of its direct interaction with the immune system. Reviews of mathematical models for the transmission of HIV and AIDS were given by Isham (1988) and Anderson (1988b). Statistical issues arise in the analysis of these mathematical models, especially in the drawing of inferences from real data, either in the generation of predictions or in the estimation of key parameters. It is thus natural that statistical methodology plays an important role in research on HIV/AIDS. An annotated bibliography of quantitative methodology related to HIV/AIDS was given by Fusaro *et al.* (1989). It emphasized mathematical and statistical models of the magnitude of the AIDS epidemic, and statistical techniques for estimating key aspects of the disease process.

Statistics attempts to discover the underlying structure of a process from observed data in the presence of random variability. Statistical techniques have been developed to accomplish several tasks addressing this objective. Estimation is perhaps the best known of these. There are two standard approaches, parametric and nonparametric estimation.

Parametric estimation proceeds from the assumption that the distributional form of a randomly varying quantity, or random variable, is known. A particular distribution of this form is determined by the value of a parameter, consisting of one or more quantities associated with the distributional form. For example, an incubation time may be known (or assumed) to have a gamma distribution, with probability density function $f(x;r,\lambda) = \lambda^r \Gamma(r)^{-1} x^{r-1} e^{-\lambda x}$ for $x > 0$; the parameter is the vector (r,λ), which completely determines one member of this family. Estimation procedures seek to determine a single value (point estimate), or a range of values (confidence interval or region), representing our best judgment about the true value of the unknown parameter. Several standard methods of estimation have been developed, including maximum likelihood and least squares, each with properties that make it a good choice under certain circumstances. Maximum likelihood estimators, or MLEs, are the most commonly used because of their desirable theoretical properties: under broad regularity conditions, MLEs are consistent, asymptotically normal, and asymptotically efficient. It may be that only some, but not all, of the components of the parameter are of primary importance; the rest are then called nuisance parameters. Another possibility is that a function of the parameters, such as r/λ, is of special interest, perhaps because of its epidemiological interpretation. Both of these situations can be handled by appropriate estimation techniques. A general treatment of parametric estimation has been given by Mood, Graybill, and Boes (1974); a fuller treatment of parametric point estimation has been given by Lehmann (1983).

Nonparametric estimation, in contrast, seeks to obtain results when the distributional form of a random variable is not known. Nonparametric estimation methods must therefore perform well over a broad range of distributional forms. For example, we may want to estimate the mean of a distribution whose form cannot be specified because we lack sufficient information. This is inherently more difficult than parametric estimation because of the greater generality of the problem: many families of distributional forms may be consistent with the observed data, and nonparametric estimates must be appropriate for this whole range of families. Nonparametric estimation has been treated by Conover (1980) and Lehmann (1975).

There is an intermediate approach, semiparametric estimation, in which the unknowns include both parameters and functions. The parameters in the model are usually of primary interest, with the unknown function(s) serving as extremely flexible nuisance parameter(s). The proportional hazards model (Cox 1972) is a semiparametric model useful in AIDS and other epidemiological research.

It is important to distinguish between estimation of a parameter or other quantity associated with a distribution and estimation of the distribution itself. For example, the distribution of incubation times or reporting lags of AIDS cases may carry important information not retained by the mean and variance of this distribution. Distributions can be estimated by both parametric and nonparametric approaches. Parametric estimation of the distribution is closely related to testing distributional goodness of fit. This will be discussed shortly. Nonparametric density estimation techniques have developed along several lines. The most commonly used is the smoothing kernel approach, which spreads the atom of probability mass of each observation continuously across a neighborhood of its location. Splines and other methods have also been used. Details can be found in Silverman (1986) and Eubank (1988).

The testing of hypotheses is another major statistical activity related to mathematical modeling, as it seeks to determine whether observed data are consistent with proposed hypotheses about the underlying mechanism. In the usual testing formulation, we specify a null hypothesis H_0 of "no difference" or "no effect" and an opposing alternative hypothesis H_1. Then we compute a test statistic that quantifies the strength of the evidence in the observed data against the null hypothesis. For example, a null hypothesis might claim that the mean length of the incubation time does not differ for various routes of exposure to HIV; the alternative hypothesis might be very broad, e.g., that there are some differences among routes, or more narrow, e.g., that routes of exposure differ in a highly specified pattern (mean incubation time – latent period plus asymptomatic infectious period – is greater for sexual contact than for blood transfusion, greater for blood transfusion than for IV drug use, and so on), as suggested by the researcher's knowledge of the process. Statistical methodology for hypothesis testing is well developed, although there are still many specialized questions that need further investigation. For details, see Mood, Graybill, and Boes (1974) and Lehmann (1986).

An important class of hypothesis tests deals with the question of whether or not an observed set of data is consistent with a specified distribution. This class of procedures, called goodness-of-fit tests, can be illustrated by considering a test of the null hypothesis H_0: data came from a gamma population with (r,λ) unknown. The alternative hypothesis may be either very general, e.g., H_1: data came from other than a gamma population, or more specific, e.g., H_1: data came from a contaminated gamma population, or H_1: data came from a mixture of gamma distributions. Some or all of the parameter values may be known in either the null or the alternative hypothesis, or both.

Predictions of the future course of the AIDS epidemic provide important information for public policy formulation. Anderson (1988a) listed several key questions for government and health planners, i.e., the likely magnitude of the epidemic and the level of change in the population's sexual behavior needed to affect this magnitude. Various aspects of the disease are of interest, i.e., the prevalence and incidence of HIV infection, the number of AIDS cases, and the number of deaths of patients diagnosed as having AIDS. We need estimates of the future values of these and other aspects of the epidemic. With sufficient data, short-term predictions for 1-3 years into the future can be made with reasonable accuracy. Prediction over a longer period (using statistical approaches) appears to be much more difficult owing to the greater uncertainties involved. At present, transmission models may provide us with the best approach to the generation of mid- to long-term predictions. Three approaches have been applied to prediction of various features of the course of HIV and AIDS: direct extrapolation of the recent data by empirical curve fitting; the back-calculation approach, which combines AIDS incidence data with an estimate of the incubation period to obtain an estimate of the pattern of HIV seroincidence over time, leading to extrapolations for future levels of HIV seroprevalence and AIDS incidence; and dynamic transmission models, based on systems of differential or difference equations quantifying the rates of transition between disease states, including susceptible, infected by HIV, and diagnosed as having AIDS. These will be discussed in detail below. Many aspects of short-term prediction of HIV infection and AIDS were treated in the report of the British Working Group chaired by Cox (Working Group 1988, see Chapters 3, 4, Appendices 3, 6).

The main body of this paper is organized as follows. Section 2 describes some special difficulties that occur in the analysis of AIDS data. Section 3 discusses the short-term prediction of various aspects of the HIV/AIDS epidemic. Section 4 treats the estimation of epidemiological parameters and distributions. Section 5 briefly reviews some of the literature on dynamic models for HIV/AIDS. We do not review the literature on models for the immune system; however, relevant references can be found in the articles by Perelson (1989), Merrill (1989), Hoffman and Grant (1989), and Layne *et al.* (1989) in this volume, and in the recent work of Anderson and May (1989).

2. Special problems of AIDS data analysis

Several special problems must be dealt with in the analysis of data on HIV infection and AIDS. These are rooted in the current state of knowledge about the disease and its modes of transmission. Many aspects of the biological mechanism underlying the disease and of the social and behavioral processes through which HIV and AIDS are spread are not well understood. As can be seen from the articles in this volume, researchers have begun to identify these mechanisms through the use of dynamical systems. Nevertheless, until further progress is made in these areas, statistical methodology must be applied in the presence of fundamental uncertainties, making analysis considerably more difficult. Not surprisingly, the interplay between dynamic models of disease transmission and statistical analysis is playing a leading role in elucidating the unknown aspects of the disease and its transmission mechanisms.

There are substantial difficulties related to the availability and quality of AIDS data suitable for statistical analysis. The report of a workshop on modeling AIDS epidemiology (Workshop 1988, Sec. 4) discussed data availability and quality and made recommendations about meeting the data needs of AIDS research. A statement by the Royal Statistical Society (1988) on data requirements and collection addressed the same issues. Layne *et al.* (1988) suggested that governments should establish national HIV databases for the use of researchers and public health officials. Data come from sample surveys which seek to determine specified features of a chosen population and from the operation of health organizations such as hospitals. The population of interest may be national, regional, or local, and the sample may range from a carefully designed probability sample to a convenience sample or a group of volunteers. The workshop report noted the need for national representative data on HIV prevalence, HIV and AIDS incidence, and prevalence of risk behaviors and size of risk groups. The collection of such data is complicated by numerous problems that make many important epidemiological parameters extremely difficult to estimate. Several of these problems will now be mentioned; the need to develop methods for overcoming them is urgent.

Parameters like the average incubation period of AIDS, duration of infectiousness, and time to death of AIDS patients involve long periods of time. The lengths of some of these periods are much greater than can be satisfactorily estimated from the eight years of observational data currently available. (State and local health officials in the U.S. have been reporting AIDS cases to the CDC since 1981, and the definition of AIDS has changed over the course of the epidemic.) Until data have accumulated over a longer interval, providing observations close to the upper extremes of the incubation period and other periods of interest, analysis will inevitably be incomplete and inaccurate. Medley *et al.* (1987, 1988), using data on transfusion-associated cases of AIDS in the U.S., noted the strong dependence of the estimated average incubation period of AIDS on the parametric model chosen and judged their work on characterizing the incubation period as "tentative until more of the incubation period is observed."

Reporting of AIDS cases often involves a time lag between the diagnosis and the receipt of the report by the central public health agency (the Centers for Disease Control in the U.S.A., the Communicable Disease Surveillance Centre in the United Kingdom, etc.). This lag can range from a few weeks to 1-2 years. Anderson (1988b, p.242) described the lag as "increasing and variable," and Harris (1987) said that the distribution of delays has been shifting to the right, with median delay up 0.6 months from mid-1986 to March 1987. The British report, however, hedged (Working Group 1988, p.31), and its Appendix 8 tends weakly to support the opposite view.

Underreporting of AIDS cases is also a major concern. This may stem either from failure to diagnose a case or from failure to report a case that has been diagnosed. One aspect of this is self-selection bias in the medical observation process: many patients who are at high risk choose to avoid diagnosis and treatment, and thus remain undetected. This often occurs even when HIV antibody testing has been completed; see McCusker *et al.* (1988) and Lyter *et al.* (1987).

A related issue is the presence of cases that do not satisfy the clinical criteria of AIDS (which have evolved over time) but whose condition is influenced by HIV infection. Some individuals may not develop "full-blown" AIDS but may nevertheless die as a result of HIV infection, perhaps indirectly; some physicians have reported seeing about three times as many cases of non-AIDS HIV-associated illness as cases of AIDS (Working Group 1988, p.37).

Incomplete data can arise in numerous ways. There can be a failure to collect information that subsequently turns out to be necessary for analysis. The attempt to collect information can result in missing values, for example, laboratory measurements not made or questions not answered by the patient. Patients can (and often do) drop out of clinical trials and other observational studies prematurely.

The quality of data can be adversely affected by biases of several kinds. The self-selection bias described above and other refusals by patients at risk for HIV infection and AIDS to provide information are forms of nonresponse bias. Another possibility is the misreporting, either accidentally or intentionally, of medical and behavioral information. This response bias has many causes, ranging from the phrasing of questions (Schuman and Presser 1981) to some respondents' selecting answers to gain social approval (Bradburn 1983). Fox and Tracy (1984) cited many examples of both response and nonresponse bias on sensitive questions.

The behavioral and sociological processes related to the spread of AIDS must be addressed. Some work of this kind has been done. Baldwin and Baldwin (1988) studied factors associated with AIDS-related sexual high-risk behavior among Southern California college students. McCusker *et al.* (1988) reported that HIV antibody testing reduced the level of sexual activity of a group of homosexuals in Boston. Johnson (1988) reviewed research on sexual and drug-use behavior in the population and considered future research on the social determinants and prevention of HIV transmission. Kaplan *et al.* (1987) surveyed the sociological literature on AIDS and suggested a research agenda based on models for the social factors related to the onset and the course of AIDS. In this volume, Aron and Sarma (1989) use behavioral data from a 1988 U.S. survey on sexual partners to examine the risk of HIV spread in the population.

The profile of HIV infection and AIDS incidence is changing over time. Anderson (1988b, p.242) cited "the changing shape of the epidemic as saturation effects occur and the infection moves from high-risk group into the general population" as one of the two major problems with exponential extrapolation. The behavioral patterns of high-risk activity in the population are evolving, partially in reaction to the epidemic. Estimation under these conditions is an attempt to hit a moving, rather than a stationary, target.

A final complicating factor is the recent modification in the clinical definition of AIDS. For full details, see Centers for Disease Control (1987); Karon *et al.* (1988) summarized the changes. The classification of a patient as having or not having AIDS is consequently time-dependent; two identical patient histories, one before and one after the change, could result in different diagnoses. This problem affects many aspects of the statistical analysis of data on HIV infection and AIDS.

If mathematical models of the AIDS epidemic are to provide reliable results, they must factor in the limitations of the data in sample size and accuracy of observed values. In this volume, De Gruttola and Lagakos (1989b) examine how these limitations can affect the uncertainty of estimation using models.

3. Short-term Prediction of HIV Infection and AIDS

Three approaches that have been applied to forecasting the course of the AIDS epidemic are direct extrapolation (see Morgan and Curran 1986; Karon *et al.* 1989; and references therein), back-calculation (see Brookmeyer and Gail 1986, 1988; Brookmeyer and Damiano 1989; Colgate *et al.* 1989; and references therein), and dynamic transmission models (see Anderson 1988b and references therein). These have been used to predict the prevalence of HIV infection, the incidence of new cases of AIDS, and the number of deaths associated with HIV and AIDS. These methods require data on the quantity of interest over at least the past few time periods. Information about a greater number of time periods allows for more accurate analysis; for example, it helps in choosing which mathematical function to use in the extrapolation approach. Data on the values of related quantities are needed in the back-calculation and dynamic transmission model approaches. Partitioning the population into subgroups, analyzing each of these separately, and then combining the resulting predictions into an overall population prediction is often effective when the available data make this possible.

Prediction involves four broad kinds of errors: model errors, caused by inadequacy of the model in representing the actual process; shift errors, caused by future changes in the nature of the process; estimation errors, caused by the estimation of the unknown parameters in a specified prediction model; and random errors or statistical fluctuations, caused by the variability present in any stochastic process even when model and estimation errors do not occur (Gilchrist 1983). The transmission models described in Section 5 provide a framework that can be used to generate short- and mid-term predictions for HIV and AIDS seroincidence, and therefore will not be discussed in this section. We proceed with the description of the extrapolation and back-calculation approaches.

3.1. Direct Extrapolation

The direct extrapolation approach involves extending a chosen mathematical function into the future. It is based on the assumption that the observed trend will continue into the future. A specified family of functions consistent with the observed data is selected, for example, the exponential (a exp(bt)), the logistic (1/[1 + a exp(-bt)]), or the damped exponential (a exp(bt^c)). The parameters are estimated from past data, usually by the method of weighted nonlinear least squares, and the resulting curve provides estimated future values. These estimated values may be modified to reflect reporting delays, underreporting, and other difficulties mentioned earlier. A commonly used technique for obtaining overall population estimates is to divide the population into subgroups, analyze each separately, and amalgamate the results. This kind of extrapolation, or trend analysis, gives reasonably accurate estimates for 1-3 years into the future when based on sufficient data. Such estimates are critical to our understanding of the course of the disease in the short run, since it is on this basis that current policy decisions must be made.

Extrapolation is used by the CDC for short-term projections of AIDS case incidence in the U.S. Details were given by Karon *et al.* (1988) who estimated that 365,000 AIDS cases will be diagnosed in the U.S. by 1992, with a 68% prediction interval of 205,000 to 440,000 cases. Healy and Tillett (1988) extrapolated monthly figures to the end of 1986 to estimate the number of AIDS cases in the U.K. two years into the future using several different model assumptions. Both normal and Poisson error models resulted in a roughly exponential rate of increase, with doubling time of about 14 months having remained nearly constant since mid-1985. Downs *et al.* (1987) fitted exponential functions to European AIDS surveillance data after adjusting reported case numbers through June 1986 for the estimated delays between diagnosis and report (but not for under-reporting). They estimated a wide range of doubling times (4.3 to 17.7 months) and predicted numbers of AIDS cases through mid-1988 for various European countries. In Morgan and Curran (1986), a quadratic polynomial was fitted, using weighted linear regression, to adjusted AIDS case counts transformed by the modified Box-Cox method. The resulting polynomial was extrapolated to 1991. In this volume, Karon *et al.* (1989) base their projections on the Box-Cox procedure, modeling the proportions of AIDS cases in population subgroups over time.

The extrapolation approach, although relatively straightforward to apply, has several important drawbacks; some are related to its simplicity. It is unlikely to give realistic results beyond a few years into the future, since it takes into account neither the changing pattern of the epidemic as high-risk groups become saturated and the infection expands into the general population (Anderson 1988b, p.242) nor changes in the behavior of the population. Moreover, the extrapolation method provides very little understanding of the epidemiological processes involved in HIV and AIDS, not being based on biological or behavioral mechanisms. Thus, it cannot be used to predict the effects of biological, behavioral, or social changes in the population or any of its subgroups. Nevertheless, it is useful insofar as it provides those who must make policy decisions with a baseline on which to plan for the immediate future.

Choosing the mathematical function to fit historical data is complicated by the agreement of many different functional forms with the data (see DeGruttola and Lagakos 1989, in this volume); these forms can produce very different predictions over even a short time period. The fit to the data can be improved by increasing the number of parameters in the chosen mathematical function, but this improved fit may actually decrease the predictive power of the model (Workshop 1989, p. 10). When subgroups within the population are considered separately and then amalgamated, lack of accurate knowledge of the sizes of high-risk subgroups, such as homosexuals, IV drug users, and prostitutes, can lead to difficulties.

In the Working Group (1988) report on short-term prediction of HIV infection and AIDS in England and Wales, direct extrapolation was used to estimate the prevalence of HIV infection and the incidence of new cases of AIDS. In the discussion of new cases of AIDS, several different mathematical functions were examined, including the exponential, the quadratic exponential, and the linear logistic. All three of these functional forms were consistent with historical data; however, this was not surprising as the abundance of parameters makes this historical agreement easy to achieve. We note, though, that the exponential produced a 1992 estimate nearly five times as great as the other two functions. The transmission models to be discussed in Section 3.3 provide us with a systematic approach for the evaluation of parametric models.

3.2. Back-calculation

The back-calculation, or back-projection, approach combines data on the incidence of AIDS cases with an estimate of the distribution of the length of the incubation period. The cumulative incidence of AIDS at time t is the summation up to time t of the product of the incidence of HIV at time τ and the probability of developing AIDS within t - τ years after infection (given that AIDS will eventually develop). If the incidence of AIDS up to time t and the distribution of the AIDS incubation period are known, it is possible to calculate the incidence of HIV up to time t. In other words, since the cumulative incidence of AIDS is a convolution, the incidence of HIV can be found by deconvolution. Therefore, the incidence of HIV can be estimated by deconvolution from data on AIDS incidence adjusted for reporting lags and underreporting, and the estimated distribution of the length of the incubation period. This leads to extrapolations for future levels of HIV infection and AIDS incidence.

Back-calculation yields predictions for homosexuals and IV drug users that are reliable for 1-3 years into the future. However, for the general population, there is more uncertainty: AIDS incidence data are currently much more limited, and the estimated distribution of the incubation period comes from studies of high risk groups, raising doubts about its validity for the general population (Workshop 1988, p. 10). The accuracy of the estimated distribution of the incubation period is critical; the back-calculation method is very sensitive to the distribution assumed for the incubation period (Brookmeyer and Gail 1986, 1988, Brookmeyer and Damiano 1989). This is especially troublesome because it is currently necessary to assume a functional form and to estimate the parameters of this distribution, and data are available only for a limited range of values of t; thus, we know much about the lower tail of the distribution of the incubation period but little about the upper tail. Back-calculation "can establish a range of plausible estimates of HIV seroprevalence, but the error range is wide and confidence limits are not available" (Workshop 1988, p. 10).

Brookmeyer and Gail (1986, 1988) used back-calculation to estimate the minimum size of the AIDS epidemic in the U.S. They used the Weibull distribution with a median of 4.3 years, obtained earlier by other authors, to estimate the incidence of HIV before 1986, and then estimated the number of AIDS cases from 1986 to 1991 in people infected before 1986. However, Hyman and Stanley (1988) found such estimates to be very sensitive to the assumed nature of the probability distribution of the length of the incubation period; considering the continuous analog of the back-calculation process, they determined that the confidence intervals on the forecasts were very wide. The sensitivity of model predictions to assumptions about the distribution of the incubation period was also noted by Anderson *et al.* (1987) and Anderson (1988a).

4. Estimation of Epidemiological Parameters and Distributions

The epidemiology of HIV infection and AIDS is characterized by the distributions of various quantities associated with the disease. Some of these are intervals of time, e.g., the incubation period, others are probabilities, e.g., the probability of transmission per sexual contact and rates, e.g., the rate of change of sexual partners. A simple approach is to treat these as unknown constants, or parameters of the disease model, which we seek to estimate from observed data. A more realistic approach, though, is to view these as random quantities, each varying from individual to individual according to an unknown probability distribution. For some purposes, knowing (or estimating) some particular numerical aspect or parameter of one of these distributions will suffice, while for other purposes, knowing (or estimating) the entire probability distribution or probability density function is necessary. Whether we need to estimate quantities or distributions is closely related to the type of questions that we wish to address. These issues are intimately connected to dynamic models. (See the contributions in this volume by Castillo-Chavez *et al.* 1989a, Thieme and Castillo-Chavez 1989a; Jacquez *et al.* 1989; Koopman *et al.* 1989; Kaplan *et al.* 1989; Cardell and Kanouse 1989; or see Huang *et al.* 1989 and Thieme and Castillo-Chavez 1989b).

For example, the mean length of the AIDS incubation period is an important piece of information, so we may seek to estimate this parameter. The standard deviation of the incubation period is another parameter we may want to estimate. But these two values do not give information about the distribution of the length of the incubation period. Rather than estimating the mean and standard deviation directly, a different approach is to estimate its entire probability distribution, from which the mean, standard deviation and other parameters can be found. Lui *et al.* (1988) and Giesecke *et al.* (1988) are among those who have modeled the incubation period distribution with parametric families. In this volume, Longini *et al.* (1989) model the incubation period as a sum of a two-parameter (time-delayed) exponential variable and three time-homogeneous Markov process waiting times, which gives a generalized gamma distribution.

A nonparametric approach to estimating the distribution of the incubation period was taken by Lagakos *et al.* (1988). They handled the problem of right truncation of the data by transforming to reverse time, obtaining left truncated survival data. They developed nonparametric methods for estimating and comparing identifiable aspects of incubation period distributions for several population groups. De Gruttola and Lagakos (1989a) developed nonparametric methods for doubly censored survival data in which both the time of infection and the onset of AIDS can be truncated. These nonparametric methods constitute a response to the fact that the distribution of the incubation period is not identifiable outside the range of incubation times spanned by the observed (truncated) data.

The focus of the inference process is on this range. To estimate the entire distribution for use in epidemic models for the spread of AIDS and other purposes, it is necessary to specify a parametric model and to use likelihood or similar methods. Lagakos *et al.* (1988) pointed out the fundamental problem of the parametric approach through an example in which Weibull distributions with medians of 8.5 years and 210 years both agreed well with the data. This demonstrated the inherent weakness of parametric estimates of quantities related to the unobserved portion of the distribution. A comprehensive discussion of the use, strengths, and weaknesses of nonparametric approaches appears in this volume (De Gruttola and Lagakos, 1989b). We note, however, that some of the difficulties pointed out by the example in Lagakos *et al.* (1988) can be overcome through the use of dynamic models. The simplest approach is to feed these parametric representations for the incubation period into a dynamic model and then to require realistic predictions not only of the number of AIDS cases but also of the number of HIV infected. The theoretical basis for this approach has been developed and has been applied to fit models optimally for the dynamics of interacting populations (see Banks *et al.* 1989 and references therein).

Kalbfleisch and Lawless (1989) considered both nonparametric and parametric estimation from data on transfusion-related AIDS. The data were compiled by the Centers for Disease Control using retroactive ascertainment: when an individual is diagnosed as having AIDS, often the time of the initiating event, infection with HIV by blood transfusion, can be determined exactly, or nearly so. Kalbfleisch and Lawless constructed the likelihood function of the data, noting that it had been used by Brookmeyer and Gail (1988), Lagakos *et al.* (1988), Lui *et al.* (1986), and Medley *et al.* (1987, 1988). They examined nonparametric estimation based on the occurrence of initiating events as a Poisson process. Neither the distribution of the incubation period nor the Poisson process cumulative intensity function is estimable, although time-truncated versions of them are. This identifiability problem was pointed out by Lagakos *et al.* (1988). Adopting a parametric model seems to solve the problems inherent in nonparametric estimation by making the quantities of interest functions of the parameters which can be estimated by maximum likelihood from the data; however, these functions may be estimated very poorly. Kalbfleisch and Lawless showed that this happens with the transfusion data, reflecting the fact, clearly visible in the nonparametric analysis, that these data have virtually no information on percentiles of the distribution of the incubation period, expected number of infections leading to a diagnosis of AIDS, and other quantities of interest. Consequently, the parametric model point estimates for these are imprecise.

The term "parameter" has two slightly different meanings. A probability distribution in a specified family is characterized by a vector of parameter values; the probability density function is an expression involving these parameters. For example, a normal distribution is characterized by its mean and variance (μ,σ^2), a binomial distribution by the pair (n,p). A considerable amount of statistical literature is devoted to methods of estimating these parameters, which we can call "statistical model parameters," and to criteria for comparing competing estimation methods. An "epidemiological parameter," on the other hand, is any quantity whose value is useful in understanding the epidemiology of the situation. Epidemiological parameters may or may not be statistical model parameters, and vice versa. For example, Anderson (1988b) described models of HIV spread in different population subgroups for which the "effective average rate of partner change" should be defined as $c = m + v/m$ where m is the mean rate of partner change and v is the variance; c is an epidemiological parameter here but probably not a statistical model parameter in the usual sense.

Estimation is often accompanied by related analyses. When estimating a vector of statistical model parameters, we are frequently interested in testing the hypothesis that some of them take on special values. These values often reduce the model to a simpler special case. For example, in modeling a Weibull distribution with a time delay, Longini *et al.* (1989) test the hypothesis that the Weibull shape parameter α equals 1, reducing the distribution to an exponential. Another type of analysis related to parameter estimation is testing whether the distribution being fitted is consistent with the observed data by using a goodness-of-fit test. Still another type of analysis is testing the dependence among parameters, e.g., the effects of cofactors and markers (other STD's, age, health status, etc.) on the distributions of time spent in the stages of HIV infection. Brookmeyer *et al.* (1987) pointed out several potential sources of bias in an AIDS prevalent cohort study of cofactors and markers under a proportional hazards model. Other recent studies of cofactors and markers were reported by Goedert *et al.* (1987) and Padian *et al.* (1987). A general discussion of statistical techniques for addressing many of these issues can be found in Neter *et al.* (1985).

5. Dynamic Models

The first epidemiological model was presented by Daniel Bernoulli (1760) to the Royal Academy of Sciences in Paris. The mathematical theory of epidemiology made no significant advances until the work of the Russian physician P. D. En'ko was published in 1889 (see Dietz 1988a). En'ko constructed the first chain binomial model (wrongly attributed to Reed, see Dietz 1988a for further details). The so-called Reed-Frost models still play a very important role in theoretical and applied epidemiology. The key concepts in the development of the mathematical foundations of theoretical epidemiology derive from the work of the Nobel laureate Sir Ronald Ross (1911), although partial credit should be given to Brownlee

(1907) and McKendrick (1912). Ross introduced the assumption that the rate of new infections is proportional both to the number of susceptibles and to the number of infectious individuals (the so-called "mass-action law"), developed the first mathematical model for the spread of a vector-transmitted disease (malaria), and concluded that, to eradicate malaria, it was sufficient to bring the vector population below a threshold level. This theoretical result, the first threshold theorem, provided the theoretical foundation for the development of control programs. Ross used this result to conclude that a successful control program for malaria did not require the elimination of the whole mosquito population. McKendrick extended these results, and in 1927, he co-authored his celebrated paper with Kermack (see Kermack and McKendrick 1927) establishing that a threshold number of susceptible individuals must be available if an epidemic is to take place.

Ross was aware of the necessity of taking into account the effects of nonhomogeneous mixing, demography, geographical distribution and other factors in order to increase the predictive and explanatory power and applicability of epidemiological models. This level of detail could only be introduced by the stratification of a population into subpopulations according to specified criteria and by a detailed description of the mixing between subpopulations. Further elaboration of these ideas had to await the dramatic increases observed in venereal diseases during the 1960's, and was finally propelled further by the AIDS epidemic.

The first mathematical model for the transmission of a venereal disease was developed by Cooke and Yorke (1973). A model for gonorrhea with an arbitrary number of randomly (proportionally mixing) interacting groups was formulated and analyzed by Lajmanovich and Yorke (1976). Hethcote (1976), by observing that modeling sexually transmitted diseases for two-sex populations is mathematically equivalent to modeling a host-vector interaction, took us back to the seminal work of Ross. Yorke, Hethcote and Nold (1978) and Hethcote and Yorke (1984) introduced concepts such as saturation and preemption, as well as the concept of core subpopulation, into gonorrhea analysis. The idea of the core subpopulation has been extremely important in theoretical epidemiology. Its importance in disease dynamics was clearly understood by Ross and was later used by MacDonald (1957) as an explanatory mechanism for the lack of success in eliminating malaria.

Many mathematical models for HIV transmission and AIDS incidence have dealt primarily with one homogeneously mixing risk group which usually consists of highly sexually-active homosexual men. Some of these modeling efforts are described below.

5.1 Single-group models

Anderson *et al.* (1986) described some preliminary attempts to use mathematical models for HIV transmission in a homosexual community. The epidemic data available on HIV infection and the incidence of AIDS was surveyed. After the risk groups and transmission mechanisms were described, doubling times for AIDS incidence were given for risk groups in various geographic locations. Some data were also given for the HIV infectious period, the proportion who develop AIDS, and measures of sexual activity. Models of the early stages of the AIDS epidemic in homosexual men were used to find the reproductive number from the distribution of the AIDS incubation period and the initial doubling time. These more complex models showed that heterogeneity in sexual behavior can greatly influence the predictions, with more heterogeneity implying decreased magnitude of the AIDS epidemic. This result is reasonable since high heterogeneity implies that the few very sexually active people are removed rapidly from the infectious pool. Anderson *et al.* (1986) emphasized that uncertainty in parameter values implies that the models are not suitable for prediction. The purpose of their modeling was to investigate the effects of various parameters and to help improve our general understanding of the transmission dynamics of HIV infection. Areas of biological uncertainty, future data needs, and public health policy implications were discussed.

Pickering *et al.* (1986) formulated a model for the spread of HIV and AIDS incidence in the homosexual male population in three large cities. They used a discrete time nonlinear model for the sexual transmission of HIV with several possible courses of progression after infection. The models used trends in anal-rectal gonorrhea incidence to determine the changes in homosexual behavior. They gave some preliminary forecasts for San Francisco, Los Angeles and New York City but concluded that there were insufficient data to choose between radically different forecasts.

May and Anderson (1987) presented some simple HIV transmission models to help clarify the effects of various factors on the overall pattern of the AIDS epidemic. They began by defining the basic reproductive number as the product of three parameters and then obtained estimates of these three parameters from various data sources. They showed that if the probability of developing AIDS increases linearly with time since infection, then the distribution of the AIDS incubation period is a Weibull distribution. Their calculations assumed that 30% of HIV infecteds eventually develop AIDS, but we now know that this percentage is too low. They considered a model for heterosexual transmission where infection comes from the homosexual male population through bisexuals and found that the doubling times would be significantly larger in the heterosexual population than in the homosexual population. At present, this is not a realistic model for the sexual transmission of HIV in the

United States, since most heterosexual transmission is to sexual partners of intravenous drug users. In their discussion, they emphasized the uncertainty of the parameter values and the need for better data in several areas.

Blythe and Anderson (1988a) considered HIV transmission models with four forms for the distribution of AIDS incubation period (exponential, Weibull, gamma, and rectangular). As in most models, the HIV infectious period was assumed to be equal to the AIDS incubation period. The impact of the four distributions on HIV transmission dynamics in male homosexual communities was assessed by examining the equilibrium states and their local stability in a model with constant recruitment of susceptibles. In their discussion of the relative merits of the four distributions of the AIDS incubation period, they concluded that, for qualitative purposes, it may be sufficient to consider only these four distributions (if their means coincided with the observed value). Castillo-Chavez *et al.* (1989a, b, c) extended the above results to arbitrary distributions and analyzed a model where the mean rate of acquisition of new partners depends on the size of the sexually active population. Their results are further described in this volume (see Castillo-Chavez *et al.* 1989d).

Blythe and Anderson (1988b) also considered an HIV transmission model that encapsulates temporal variation in the infectiousness of HIV-infected persons and variability in the incubation period for AIDS. Variable infectivity was modeled in two ways for a homogeneously mixing homosexual population. They found their first approach, based on a multi-stage classification, more useful at present. Using two infectivity peaks (one after a short latent period and the other before the onset of "full-blown" AIDS), they observed that the initial phase of the infectiousness will tend to drive the early doubling time of the epidemic, while both peaks will determine the overall magnitude of the epidemic and the magnitude of the unique endemic state. Thieme and Castillo-Chavez (1989b) have carried out the theoretical analysis of a more general model that includes Blythe and Anderson's and have shown that the exclusive existence of a single initial peak could potentially force the incidence to oscillate. These authors, however, have not yet performed numerical simulations to investigate the possibility of this type of fluctuations for realistic parameter values. A discussion of their results is included in this volume (see Thieme and Castillo-Chavez 1989a).

Bailey (1989) presented a model for HIV infection and AIDS in which infected people proceed through a sequence of stages to AIDS and then to death. The model is given by a system of m+2 nonlinear differential equations with mass-action incidence term and negative exponential waiting times in the infected stages, which correspond to a gamma distribution for the AIDS incubation period. He used data on HIV prevalence in the San Francisco City Clinic cohort of 7,000 people and the reported AIDS incidence in all San Francisco and obtained a best (minimum chi-square) fit of his model. The best fit yielded a gamma distribution with $m = 7$ for the AIDS incubation period.

A further class of models that explicitly considers the dynamics of pairs of individuals and the duration of these partnerships has been developed by Dietz (1988b) and Dietz and Hadeler (1988). Their approach consists of the superposing of an epidemic process on the demographic "marriage" models of Kendall (1949) and Fredrickson (1971). Dietz, Hadeler, and their collaborators have further clarified the process of pair-formation. Details of their most recent work can be found in Hadeler (1987), Hadeler *et al.* (1988), and Hadeler (1989a). In addition, an article that reviews this important work with a higher degree of detail and presents some new results appears in this volume (see Waldstätter 1989).

Mode *et al.* (1989) considered a stochastic population model of an AIDS epidemic in a population of male homosexuals. Computer intensive methods were used to study some properties of the model statistically. A numerical factorial experiment was used to study three factors of importance in the evaluation of the AIDS epidemic. These factors were the distribution of the latent period of HIV, the probability of infection with HIV per sexual contact with an infected individual, and the distribution of the number of contacts per sexual partner per month. They found that the latent period of HIV infection had a decisive impact, but the impact depended crucially on the other factors. Their Monte Carlo experiment showed that the deterministic, nonlinear difference equations using expected values gave more pessimistic predictions than the stochastic population process. Their latent period of HIV would more properly be called the incubation period for AIDS. They used the Weibull and gamma distributions for this AIDS incubation period. The infectivity of HIV-positive individuals was taken to be constant and then zero when they developed AIDS. Since a longer median AIDS incubation period implies a longer infectious period, their conclusion that the HIV prevalence is much higher for longer median AIDS incubation period seems reasonable.

Tan (1989) used a stochastic model for the spread of the AIDS virus in a homosexual population. In his model, susceptible (S) persons become HIV latent (L), infective (I) and then develop AIDS (A). Transitions between these groups were governed by probabilities with contact rate and two transmission rates. The probability generating functions (PGF) of the number of latent persons, infective persons, and AIDS cases were derived. The expected numbers, and variances and covariances of these persons satisfy some ordinary differential equations. These equations are solved numerically to assess the effects of various factors on AIDS spread.

Kaplan (1989) developed dynamic models that apply to needle sharing populations. He made the assumption that a susceptible individual using an infected needle removes the virus from the needle. Kaplan performed extensive simulations illustrating the sensitivity of the model to various parameters and computed the basic reproductive number for his model. He also discussed the effect of possible intervention strategies.

5.2 Multigroup models

The AIDS models described above have involved only one population. Clearly, HIV transmission takes place in populations that are heterogeneous in a variety of ways. The contacts between people can be homosexual, heterosexual, or by needle sharing among intravenous drug users; some groups have higher contact rates than others; people may have contacts primarily with others who are similar or with a wide variety of partners; and behavior is not uniform geographically or temporally. One way in which this heterogeneity can be modeled is to consider models with multiple groups. Another possibility is to use continuous distributions of behaviors instead of discrete groups with different behaviors. Some recent models of these types for sexually transmitted diseases and AIDS will now be described.

One of the first multigroup models for a sexually transmitted disease was the gonorrhea model of Lajmanovich and Yorke (1976). In this model with n groups, each group was divided into two classes: the susceptibles and the infecteds. Since people are susceptible again after they are cured of a gonococcal infection, gonorrhea is called an SIS disease. Their model was a system of n nonlinear ordinary differential equations where the incidences were quadratic mass action laws and the removal rates corresponded to negative-exponential distributed infectious periods. Lajmanovich and Yorke determined a theoretical threshold condition for this model. They proved global asymptotic stability of the trivial equilibrium point below the threshold. No attempt was made to estimate parameters or to apply the model.

Nold (1980) proved similar results for a generalization of the Lajmanovich and Yorke SIS model. Similar results for an analogous SIR model were proved in Hethcote (1978), Hethcote and Thieme (1985), and Hethcote and Van Ark (1987). Nold (1980) also introduced the ideas of proportionate mixing and a convex combination of internal and proportionate mixing (named preferred mixing by Jacquez *et al.* 1988 and biased mixing by Hyman and Stanley 1988, 1989). Note, however, that different results have been obtained for an SIR model with variable population size for these two types of mixing by Castillo-Chavez *et al.* (1989c) and Huang *et al.* (1989). For further details see Castillo-Chavez *et al.* (1989d) in this volume.

The results of a long-term gonorrhea modeling project have been described in the book by Hethcote and Yorke (1984). The n-group model used was

$$\frac{dN_iI_i}{dt} = \left[\sum_{j=1}^{n} \lambda_{ij} N_i I_i\right] (1 - I_i) - N_i I_i / d_i,$$

where N_i is the group i population size (assumed constant), λ_{ij} is the average number of adequate contacts per unit time of a person in group j with all people in group i, and d_i is the average duration of infection in group i. The concept of a core group was introduced and control strategies were compared in a core-noncore model. Also, seasonal oscillations were analyzed in a female-male model. Six contact methods were compared in an eight-group model where people were divided by sex, sexual activity level, and whether infection was symptomatic or asymptomatic. Many of the multigroup models for HIV transmission and AIDS are similar in some ways to the gonorrhea model of Hethcote and Yorke (1984).

A multigroup model with both local and broader mixing was developed by Sattenspiel (1987) for the spread of Hepatitis A among day care centers in Albuquerque, New Mexico. This model included neighborhood play groups whose members mixed together by going to day care centers. This model was analyzed mathematically in Sattenspiel (1987) and Sattenspiel and Simon (1988).

Recently, multigroup models have been used for AIDS by several different authors. Instead of attempting to describe the chronological development of all of these models, the work of several authors or working groups is described. The selection is biased by our viewpoints and interests; no attempt is made to include all modeling efforts.

A working group at Los Alamos National Laboratory has analyzed models for HIV transmission and AIDS which include heterogeneity in sexual activity and mixing. In these models, which could be called continuous models, heterogeneity is introduced as continuous distributions of sexual behavior instead of as discrete groups with different behaviors. Hyman and Stanley (1988, 1989) formulated and used several models to study questions related to the AIDS epidemic. Their τ-dependent model, where τ denotes time since infection, includes variable infectivity as a function of τ. This model is given by a system of nonlinear integro-differential equations for the distribution of infecteds and AIDS cases as a function of time and age since infection. Sample calculations showed that the infectivity profile could dramatically change the rate at which the susceptible population is infected. In their models, they used a Weibull distribution for the AIDS incubation period, and initial cubic growth of the AIDS cases and inverse quartic distributions for the number of sexual partners per unit time. They also used risk-based models with random (proportionate) mixing and biased (preferred) mixing. With random mixing, their numerical simulations showed that the disease progresses rapidly in both the high and low risk populations, but with biased (like-with-like) mixing, the disease progresses rapidly in the high risk populations and much more slowly in the low risk populations. The random mixing result seems inconsistent with data. They also noted that if the difference between the male-to-female and female-to-male infectivities is large, then the lower of these two infectivities tends to determine heterosexual spread. The number of infected people as a function of time can be determined by a convolution integral from the AIDS incidence as a function of time and the distribution of the AIDS incubation period. Back-calculation (discussed in Section 3.2) estimated the HIV incidence as a function of time from the AIDS incidence and as an assumed distribution of the AIDS incubation period. Hyman and Stanley analyzed the accuracy of this procedure and estimated confidence intervals on forecasts based on the accuracy of AIDS data and the incubation time. Recently, Hyman and Stanley (1989) explored the sensitivity of an HIV transmission model to different social mixing patterns. This model was more general than that in Hyman and Stanley (1988) since it simultaneously included both continuous distributions for sexual partner change rates and also variable infectivity as a function of time since infection. A Weibull distribution was used for the AIDS incubation period. An acceptance (or preference) function determined which partners are acceptable to an individual and defined the mixing between groups with different partner change rates. Hyman and Stanley found that, if people select partners with very similar risk behavior, then the epidemic grows much more slowly than if they were more random in selecting partners. This reinforces the results in the previous paper.

Busenberg and Castillo-Chavez (1989b) have generalized this model to include age-structure. Furthermore, Busenberg and Castillo-Chavez (while generalizing the mixing framework of Blythe and Castillo-Chavez 1989) have found an explicit formula – the mixing function – that includes all mixing patterns for a homosexually active age-structured population as a function of an arbitrary preference (acceptance) function. Furthermore, they have determined an explicit formula for the reproductive number, in the case of proportionate mixing, for this very general model. A brief article discussing these results (which also generalize those of the Michigan group, described below) appears in this volume (see Busenberg and Castillo-Chavez 1989a).

Colgate *et al.* (1989) observed that the cumulative number of AIDS cases in the United States has grown as the cube of time rather than exponentially. They used a risk behavior model in which individuals tend to mix with people in their own risk group to explain that cubic growth is the result of a saturation wave of infection moving from the high to the low risk groups. Thus they claim that the observed decreasing growth rate in AIDS cases is due to the mixing pattern of the risk groups rather than to changes in behavior.

A primary focus of a working group centered at the University of Michigan has been to analyze the effects of various mixing patterns in discrete multigroup models for HIV and AIDS. In Jacquez *et al.* (1989), they presented a compartmental model for the spread of HIV in a homosexual population divided into subgroups by level of sexual activity. Their model included constant recruitment into the susceptible classes and variable infectivity in the stages of infection leading up to AIDS. They introduced the term "preferred mixing" for the situation in which a fraction of each group's contacts are internal and the balance is distributed using proportionate mixing among all groups. This convex combination approach was not given a name by Nold (1980) and is similar to "biased mixing" in Los Alamos working group models. Both types of mixing are special cases of the like-with-like mixing of Blythe and Castillo-Chavez (1989), and they are included in the representation theorem of Busenberg and Castillo-Chavez (1989a, b). The Michigan group determined a threshold for their model involving the mean number of contacts per infective, which determines whether or not there exists a unique endemic equilibrium (under some special conditions) in addition to the trivial (infection-free) equilibrium. For special cases, they were able to analyze the local stability of these equilibria. For a five-group model, numerical simulations revealed certain features. Increasing contacts between the groups greatly increased the rate of spread of the epidemic in the low activity level groups and also increased the fractions within those groups eventually infected. The conclusions of the Los Alamos working group and the Michigan working group are similar even though the former used continuously distributed models (and based its conclusions mostly on numerical simulations) and the latter used multigroup models and provided a local stability analysis of their model. They both found, through numerical simulations, that the mixing patterns between people with different sexual activity levels influenced the speed and asymptotic behavior of the epidemic.

A discrete n-group model that includes the Michigan model (Jacquez *et al.* 1988) has been analyzed recently by Castillo-Chavez *et al.* (1989c, d) and Huang *et al.* (1989) in the case of biased or preferred mixing and in the case of proportionate mixing. These researchers have found that the incorporation of a less restrictive incidence term allows for the possibility of two endemic equilibria. The bifurcation parameter is given by the average length of sexual activity, and non-symmetric mixing appears to play a very important role in the bifurcation two multiple equilibria. The article by Castillo-Chavez *et al.* (1989c) in this volume discusses these results in further detail, and provides two artificial examples, using proportionate and preferred mixing, for which asymmetry in epidemiological or mixing parameters leads to the existence of at least two endemic equilibria.

Jacquez *et al.* (1989, this volume) examined a model with mixing occurring in mixing subgroups that cut across "structural" subgroups. A mixing group matrix specifies the allocation of structural subgroups to the mixing subgroups. They also defined contact matrices for the mixing subgroups and gave examples. They called this "structured mixing".

Koopman *et al.* (1989, this volume) consider selective mixing which specifies the selection of contacts within a mixing group. The contact matrix involves conversation contact activity levels, the mutual acceptability of conversation contacts for sex, and the proportion of mutually acceptable encounters which result in new sexual partnerships. An example for a homosexual male population shows the difficulty of estimating the relative risk of HIV infection during anal and oral sex.

Knox (1986) used a multigroup model for transmission of AIDS. The twelve groups considered included male homosexuals divided into anal penetrative, anal receptive or both, and divided into promiscuous and not promiscuous. Equilibrium levels were predicted for the groups, and the times necessary to reach these levels were determined. Because of the uncertainties of his plausible parameter set, he also analyzed forecasts using parameter sets from the surrounding parameter spaces.

In contrast to the many models for a homosexual male population, De Gruttola and Mayer (1987) considered a model for two interacting groups: a small population of individuals rapidly infected by high risk activity and a large population of individuals at risk only from heterosexual contact. The model was a system of differential equations in the male and female risk groups of intravenous drug users and their heterosexual partners. Individuals were either susceptible, asymptomatically infected or symptomatically infected. Fitted parameter values were restricted to a range consistent with findings from partner studies. Their modeling showed that the interpretation of existing data on heterosexual transmission depends strongly on the infectiousness over time of HIV infecteds. Moreover, they showed that epidemics of widely varying severity among heterosexuals are consistent with the available epidemiological data.

Gail *et al.* (1989) developed a model for AIDS in order to evaluate the potential benefits of voluntary confidential screening for HIV. The model includes very active homosexuals, active homosexuals, bisexuals, heterosexual males, and heterosexual females. The contact matrix is determined by minimizing the discriminant information which is different from proportionate mixing. Conclusions are drawn about the usefulness of voluntary confidential screening in the high and low risk groups in a population of about 100,000 over a period of 5 to 15 years. The economic ratio (ER) is defined as the number of tests required to prevent one case. Voluntary confidential testing (VCT) prevents many cases in isolated high risk populations where ER values are less than 100. VCT prevents only a few cases in isolated low risk populations with ER values over 2,000 when the initial prevalence is below 0.1%, but prevents many more cases when the initial prevalence is above 1%. This paper quantifies the conclusion that screening is more effective in high risk populations than in low risk.

A general model for HIV transmission and AIDS has been formulated by Hethcote (1987, 1989a). The comprehensive model proposed contains all known transmission routes including homosexual and heterosexual intercourse, needle sharing among intravenous drug users, blood transfusions, blood factor concentrates to hemophiliacs, and perinatal infections. The primary risk groups in the model were sexually active homosexual and bisexual men, prostitutes, sexually active heterosexual women and men, and intravenous drug using women and men. The secondary risk groups were transfusion recipients, hemophiliacs, monogamous partners and children born to women in a previous risk group. For each risk group there was a differential equation incorporating the inflow and outflow. The progression from HIV infection to AIDS was modeled by a unidirectional flow in a sequence of stages. No attempt was made in Hethcote (1987, 1989a) to estimate parameter values or to apply the model.

In Hethcote (1989b), an HIV transmission and AIDS model was formulated as a system of nonlinear difference equations with a time step of one month. A priori estimates of the parameters were obtained from the literature. Parameters were estimated for group population sizes, migration, mortality, sexual activity levels and contact rates, needle sharing behavior, and state transition rates. Because of the uncertainty in some of these parameter estimates, more focused models have been used in specific geographic locations. Because both HIV prevalence and AIDS incidence data are available for homosexual males in San Francisco, Hethcote (1989c) focused on this population. After presenting the data, parameters related to the stages leading to AIDS and also to homosexual behavior were estimated. A best fit which optimized the fit criterion was obtained, and the sensitivity of the patterns to parameter changes was analyzed. The data and the model yielded a distribution of the AIDS incubation period which gave the best fit. A forecast based on the best fit was given. Hethcote (1989c) also concluded that the observed HIV prevalence and AIDS incidence in San Francisco were due to changes in sexual behavior and not due solely to saturation in high risk groups.

5.3 Demographic models

One of the most pressing issues in developing nations is that of determining what are the demographic consequences of the AIDS epidemic. Noticeable changes in the age-structure of a population can affect social and economic structure significantly even without observable reductions in population growth rates. Models help to outline possible scenarios, sort out the possibilities, reject or support hypotheses and identify specific data needs.

The history of epidemiological models that incorporate age-structure goes back to the influential paper of Hoppensteadt (1974). Hoppensteadt's article has generated a tremendous amount of activity in mathematical epidemiology and has influenced the field of theoretical biology. For some of the most recent applications see Castillo-Chavez *et al.* (1988, 1989e) and references therein.

Until recently, most of the demographic models of HIV transmission were developed and analyzed by May, Anderson, and their collaborators. May *et al.* (1988, 1989b) and Anderson *et al.* (1988c) introduced some of the first age-structured models for the sexual transmission of HIV. Conventional demographic models (see Hoppensteadt 1974, 1975; Castillo-Chavez 1989) were combined by May, Anderson and McLean with simple epidemiological models in order to explore the effects of horizontally- and vertically-transmitted AIDS upon total population growth rates as well as upon age-profile growth rates. The main objective of these papers was to use simple models to gain some qualitative understanding for reference in numerical simulations of more realistic models. Model results suggest that AIDS is capable of changing population growth rates from positive to negative over a period of a few decades. Further results suggest that AIDS may have a minimal impact on the dependency ratio (the number of individuals below age 15 and above age 64 divided by the number of individuals in the complementary age classes).

The explosion of theoretical work on mixing (see Castillo-Chavez and Blythe 1989, Busenberg and Castillo-Chavez 1989a, and references therein) has demonstrated that further understanding of HIV transmission depends heavily on a better understanding of social/sexual mixing patterns. Progress is, therefore, limited by the lack of accurate data on sexual/social mixing patterns. The recent work of Gupta *et al.* (1989) and Anderson *et al.* (1989a) begins to look systematically at mixing patterns and their relationship to dynamic models. The representation theorem of Busenberg and Castillo-Chavez of all mixing patterns for a risk-based and age-structured homosexually-active population via a preference or acceptance function has provided a solid mathematical foundation upon which the effects of social/sexual mixing can be systematically analyzed.

Most of the models described above do not take into consideration the temporary periods of immunity that are naturally provided by short or long-term monogamous relationships. These effects can only be considered through models that follow the dynamics of pairs, i.e., models that explicitly take into consideration the processes of pair formation and pair dissolution. Demographic models that consider the age structure of a population and follow the dynamics of pairs were introduced by Fredrickson (1971). The first epidemiological model incorporating pairs was formulated in Dietz and Hadeler (1988) and Dietz (1988). Extensions of these models to age-structured populations were introduced and partially analyzed by Hadeler (1989a b). As stated earlier, the work of Dietz, Hadeler and collaborators suggests that the incorporation of the processes of pair formation and pair dissolution have a significant downward effect on the magnitude of the AIDS epidemic, when compared with the results of classical models.

Although these modeling approaches provide us with valuable insights, it is clear that they represent two extremes, and therefore the development and analysis of hybrid models is of extreme importance (see Waldstätter 1989). An alternative approach for the construction of hybrid two-sex models starts by postulating the existence of two mixing functions (one for females, the other for males) that satisfy appropriate mixing axioms. Solutions to these axioms — or mixing functions — can be incorporated into models with pairs and models without pairs, and possibly to hybrid models. Some specific cases are being studied by Castillo-Chavez and Busenberg (1989) but further work is needed.

6. Conclusion

This paper presents a partial review of the literature on mathematical and statistical approaches to AIDS epidemiology . Mathematical models for AIDS cannot be built in a vacuum. They have to be guided and motivated by data. Unfortunately, data is not readily available and there are many difficulties when dealing with the analysis of the available AIDS data (see Section 2). Models have been used quite successfully for short-term predictions of AIDS incidence and, with some degree of success, in estimating the number of infected individuals and the incubation period distribution. Dynamic models can be very useful in reducing the uncertainties in many of these estimates (see Section 3). Further, they allow us to see the effects that of a varying environment (due to changes in behaviors, medical treatment, etc.) on key parameters. Therefore, models can be irreplaceable in the evaluation of the relative merits of preventive strategies.

There is strong agreement that variable infectivity, the nature and type of the social/sexual mixing structures, and the long and variable period of infectiousness are key factors that must be understood if we expect to have some degree of success in the fight against this epidemic. Although there will always be the need for further mathematical studies, it is clear that in order to have an immediate impact in the fight against AIDS, we need to tie models to data and we need more quality data. Especially urgently required is data on mixing patterns and variable infectivity.

Mathematical epidemiology has shown a tremendous growth over the last two to three years. The challenging questions posed by the AIDS epidemic have focused the research of several scientists and have opened new directions of research, many of which are illustrated in this volume. Unfortunately, the scientific growth spurred by this epidemic may be one of the very few positive consequences of an otherwise frightful situation. This epidemic has created world-wide fear and pain, and it has just begun to affect significantly the economies of developed and developing nations through severe taxing of their medical services. At present it appears that this epidemic will eventually affect the lives of all individuals. We must keep this situation in mind as we continue to test and develop mathematical and statistical models for AIDS.

ACKNOWLEDGMENTS

This research has been partially supported by NSF grant DMS-8906580, NIAID grant RO1 A129178-01, and Hatch project grant NYC 151-409, USDA awarded to C. C.-C. We thank S.A. Colgate, K.L. Cooke, C.M. Crawford, K. Dietz, J.M. Hyman, A. Levin, E.A. Stanley, and R. Waldstätter for their stimulating conversations.

REFERENCES

Anderson, R.M. (1988a). The epidemiology of HIV infection: variable incubation plus infectious periods and heterogeneity in sexual activity. *J. R. Statist. Soc. A*, 151, 66-93.

Anderson, R.M. (1988b). The role of mathematical models in the study of HIV transmission and the epidemiology of AIDS. *J. AIDS* 1, 241-256.

Anderson, R.M. (1989). Mathematical and statistical studies of the epidemiology of HIV. *AIDS* 3, 333-346.

Anderson, R.M., S.P. Blythe, G.F. Medley, and A.M. Johnson. (1987). Is it possible to predict the minimum size of the acquired immunodeficiency syndrome (AIDS) epidemic in the United Kingdom? *Lancet* 1073-1075, May 9.

Anderson, R.M., S.P. Blythe, S. Gupta, E. Konnings. (1989a). The transmission dynamics of the human immunodeficiency virus type 1 in the male homosexual community in the United Kingdom: the influence of changes in sexual behavior. (Manuscript.)

Anderson, R.M. and R.M. May. (1989). Complex dynamical behaviour in the interaction between HIV and the immune systems. In *Cell to Cell signalling: from experiment to theoretical models*, Academic Press, 355-349.

Anderson, R.M., R.M. May, A.R. McLean. (1988). Possible demographic impact of AIDS in developing countries. *Nature* 332, 228-234.

Anderson, R.M., G.F. Medley, R.M. May, and A.M. Johnson. (1986). A preliminary study of the transmission dynamics of the human immunodeficiency virus (HIV), the causative agent of AIDS. *IMA J. of Mathematics Applied in Med. and Biol.* 3, 229-263.

Aron, J.L. and P.S. Sarma. (1989). Assessment of the risk of HIV spread via non-steady heterosexual partners in the U.S. population. (This volume.)

Bailey, N.T.J. (1989). The modeling and prediction of HIV/AIDS. (Manuscript.)

Baldwin, J.D. and J.I. Baldwin. (1988). Factors affecting AIDS-related sexual risk-taking behavior among college students. *J. Sex Research* 25, 181-196.

Banks H.T., and B.G. Fitzpatrick. (1989). Inverse problems for distributed systems: statistical tests and ANOVA. In *Mathematical approaches to problems in resource management and epidemiology.* C. Castillo-Chavez, S.A. Levin, and C. Shoemaker (eds.). Lecture Notes in Biomathematics 81, Springer-Verlag, Berlin, Heidelberg, New York, Tokyo. (In press.)

Bernoulli, D. (1760). Essai d'une nouvelle analyse de la mortalité causée par la petite vérole et des advantages de l'inoculation pour la prévenir. *Mém. Math. Phys. Acad. Roy. Sci.*, Paris, pp. 1-45.

Blythe, S.P. and R.M. Anderson. (1988a). Distributed incubation and infectious periods in models of transmission dynamics of human immunodeficiency virus (HIV). *IMA. J. of Mathematics Applied in Med. and Biol.* 5, 1-19.

Blythe, S.P. and R.M. Anderson. (1988b). Variable infectiousness in HIV transmission models. *IMA J. of Mathematics Applied in Med. and Biol.* 5, 181-200.

Blythe, S.P. and C. Castillo-Chavez. (1989). Like-with-like preference and sexual mixing models. *Math. Biosci.* 96, 221-238.

Bradburn, N.M. (1983). Response effects. In: *Handbook of Survey Research,* P.H. Rossi, J.D. Wright, and A.B. Anderson (Eds.). Quantitative Studies in Social Relations, Academic Press, New York.

Brookmeyer, R. and A. Damiano. (1989). Statistical methods for short term projections of AIDS incidence. *Statis. Med.* 8. (In press.)

Brookmeyer, R. and M.H. Gail. (1986). Minimum size of the acquired immunodeficiency syndrome (AIDS) epidemic in the United States. *Lancet* 1320-1322, December 6.

Brookmeyer, R. and M.H. Gail. (1988). A method for obtaining short-term projections and lower bounds on the size of the AIDS epidemic. *J. Amer. Stat. Assn.* 83, 301-308.

Brookmeyer, R., M.H. Gail, and B.F. Polk. (1987). The prevalent cohort study and the acquired immunodeficiency syndrome. *Amer. J. Epidem.* 126, 14-24.

Brownlee, J. (1907). Statistical studies in immunity. The theory of an epidemic. *Proc. Soc. Edinburgh* 26, 484-521.

Busenberg, S. and C. Castillo-Chavez. (1989a). Interaction, pair formation and force of infection terms in sexually transmitted diseases. (This volume.)

Busenberg, S. and C. Castillo-Chavez. (1989b). Risk and age-dependent mixing functions and force of infection terms in sexually transmitted diseases. (Submitted.)

Cardell, N.S. and K.E. Kanouse. (1989). Population heterogeneity in a model of the spread of HIV infection. (This volume.)

Castillo-Chavez, C. (1989). Some applications of structure models in population dynamics. In *Applied Mathematical Ecology.* S.A. Levin, T.G. Hallam, and L.J. Gross (eds.). *Biomathematics* 18, 450-470. Springer-Verlag, Berlin, Heidelberg, New York, Tokyo. (In press.)

Castillo-Chavez, C. and S.P. Blythe. (1989). Mixing framework for social/sexual behavior. (This volume.)

Castillo-Chavez, C. and S. Busenberg. (1989). Pair formation in age- and risk-structured populations. (Manuscript in preparation.)

Castillo-Chavez, C., K. Cooke, W. Huang, and S.A. Levin. (1989a). On the role of long periods of infectiousness in the dynamics of acquired immunodeficiency syndrome (AIDS). In *Mathematical approaches to problems in resource management and epidemiology.* C. Castillo-Chavez, S.A. Levin, and C. Shoemaker (eds.). Lecture Notes in Biomathematics 81, Springer-Verlag, Berlin, Heidelberg, New York, Tokyo. (In press.)

Castillo-Chavez, C., K. Cooke, W. Huang, and S.A. Levin. (1989b). On the role of long incubation periods in the dynamics of acquired immunodeficiency syndrome (AIDS), Part 1. Single population models. *J. Math. Biol.* 27, 373-398.

Castillo-Chavez, C., K. Cooke, W. Huang, and S.A. Levin. (1989c). Results on the dynamics for models for the sexual transmission of the human immunodeficiency virus. *Applied Mathematics Letters.* (In press.)

Castillo-Chavez, C., K. Cooke, W. Huang, and S.A. Levin. (1989d). On the role of long incubation periods in the dynamics of acquired immunodeficiency syndrome (AIDS), Part 2. Multiple group models. (This volume.)

Centers for Disease Control. (1987). Revision of the CDC surveillance case definition for acquired immunodeficiency syndrome. *MMWR* 36, 3S-15.

Colgate, S.A., E.A. Stanley, J.M. Hyman, S.P. Layne, and C. Quails. (1989). A risk based model for explaining the cubic growth of AIDS cases. LA-UR-873412. (Los Alamos technical report.)

Conover, W.J. (1980). *Practical Nonparametric Statistics*, 2nd edition. John Wiley & Sons, New York.

Cooke, K.L. and J.A. Yorke. (1973). Some equations modeling growth processes and gonorrhea epidemics. *Math. Biosci.* 16, 75-101.

Cox, D.R. (1972). Regression models and life tables. *J. R. Statist. Soc. B*, 34, 187-220.

De Gruttola, V. and S.W. Lagakos. (1989a). Analysis of doubly-censored survival data, with application to AIDS. *Biometrics* 45, 1-11.

De Gruttola, V. and S.W. Lagakos. (1989b). Epidemic models, empirical studies, and uncertainty. (This volume.)

De Gruttola, V. and K.H. Meyer. (1987). Assessing and modeling heterosexual spread of human immunodeficiency virus in the United States. *Reviews of Infectious Diseases,* 10(1), 138-150.

Dietz, K. (1988a). The first epidemic model: a historical note on P. D. E'nko, *Austral. J. Statist.* 30(A), 56-65.

Dietz, K. (1988b). On the transmission dynamics of HIV. *Math. Biosci.* 90, 397-414.

Dietz, K. and K.P. Hadeler. (1988). Epidemiological models for sexually transmitted diseases. *J. Math. Biol.* 26, 1-25.

Downs, A.M., R.A. Ancelle, H.J.C. Jager, and J-B. Brunet. (1987). AIDS in Europe: current trends and short-term predictions estimated from surveillance data, January 1981 – June 1986. *AIDS* 1, 53-57.

Eubank, R. (1988). *Spline Smoothing and Nonparametric Regression.* Marcel Dekker, Inc. New York.

Fredrickson, A.G. (1971). A mathematical theory of age structure in sexual populations: random mating and monogamous marriage models. *Math. Biosci.* 10, 117-143.

Fox, J.A. and P. Tracy. (1984). *Randomized Response.* Sage, Beverly Hills, CA.

Fusaro, R.E., N.P. Jewell, W.W. Hauck, D.C. Heilbron, J.D. Kalbfleisch, J.M. Neuhaus, and M.A. Ashby. (1989). An annotated bibliography of quantitative methodology relating to the AIDS epidemic. *Statistical Science* 4, 264-281.

Gail, M.H., D. Preston, and S. Piantadosi. (1989). Disease prevention models of voluntary confidential screening for human immunodeficiency virus (HIV) in isolated low risk and high risk populations and in mixed gay/heterosexual populations. *Statistics in Med.* 8. (In press.)

Giesecke, J., G. Scalia-Tomba, O. Berglund, E. Berntorp, S. Schulman, and L. Stigendal. (1988). Incidence of symptoms and AIDS in 146 Swedish hemophiliacs and blood transfusion recipients infected with human immunodeficiency virus. *Br. Med. J.* 297, 99–102.

Gilchrist, W. (1983). Forecasting. In *Encyclopedia of Statistical Sciences.* S. Kotz, N.L. Johnson, and C.B. Read (eds.). Volume 3, John Wiley & Sons, New York.

Goedert, J.J., R.J. Biggar, M. Melbye, D.L. Mann, S. Wilson, M.H. Gail, R.J. Grossman, R. A. DiGioia, W.C. Sanchez, S.H. Weiss, and W.A. Blattner. (1987). Effect of T4 count and cofactors on the incidence of AIDS in homosexual men infected with human immunodeficiency virus. *J. Amer. Med. Assn.* 257, 331-334.

Gupta, S., R.M. Anderson, and R.M. May. (1989). Networks of sexual contacts: implications for the pattern of spread of HIV. (Manuscript.)

Hadeler, K.P. (1987). Pair formation in age structured populations. *Proceedings, Workshop on Selected Topics in Biomathematics,* IIASA. Kurzhanshij, A. and K. Sigmund (eds.). Laxenburg, Austria.

Hadeler, K.P. (1989a). Pair formation in age-structured populations. *Acta Applicandae Mathematicae* 14, 91-102.

Hadeler, K.P. (1989b). Modeling AIDS in structured populations. (Manuscript.)

Hadeler, K.P., R. Waldstätter, and A. Wörz-Busekros. (1988). A model for pair formation in bisexual populations. *J. Math. Biol.* 26, 635-649.

Harris, J.E. (1987). Delay in reporting acquired immune deficiency syndrome (AIDS). Working paper 452, Department of Economics, MIT. Cambridge, Mass.

Healy, M.J.R. and H.E. Tillett. (1988). Short-term extrapolation of the AIDS epidemic. *J. R. Statist. Soc. A*, 151, 50-61.

Hethcote, H.W. (1976). Qualitative analyses for communicable disease models, *Math. Biosci.* 28, 335-356.

Hethcote, H.W. (1978). An immunization model for a heterogeneous population. *Theor. Pop. Biol.* 14, 338-349.

Hethcote, H.W. (1987). AIDS modeling work in the USA. In *Future Trends in AIDS.* Her Majesty's Stationery Office, London, 35-40.

Hethcote, H.W. (1989a). A model for HIV transmission and AIDS. In *Mathematical approaches to problems in resource management and epidemiology.* C. Castillo-Chavez, S. A. Levin, and C. Shoemaker (eds.). Lecture Notes in Biomathematics 81, Springer-Verlag, Berlin, Heidelberg, New York, Tokyo. (In press.)

Hethcote, H.W. (1989b). Model formulation and parameter estimation, phase 1 progress report to CDC. (Unpublished report.)

Hethcote, H.W. (1989c). HIV prevalence and AIDS in San Francisco, phase 2 progress report to CDC. (Unpublished report.)

Hethcote, H.W. and H.R. Thieme. (1985). Stability of the endemic equilibrium in epidemic models with subpopulations. *Math. Biosci.* 75, 205-227.

Hethcote, H.W. and J.A. Van Ark. (1987). Epidemiological models for heterogeneous populations: proportionate mixing, parameter estimation and immunization programs. *Math. Biosci.* 84, 85-118.

Hethcote, H.W. and J.A. Yorke. (1984). *Gonorrhea transmission dynamics and control.* Lecture Notes in Biomathematics 56, Springer-Verlag, Berlin, Heidelberg, New York, Tokyo.

Hoffman, G.W. and M.D. Grant. (1989). When HIV meets the immune system: network theory, alloimmunity and AIDS. (This volume.)

Hoppensteadt, F. (1974). An age dependent epidemic model. J. Franklin Instit. 297, 325–333.

Hoppensteadt, F. (1975). Mathematical Theories of Populations: demographics, genetics and epidemics. *SIAM* Regional Conference Series in Applied Math., No. 20. Philadelphia.

Huang, W., K. Cooke, and C. Castillo-Chavez. (1989). Stability and bifurcation for a multiple group model for the dynamics of HIV/AIDS. (Manuscript.)

Hyman, J.M. and E.A. Stanley. (1988). Using mathematical models to understand the AIDS epidemic. *Math. Biosci.* 90, 415-473.

Hyman, J.M. and E.A. Stanley. (1989). The effect of social mixing patterns on the spread of AIDS. In *Mathematical approaches to problems in resource management and epidemiology.* C. Castillo-Chavez, S.A. Levin, and C. Shoemaker (eds.). Lecture Notes in Biomathematics 81, Springer-Verlag, Berlin, Heidelberg, New York, Tokyo. (In press.)

Isham, V. (1988). Mathematical modeling of the transmission dynamics of HIV infection and AIDS: a review. *J. R. Statist. Soc. A*, 151, 5-30.

Jacquez, J.A., C.P. Simon, and J. Koopman. (1989). Structured mixing: heterogeneous mixing by the definition of mixing groups. (This volume.)

Johnson, A.M. (1988). Social and behavioural aspects of the HIV epidemic - a review. *J. R. Statist. Soc. A*, 151, 99-114.

Kalbfleisch, J.D. and J.L. Lawless. (1989). Inference based on retrospective ascertainment: an analysis of the data on transfusion-related AIDS. *J. Amer. Stat. Assn.* 84, 360-372.

Kaplan, E.H. (1989). Needles that kill: modeling human immunodeficiency virus transmission via shared drug injection equipment in shooting galleries. *Rev. of Inf. Diseases.* (In press.)

Kaplan, E.H., P.C. Cramton, and A.D. Paltiel. (1989). Nonrandom mixing models of HIV transmission. (This volume.)

Kaplan, H.B., R.J. Johnson, C.A. Bailey, and W. Simon. (1987). The sociological study of AIDS: a critical review of the literature and suggested research agenda. *J. Health and Social Behavior* 28, 140-157.

Karon, J.M., O.J. Devine, and W.M. Morgan. (1989). Predicting AIDS incidence by extrapolating from recent trends. (This volume.)

Karon, J.M., T.J. Dondero, Jr., and J.W. Curran. (1988). The projected incidence of AIDS and estimated prevalence of HIV infection in the United States. *J. AIDS* 1, 542-550.

Kendall, D.G. (1949). Stochastic processes and population growth. *Roy. Statist. Soc., Ser. B* 2, 230-264.

Kermack, W.O. and A.G. McKendrick. (1927). A contribution to the mathematical theory of epidemics. *Proc. Roy. Soc. London, Ser. A* 115, 700-721.

Knox, E.G. (1986). A transmission model for AIDS. *Eur. J. Epidemiol.* 2, 165-177.

Koopman, J.S., C.P. Simon, and J.A. Jacquez. (1989). Selective contact within structured mixing groups; with an application to the analysis of HIV transmission risk from oral and anal sex. (This volume.)

Lagakos, S.W., L.M. Barraj, and V De Gruttola. (1988). Nonparametric analysis of truncated survival data, with application to AIDS. *Biometrika* 75, 515-523.

Lajmanovich, A. and J.A. Yorke. (1976). A deterministic model for gonorrhea in a nonhomogeneous population. *Math. Biosci.* 28, 221-236.

Layne, S.P., T.G. Marr, S.A. Colgate, J.M. Hyman, and E.A. Stanley. (1988). The need for national HIV databases. *Nature* 333, 511-512.

Layne, S.P., J.L. Sponge, and M. Dembo. (1989). Measuring HIV infectivity. (This volume.)

Lehmann, E. L. (1975). *Nonparametrics.* Holden-Day, San Francisco.

Lehmann, E. L. (1983). *Theory of Point Estimation.* John Wiley & Sons, New York.

Lehmann, E.L. (1986). *Testing Statistical Hypotheses,* 2nd edition. John Wiley & Sons, New York.

Longini, I.M., Jr., W.S. Clark, M. Haber, and C.R. Horsburgh, Jr. (1989). The stages of HIV infection: waiting times and infectious contact rates. (This volume.)

Lui, K-J., W.W. Darrow, and G.W. Rutherford III. (1988). A model based estimate of the mean incubation period for AIDS in homosexual men. *Science* 240, 1333-1335.

Lui, K.J., D.N. Lawrence, W.M. Morgan, T.A. Peterman, H.W. Haverkos, and D.J. Bragman. (1986). A model-based approach for estimating the mean incubation period of transfusion-associated acquired immunodeficiency syndrome. *Proc. National Acad. Science, USA* 83, 3051-3055.

Lyter, D.W., R.O. Valdiserri, L.A. Kingsley, W.P. Amoroso, and C.R. Rinaldo. (1987). The HIV antibody test. Why gay and bisexual men want or do not want to know their results? *Public Health Rep* 102, 468-474.

MacDonald, N. (1957). *The Epidemiology and Control of Malaria.* Oxford University Press, London.

May, R.M. and R.M. Anderson. (1987). Transmission dynamics of HIV infection. *Nature* 326, 137-142.

May, R.M. and R.M. Anderson, and A.R. McLean. (1988). Possible demographic consequences of HIV/AIDS: I. Assuming HIV infection always leads to AIDS. *Math. Biosci.* 90, 475-506.

May, R.M. and R.M. Anderson, and A.R. McLean. (1989). Possible demographic consequences of HIV/AIDS: II. Assuming HIV infection does not necessarily leads to AIDS. In *Mathematical approaches to problems in resource management and epidemiology.* C. Castillo-Chavez, S.A. Levin, and C. Shoemaker (eds.). Lecture Notes in Biomathematics 81, Springer-Verlag, Berlin, Heidelberg, New York, Tokyo. (In press.)

McCusker, J., A.M. Stoddard, K.H. Mayer, J. Zapka, C. Morrison, and S.P. Saltzman. (1988). Effects of HIV antibody test knowledge on subsequent sexual behaviors in a cohort of homosexually active men. *Amer. J. Public Health* 78, 462-467.

McKendrick, A.G. (1912). On certain mathematical aspects of malaria. In *Proc. Imperial Malaria Com.* pp. 54-66.

Medley, G.F., R.M. Anderson, D.R. Cox, and L. Billard. (1987). Incubation period of AIDS in patients infected via blood transfusion. *Nature* 328, 719-721.

Medley, G.F., L. Billard, D.R. Cox, and R.M. Anderson. (1988). The distribution of the incubation period for the acquired immunodeficiency syndrome (AIDS). *Proc. R. Soc. Lond. B*, 233, 367-377.

Merrill, S.J. (1989). Modeling the interaction of HIV with cells of the immune response. (This volume.)

Mode, C.J., H.E. Gollwitzer, and W. Herrman. (1989). A methodological study of a stochastic model of an AIDS epidemic. *Math. Biosci.* 92, 201-229.

Mood, A.M., F.A. Graybill, and D.C. Boes. (1974). *Introduction to the Theory of Statistics*, 3rd edition. McGraw-Hill Book Company, New York.

Morgan, W.M. and J.W. Curran. (1986). Acquired immunodeficiency syndrome: current and future trends. *Public Health Rep* 101, 459-465.

Neter, J., W. Wasserman, and M.H. Kutner. (1985). *Applied Linear Statistical Models*, 2nd edition. Richard D. Irwin, Inc., Homewood, IL.

Nold, A. (1980). Heterogeneity in disease-transmission modeling. *Math. Biosci.* 52, 227–240.

Padian, N., L. Marquis, D.P. Francis, R.E. Anderson, G.W. Rutherford, P.M. O'Malley, and W. Winkelstein. (1987). Male-to-female transmission of human immunodeficiency virus. *J. Amer. Med. Assn.* 258, 788-790.

Perelson, A.S. (1989). Modeling the interaction of the immune system with HIV. (This volume.)

Pickering, J., J.A. Wiley, N.S. Padian, L.E. Lieb, D.F. Echenberg, and J. Walker. (1986). Modeling the incidence of acquired immunodeficiency syndrome (AIDS) in San Francisco, Los Angeles and New York. *Mathematical Modeling* 7, 661-698.

Ross, R. (1911). *The prevention of malaria*, 2nd edition. John Murray, London.

Royal Statistical Society. (1988). Statistical requirements of the AIDS epidemic. *J. R. Statist. Soc. A* 151, 127-130.

Sattenspiel, L. (1987). Population structure and the spread of disease. *Human Biol.* 59, 411-438.

Sattenspiel, L. and C.P. Simon. (1988). The spread and persistence of infectious diseases in structured populations. *Math. Biosci.* 90, 341-366.

Schuman, H. and S. Presser. (1981). *Questions and Answers in Attitude Surveys.* Quantitative Studies in Social Relations, Academic Press, Inc., New York.

Silverman, B.W. (1986). *Density Estimation for Statistics and Data Analysis.* Chapman and Hall, New York.

Tan, W. Y. (1989). Some stochastic models of AIDS spread. *Stat. in Med.* 8, 121-136.

Thieme, H.R. and C. Castillo-Chavez. (1989a). On the role of variable infectivity in the dynamics of the human immunodeficiency virus. (This volume.)

Thieme, H.R. and C. Castillo-Chavez. (1989b). On the possible effects of infection-age-dependent infectivity in the dynamics of HIV/AIDS. (Manuscript.)

Waldstätter, R. (1989). Pair formation in sexually-transmitted diseases. (This volume.)

Working Group. (1988). *Short-term prediction of HIV infection and AIDS in England and Wales.* Her Majesty's Stationery Office, London.

Workshop. (1988). *A National Effort to Model AIDS Epidemiology.* Office of Science and Technology Policy, Executive Office of the President, Washington, D.C.

Yorke, J.A., H.W. Hethcote, and A. Nold. (1978). Dynamics and control of the transmission of gonorrhea. *Sexually Transmitted Diseases* 10, 72-76.

1. Statistical Methodology and Forecasting

EPIDEMIC MODELS, EMPIRICAL STUDIES, AND UNCERTAINTY

Victor De Gruttola and Stephen Lagakos
Department of Biostatistics
Harvard School of Public Health
Boston, MA 02115 U.S.A.

Abstract

Mathematical models of the AIDS epidemic require information from a variety of sources. To produce reliable results, these models must take into account the limitations of each data source regarding sample size, accuracy of actual data values, and data structure. Because these limitations determine what can be estimated from each source and how precisely this can be estimated, they affect the quality of model results. Therefore, it is important to consider the effect of uncertainty of estimation in interpreting models.

1. Introduction

Modeling the Human Immunodeficiency Virus (HIV) is one of the most important challenges currently facing quantitative scientists. Because of the complexity of the biology and population dynamics that determine the spread of HIV, there are many features of the epidemic which must be considered when included in models. Modelers must locate different sources of information about these features and characterize their quality and limitations. Since there are more features than can be handled practically, it is necessary to decide which ones are of primary importance to the modeling exercise and which ones can be safely excluded. One must then interpret the results of models in light of these uncertainties.

Sources of information about the AIDS epidemic include epidemiological studies, population surveillance, and laboratory research. In making use of these sources, models must take their limitations into account. These limitations are related to the type of sampling that produced the data, the uncertainty in the observations themselves, and the specificity of the models used to describe the data. Often the features of interest cannot be estimated from these sources without parametric assumptions. For example, a popular assumption in several models that have been proposed for projecting the epidemic is that the distribution of the latency period between infection with HIV and the onset of AIDS is Weibull with a mean of about eight years. However, closer examination of the data on which this assumption is based reveals that a broad range of alternative distributions are also plausible and fit the available data equally well. Thus, for a proper interpretation of the model results, it is not enough to simply check model fit. In addition, one should give an indication of the range of alternative explanations that fit the data equally well.

To determine the degree to which data from a study can be generalized to other populations is crucial for model development. This depends in part on identifying the important covariates that affect distributions or parameters. When the effect of covariates on estimates of epidemic features can be accurately estimated, this information can be included in models. Modelers often describe individual differences in epidemic features as forms of heterogeneity. Observational studies can provide guidance about which sources of heterogeneity to include in models; but when the sensitivity of model results to a form of heterogeneity is low, it may not be important to include it in the model.

Just as modelers should pay attention to the limitations of observational data and other sources of uncertainty, those who conduct epidemiological studies can receive guidance from investigations of models concerning the importance of different sources of heterogeneity. For example, as shown in Section 2, studies of the efficacy of different control strategies depend heavily on the variability of infectivity across individuals. This argues that epidemiological studies should be conducted to characterize such variability.

This paper focuses on some of the important sources of information that are available for use in AIDS modeling, as well as the limitations of these data. The data structures themselves often determine the kinds of methodological development that is required for estimation. Section 2 describes how models are affected by uncertainty in different epidemic features and how model sensitivity can help indicate the types of studies that should be conducted. Section 3 describes the sources of information for characterizing the latency distribution, the ways in which the data structures determine the estimable aspects of the latency distribution, and the precision of estimation. Similary, Section 4 reviews the usefulness and limitations of available information for characterizing the infectiousness of persons infected with HIV.

2. Models, Estimation, and Robustness

With advances in high speed computing, models of enormous complexity can now be numerically evaluated and analyzed. Their ultimate usefulness depends on several factors, including: 1) precision of the input parameters, 2) model sensitivity to uncertainty in model specification and to parameter estimates, and 3) validation of model results by comparison with direct observation in special settings where detailed information is available. Since models often combine data from many sources, careful attention should be paid to the quality of parameter estimation from each of these sources. As models grow more complex, their sensitivity to uncertainty in parameter estimates may increase, and they become harder to validate; therefore, models should be made as simple as possible without ignoring the most important dynamics.

Observational studies are important for deciding which features of the AIDS epidemic need to be included in models and the level of precision with which these features can be described from available data. For example, describing the complex nature of infectiousness may require parameters on type, frequency, and duration of contact, as well as stage of HIV disease and prevalence of other sexually transmitted diseases. Because of the large number of parameters that would be required, it would be fruitless to attempt to determine the effect of all of these characteristics by fitting a model to data on AIDS surveillance or on HIV infection-time. Neither can one decide solely on the basis of model simulations that the number of contacts with an infected partner is crucial or irrelevant. Detailed analyses of studies of partners of HIV-infected people must be performed to determine which of the variables describing sexual contact and disease stage are most important in determining the risk of transmission; only such analyses can adequately characterize the variability in infectiousness within individuals over time and between individuals.

Models also require information about partner selection and the effects of illness on behavior. First we must consider the interaction of populations, since the way in which infected people of different types select their partners affects the spread of HIV. One can begin to address this issue by analyzing data from cohort studies to estimate the effect of promiscuity or place of meeting sexual partners on the time of infection with HIV (Darrow et al. 1988). As we demonstrate, establishing the importance of these covariates often requires methodological development. With appropriate methods, these analyses can also be used to validate the projections of certain models in well-studied populations, such as that of homosexually-active men in San Francisco.

Observational studies can tell much about the effect of different parameters on risk of infection, but successful modeling also requires sensitivity analyses that indicate the degree of precision required for different parameter estimates. For example, De Gruttola and Mayer (1988) demonstrate that models that make use of AIDS incidence data to predict future heterosexual spread of HIV are highly sensitive to within-person variability in infectivity. They found that modeling the future spread of the epidemic among heterosexuals is so dependent on characterizing infectivity that even precise knowledge of sexual behavior and of the interactions of groups at risk had little value without more information on transmission.

The sensitivity of a model to parameters may depend on the way the model is used. For example, models intended for projection can be very sensitive to the latency distribution and to sizes of populations at risk, whereas models intended to demonstrate the effectiveness of interventions can be more sensitive to variability in infectiousness and to population mixing. To illustrate the latter, consider two different possibilities for infectiousness of infected persons: in the first, all infected individuals are equally capable of sexually transmitting HIV to their partners (that is, their per-contact risks of transmission are equal); in the second, some individuals are highly infectious while most others are not. We know from studies of sexual partners of HIV-infected people that the average risk of transmission of HIV per contact is low, but we do not yet know whether this is because there are relatively few "super-spreaders" of HIV, i.e. highly infectious individuals, or whether all infected individuals are about equally infectious but at a low level. Suppose we wish to examine the effect of slowing the rate of partner change on the epidemic, and we are able to persuade people who change partners after every two or three sexual contacts to modify their behavior so that they change partners only after at least 50 contacts. If all infected individuals are equally infectious with a low risk of transmission per contact, say .005, then slowing rate of partner change hardly matters; however, if there are a small proportion of super-spreaders, then reducing the number of people exposed to them might matter a great deal. Of course, the true situation is more complex, because the infectivity of infected people may vary with time from infection and/or stage of disease. Thus, the implications of such variability for policy are very important.

3. Latency Distribution

As described in Section 2, most models of the AIDS epidemic include the latency distribution between infection with HIV and the onset of symptoms. Until now, information about the latency distribution has been provided by data on three categories of HIV-infected people: recipients of contaminated blood transfusions; hemophiliacs who received contaminated blood factor; and people infected by sexual contact, for whom blood samples were collected and stored for reasons other than the AIDS epidemic. An example of such a cohort is the San Francisco Hepatitis B cohort.

a. Transfusion Data

In the United States alone, thousands of people are believed to have been infected with HIV from contaminated blood transfusions. In almost all cases, they have been identified only after their diagnosis with AIDS and subsequent evaluation for possible sources of infection. As a result, the total number of people so infected is unknown; information is only available for those who proceeded from infection to AIDS before the present time.

The analysis of these data to estimate latency is not straightforward because the process of infection and disease is right-truncated in chronological time. Thus, the original estimates of a 1-2 year mean latency, based on the average observed latencies for AIDS cases determined to have been infected by transfusion, were severely biased because they did not account for the sampling distribution by which these data arose. In a subsequent analysis, Lui et al. (1986) took appropriate account of the sampling distribution and used parametric methods to estimate a mean latency of 4-5 years. However, their approach was also misleading because they failed to communicate the extent to which their results were a consequence of the parametric model they selected. Since then, several authors have indicated the limitations of transfusion data for estimating latency and have introduced nonparametric estimators for the identifiable aspects of the latency distribution (Lagakos, Barraj, and De Gruttola 1988; Kalbfleisch and Lawless 1988; Harris 1988).

Regardless of the number of observations, the only estimable aspect of F(t), the distribution function of latency, is the conditional latency distribution, given that an infected individual will develop AIDS within a given time, say T^*, after infection. That is, transfusion data provide information about the conditional distribution $G(t)=F(t)/F(T^*)$ for $0 \leq t \leq T^*$. The proportion of persons, $p=F(T^*)$, who develop AIDS within T^* time units of being infected, as well as the distribution of times of developing AIDS after time T^*, are not estimable. Thus, since descriptors such as the mean and median latency cannot be determined solely from G(t), these quantities are not estimable from transfusion data without the additional assumptions that allow them to be extrapolated.

While extrapolation may be needed to obtain estimated latency distributions for use in epidemic models, it is important to realize that parametric models with very different predicted latencies can fit the observed data equally well. For example, although Lui et al. (1986) estimate a mean latency of 4-5 years based on a particular Weibull distribution, Lagakos, Barraj, and De Gruttola (1988) show that a Weibull distribution with a mean of over 200 years fits the observed transfusion data equally well. This example is not intended to suggest that the mean latency is over 200 years, but rather to illustrate the folly in taking seriously a parametric extrapolation of latency. Thus, while it may be necessary to fit parametric models in order to obtain estimated latencies for use in epidemic models, it is important that we understand and communicate the true uncertainty surrounding these models. Considering the limitations of latency data, the current estimates of 8-10 year mean latency are given a credibility that is undeserved.

Use of parametric models in comparing the latencies of different subgroups of transfusion AIDS cases are also subject to biases. For example, Medley et al. (1987) fitted Weibull and Gamma distributions to about 400 transfusion AIDS cases and noted that persons infected at very old ages have shorter latencies. However, using nonparametric methods to analyze an enlarged version of the same data set, Lagakos and De Gruttola (1989) do not find consistently shorter latencies in older patients except in certain circumstances, and for these the shorter latency can be explained by a higher mortality from non-AIDS death in these persons. Thus, with the exception of infants (which we discuss below), the nonparametric analyses find no differences in latency between men and women, or by age at the time of infection.

There has been considerable disagreement in the scientific literature about the latency distribution of infants. Medley et al. (1987) reported a very short latency period; but these estimates were based upon a model which assumes a unimodal density for the underlying latency distribution. If untrue, these assumptions result in underestimates of median latency. Recent nonparametric analyses of transfusion-related AIDS (Lagakos and De Gruttola 1989) and of maternally-acquired AIDS (Auger et al. 1988) suggest that the latency distribution could reflect a mixed population consisting of one subgroup of children who develop AIDS within a year or two and another subgroup whose latency distribution is more similar to that of adults. The analyses of maternally-acquired AIDS demonstrate that about 20% of children who will develop AIDS within 10 years do so within the first year of life; the remainder develop AIDS at a fairly constant rate of 8% per year. The median age for those who develop AIDS within 10 years is 4.8 years. These estimates are very similar to those for infants infected by blood transfusion within the first year of life (Lagakos and De Gruttola 1989). Although the actual latency distribution of infants is still unknown, the relationship $F(t)=p \cdot G(t)$ implies that estimates of the location of the conditional distribution $G(t)$ provide a lower bound for those of $F(t)$. Therefore, nonparametric analyses produce estimates of latency period for infants that are substantially greater than parametric analogues. Clearly this information would be critical in a modeling effort which, for example, attempted to predict the number of AIDS cases in children that will occur in the next few years.

b. Hemophilia Data

Another important source of information for estimating the latency distribution arises from studies of hemophiliacs who became infected with HIV from infusion with contaminated blood factor. Because blood samples were routinely collected and stored for many hemophiliacs, it is possible to test these samples retrospectively to determine the date at which infected hemophiliacs first showed evidence of HIV infection. An unusual property of these data is that both the time of infection with HIV and time of onset of symptoms are censored — a situation referred to as doubly censored data. Since the time of seroconversion can never be known exactly, it is always interval censored, even in prospective studies. In some studies, the intervals are often short enough to be ignored; but for retrospective studies, the interval may be quite long compared to the mean latency. Therefore, ad hoc methods for analysis, such as using midpoints of intervals as times of events, may yield poor approximations. De Gruttola and Lagakos (1989) propose nonparametric and weakly structured parametric methods for analyzing survival data in which both the time, origin and the failure event can be right- or interval-censored. The methods generalize the self-consistency algorithm proposed by Turnbull (1976) for singly censored data. A byproduct of these methods is that they also produce estimates of the distribution of the chronological time of sero-conversion of the population.

One covariate that may be important for time of infection and latency is the amount of blood factor that hemophiliacs received from 1980 to 1985 (De Gruttola and Lagakos 1989). They analyzed separately two groups of patients treated at a hematology center in Paris who were defined by their level of treatment. This analysis revealed that the higher incidence of AIDS among the more heavily treated hemophiliacs resulted more from earlier infection with HIV than from a higher risk of AIDS after infection. Although the risk of the first symptom of HIV infection (including lymphadenopathy syndrome, ARC, AIDS, and leukopenia) is slightly elevated for the most heavily treated, the effect appears to be small.

Because of the problems of identifiability in nonparametric estimation of doubly interval-censored data, incorporation of covariates into analyses requires more parametric structure. One approach is to use the nonparametric analysis to suggest parametric shapes, and then incorporate the covariates into a parametric model. Brookmeyer and Goedert (1989) have suggested a parametric approach to considering the effect of covariates on interval-censored data regarding AIDS in hemophiliacs. They assumed a Weibull distribution for the time to AIDS and a piecewise exponential for the infection-time distribution. This analysis showed geographical differences in the risk of infection as well as differences related to type of hemophilia. They also found that hemophiliacs over 20 had an increased risk of clinical AIDS compared to younger hemophiliacs.

It would be interesting to compare, by age at infection, the latency distribution of hemophiliacs with that of people infected by blood transfusion. Unfortunately, the differences in the sampling for these two groups make it difficult to establish whether these distributions are equal.

c. San Francisco Hepatitis B Cohort

A sampling distribution similar to the one described for hemophiliacs also applies to a cohort of men who were recruited to participate in a trial of a hepatitis B vaccine. Between 1978 and 1980, blood samples were collected and stored for about 7000 men who were screened for the hepatitis B antibody. Men who were at risk but did not have evidence of infection with hepatitis B were invited to participate in the trial. For those who ultimately enrolled, multiple blood samples were collected; for many others who did not enroll but could subsequently be located, blood samples were obtained in the mid 1980's, after the severity of the AIDS epidemic was understood. For all of the original 7000 men, attempts have been made to determine their current status; well over 1000 have already developed AIDS.

These are perhaps the most valuable data in existence for estimating the latency distribution of homosexually-acquired AIDS; but many problems regarding their analysis remain unresolved: (1) because the censoring intervals are often long, estimates of latency that assume seroconversion took place at the midpoints of intervals may introduce severe bias. Analyses that discard persons with long intervals, in an attempt to minimize this bias, are inefficient since these reduce the sample size. A preferable approach would have been to use statistical methods designed for interval censored data; (2) the reasons for losses to follow-up in these data are hard to determine, but there is reason to suspect that they could represent informative types of censoring. If so, this can bias estimates of latency; (3) the individuals who were infected at entry into the study provide important information about people infected with HIV for longer than 10 years, but the times of infection must be imputed since no seroconversion can be documented before 1978. Bacchetti (1988) has considered the third problem, but additional methodological work is required to address all of the problems simultaneously. Only application of new methodology will make it possible to develop the best possible estimates of latency and to characterize fully the uncertainty of these estimates.

4. Infectiousness of Persons Infected with HIV

As mentioned in Section 2, epidemic models that are useful for investigating the efficacy of different interventions require characterization of the variability in per-contact probability of HIV transmission between infected and susceptible persons. In the context of sexual transmission, this probability could vary depending on the characteristics of the infected individual or on those of the susceptible individual. Thus, one might expect differences in the per-contact risk both between couples and over time within couples.

Current understanding of the biology of HIV provides some insight into the natures of infectiousness and susceptibility (Goedert et al. 1987; 1988; Osmond et al. 1988; Padian et al. 1988); however, there is still considerable uncertainty about the degree of variability of these characteristics in different populations. Sources of variability include the amount and type of contact with infected partners, the amount of virus present in genital secretions, and the presence of genital lesions. All of these factors may be related, i.e., those who have been infected longer and therefore have had more contacts with their partner subsequent to infection may also be more viremic; those with genital lesions may have more risk of transmission or infection per contact and may also be more promiscuous. Direct evidence about the variability of per-contact risk of HIV transmission is possible from observational studies of susceptible partners of an HIV-infected person, but problems of confounding complicate this research. These 'partner studies' typically involve ascertainment of the HIV sero-status of sexual partners of persons known to be infected with HIV. From this information, investigators attempt to estimate certain quantities, such as per-contact risk, and the effect on this risk of various factors characterizing the infected or susceptible person.

In this section, we review the types of partner studies that have been conducted to estimate the risk of HIV transmission. Our purpose is to identify some of the inherent limitations of these studies and to describe how their design determines what one can and cannot infer about the actual per-contact risk. We begin by describing, in generic terms, the types of sampling schemes that have been used in partner studies and then consider several plausible models for the per-contact risk. Finally, we discuss issues of statistical identifiability and estimability associated with these models and sampling schemes. For more details, see Kim and Lagakos

(1989), from which these results are condensed. See also Wiley et al. (1989) and De Gruttola et al. (1989).

a. Types of Partner Studies

Most partner studies that have been conducted involve one of three sampling designs. The simplest is a purely cross-sectional study in which the sexual partners of persons known to be HIV-positive are tested for HIV sero-positivity (cf: Seage et al. 1988). Typically, the proportions of sero-positive partners in different subgroups are then compared to assess the relative efficacy of transmission. A second type of design (cf: Peterman et al. 1988), which we refer to as a retrospective study, enrolls index cases whose times of infection with HIV are known or can be estimated, and collects retrospective information about them and their sexual partners, including the current HIV-status of the partner. A third design, which we refer to as a prospective study, enrolls and prospectively monitors the sero-status of sexual partners of persons known to be infected with HIV (Cf: Fischl et al. 1987). Of course, some studies can have both prospective and retrospective components.

Key issues in studying the ability of each of these designs to provide information about per-contact risk include: 1) what is known about the time of infection of the index case and the partner, 2) sexual contacts outside of the partnership, 3) types and frequency of sexual contacts within the partnership, and 4) characteristics of the index case and his/her partner.

Of the three designs being considered, the cross-sectional study is the simplest to conduct but the least informative. Typically, the time of infection of the index case, the frequency of sexual contacts between the index case and the partner, and details about risky behavior outside of the partnership are not known. In fact, when both individuals are found to be seropositive, it is sometimes unclear who was infected first. If a good model for progression of a marker of HIV infection becomes available, it may become possible to impute the times of infection for the partners based on the distribution of times of infections for the population from which they were sampled, from personal histories, and from serial measurements of the marker.

Retrospective studies are most capable of providing information about the per-contact risk of transmission. For example, Peterman et al. (1988) identified 80 persons infected with HIV through blood transfusion and then obtained information about their clinical symptoms, the demographic characteristics, the frequency of sexual contact, and the current sero-status of their partners. Because the index cases were infected through blood transfusions, an exact time of infection is known. Thus, if information can be obtained about the types and frequency of sexual contact between index cases and their spouses, for those couples believed to have a monogamous relationship, many of the limitations inherent to the cross-sectional design could be overcome.

Prospective studies, such as that of Fischl et al. (1987), have the inherent advantage of allowing frequent monitoring of the sero-status of spouses of infected persons who are sero-negative at enrollment. Thus, the time of sero-conversion can be determined to fall into a small time-interval. A common limitation of this type of study, however, is that the time of infection of the index case usually is not known. Thus, models for the per-contact risk of HIV transmission that allow variations in risk as a function of time since infection of the index case cannot be applied unless time of infection can be imputed from markers of disease.

With all three designs, of course, there is also considerable concern about the accuracy of the information that is collected about sexual practices, especially since this relies on self-reporting. Thus, information about frequency of specific types of sexual activity, sexual contacts outside of the partnership, and use of barrier contraceptives must always be questioned. Since it is possible that the accuracy of reporting may vary by subgroup of patients, comparisons between subgroups might be especially biased.

b. Models for Per-Contact Risk of HIV Transmission

There are many possible types of models for variability in per-contact risk of HIV transmission between and within partnerships. To illustrate some of the possibilities, we list several models that have already been used or proposed, and some that simply seem plausible. Throughout our discussion, $p_i(t,z)$ denotes the generic per-contact probability of transmission for couple i at time t after infection of the index case, and z denotes some characteristic of the index case or partner. Note that $p_i(t,z)$ is the transmission probability given that the partner was not infected prior to the current sexual contact, and that the cofactor z could be time-dependent. For example, z=1 might denote that, at the time of the contact, the index case had previously been diagnosed as having AIDS, while $z=0$ might denote that he/she had not been previously diagnosed with AIDS.

The simplest model assumes that $p_i(t,z)$ is constant in all of its arguments; that is, $p_i(t,z) = p$. Thus, the risk of transmission is assumed to be constant both within a partnership and between couples. A more general model would allow the risk to vary with time since infection of the index case in a deterministic way. For example, one might assume that $p_i(t,z)=p_1$ for $t<2$ months and $f(t)=p_2$ for $t\geq 2$ months, where p_1 and p_2 are unknown parameters that must be estimated. This specific model allows the per-contact probability of transmission to take one value (p_1) for a short time after infection and to then take a different value.

One way of generalizing the preceding models is to allow $p_i(t,z)$ to depend upon some change in the status of the index case or partner. For example, one such model would assume that $p(t,z)=p_1$ when $z=0$ and that $p_i(t,z)=1$ when $z=1$, where z denotes the AIDS status of the index case ($z=0$ indicating that the patient has not yet developed AIDS). Thus, this model assumes that the per-contact probability of transmission shifts from p_1 to p_2 when the infected partner develops AIDS. Of course, any combination of the above models could also be considered.

Until now, we have only considered models in which the per-contact risk of transmission does not vary between couples, except possibly for the factors (time since infection, AIDS status) explicitly considered. However, it may also be desirable to allow for the possibility of additional sources of variability between couples whose cause is not directly measurable. One way of doing this is to regard one or more of the parameters in these models as a random effect and to put a prior distribution on these parameters. For example, Wiley et al. (1989) assume that the per-contact risk is constant, say p, within a partnership, but then fit Beta and 2-point prior distributions to p. Such random effects models allow for the possibility that risk can vary between couples for reasons that cannot be directly related to specific cofactors. This feature makes it possible to test the hypothesis that risk varies between couples without knowledge of the source of this variability.

c. Estimability and Identifiability

Consider first the cross-sectional design. As shown by Kim and Lagakos (1989), none of the model parameters discussed previously are estimable from cross-sectional studies. For example, even with the simplest model, the parameter p is nonidentifiable unless additional assumptions are made. However, under certain circumstances, the per-contact probabilities, say p_A and p_B, of two groups can be tested for equality. The reason for this is that the cross-sectional study provides direct information about the prevalences, say π_A and π_B, of HIV in the two groups of partners. When the numbers of sexual contacts since the index case's infection have the same distribution in the two groups, then the equality of p_A and p_B implies the equality of π_A and π_B. It follows that a test of the equality of the prevalence of HIV in the two comparison groups is equivalent to a test of the quality of their corresponding p's. Thus, while the per-contact probability p cannot be estimated, one can test whether it varies across subgroups.

For prospective designs, the parameters of certain models we have described become statistically identifiable and can be estimated using standard likelihood theory. However, models for $p_i(t,z)$ that depend explicitly on time since the infection of the index case cannot be estimated since this is assumed to be unknown.

Because time of infection of the index is known with the retrospective design, each of the types of models considered in the previous section are in principal identifiable. To illustrate, we summarize the analyses presented in Kim and Lagakos (1989) of the Peterman et al. (1988) data. When the simplest model is assumed, the common value of p is estimated to be .0013 $\pm$ .0004 for male-to-female transmission and .0005 $\pm$ .0003 for female-to-male transmission. However, use of a random effects model (Wiley et al. 1988) or direct goodness-of-fit tests demonstrate that this model does not fit the data, indicating that additional sources of variation are present. For the model that allows the per-contact risk to change from p_1 to p_2 upon the onset of AIDS in the infected partner, the estimates of p_1 and p_2 for male-to-female transmission are .0009 $\pm$ .0004 and .0567 $\pm$ .034, respectively, and for female-to-male transmission, they are .0003 $\pm$ .0003 and .0032 $\pm$ .004, respectively. Note that for both directions, the point estimates of p_2 are greater than those for p_1, which supports the belief of some that persons become more infectious as they develop symptoms. However, goodness-of-fit tests show lack of fit of this model for both male-to-female and female-to-male transmission. Thus, the apparent increase in risk of transmission with the onset of symptoms may be an artifact of an inappropriate model. Even if risk does increase with the onset of symptoms, it may also depend on one or more other factors associated with this onset. This possibility could be explored further by the inclusion of cofactors into the models for $p_i(t,z)$. For example, each of the parameters in the model could be regressed onto one or more cofactors such as age of the index case at the time of infection, presence of genital ulcers in the susceptible partner, concomitant sexually-transmitted diseases, etc. A practical limitation is that it becomes difficult to discriminate between distinct models. Thus, for example, a model which assumes that the per-contact risk rises gradually with time since infection in a deterministic way and which identifies race as an important cofactor might be indistinguishable from a model in which the risk of transmission increases with the onset of AIDS and for which menopausal status is the cofactor.

Given the potential biases in these studies due to inaccuracies in the reporting of types and frequency of sexual contact, sexual contacts outside the partnership, other forms of risky behavior such as IV drug use, etc., one must be wary of drawing conclusions from partner studies. It is not surprising that some partner studies have not even established that risk of infection increases with the number of contacts with an infected partner, while others have been mistakenly cited as demonstrating a lack of association.

What can we conclude from the available evidence? It seems clear that the simplest model does not apply, and that per contact probability of transmission must vary either between couples or over time within couples. Some studies have observed an association between risk of transmission and presence of HIV-related symptoms in the index case (Osmond et al. ; Goedert et al. 1988), while other studies have shown no such association (Padian et al. 1988; De Gruttola et al. 1989). In one instance we investigated, the model that purported to show such an association did not fit the data, implying that more complex models including other sources of variability must be considered.

Our preliminary analyses imply that characterizing the variability in rates of transmission will require large studies with long follow-up times. For this reason, every effort should be made to enroll spouses of infected hemophiliacs and transfusion recipients into prospective studies. Although such individuals may not be typical of all people who become infected, they provide extremely valuable information. Most such individuals do not have other risky exposures, and the infection time of the index case is often known or can be accurately estimated. Without this information, it is not likely that the true variability in transmission risk will ever be known; and the absence of such information limits the contribution of epidemic modeling to policy decisions.

5. Discussion

Epidemic modeling requires observational studies both to suggest forms of models and to provide bases for parameter estimation. Incorporation of results from observational studies, however, is not always straightforward; one must first determine what distributions and parameters are identifiable from these studies, and then apply methods that are as robust and efficient as possible. As we have shown in Sections 3 and 4, distributions of interest are not always identifiable from available studies because of the unusual sampling schemes from which data have arisen. Without parametric assumptions, the latency distribution is not identifiable from data on transfusion-related AIDS, and the within- and between- person variability in infectivity is not identifiable from partner studies. Analyses performed under such assumptions may be unreliable because the results can depend upon the assumptions more than on the actual data. One example of this is the estimate of a very short latency period in infants. Similarly, estimates of the average rate of sexual transmission of HIV may be very misleading if the important sources of variability have not been established.

Even when the important parameters and distributions are identifiable, the variability in these estimates may be large. Appropriate estimates of this variability are required, because model results are not interpretable unless the effect of uncertainty in model parameters and specification can be assessed. Since this uncertainty must be simultaneously assessed for all parameters, it may be more useful to have simpler models. No model can fully describe a complex process, regardless of how many parameters are included. The virtue of a simple model is that one can study its properties, such as precision of estimates and robustness to assumptions, in ways that are not generally possible in complex models. Whatever type of model is used, however, it is important to emphasize the uncertainty of the resulting estimates.

The distributions we discussed in Sections 3 and 4 are useful in epidemic modeling, but they are not sufficient. Other important features of the epidemic, however, are even more difficult to characterize. One of the most important is characterization of mixing of different subpopulations of people at risk of HIV infection. Because an infection time distribution of arbitrary shape could be created by the interaction of homogeneous subpopulations, epidemic models of population dynamics must be particularly concerned with mixing. Even very precise information on the number of sexual contacts from sexual histories is not sufficient to characterize the mixing of different groups, i.e., mixing parameters are not identifiable from marginal distributions of sexual contact. Therefore, studies should be designed which include place as well as type of contact. Rather than complex diffusion models, whose parameters are not likely to be estimable from any feasible study, one might begin with simple two-population models for sexual transmission which include people who have anonymous contacts and those who do not. To fully characterize mixing would require more complex study designs, analogous to capture-recapture experiments used in ecological studies. These may never be feasible in AIDS research, but one might study pair formation by estimating the probabilities that individuals enrolled in cohort studies select others from the same studies. Further research is also need to find ways to differentiate between individual behavioral change over time that results from aging, and behavioral change of a population over time that may result from information and educational programs. These two effects are confounded in prospective cohort studies.

Just as we use individual characteristics of HIV-infected people to study the dynamics of the AIDS epidemic, we can use the epidemiological dynamics to study the individual progression of infection. Information on the infection-time distribution and the effect of measurable covariates on this distribution is very helpful in studying progression of markers of disease, since the time of infection is generally unknown for infected people enrolled in prospective studies. By estimating the distribution of the marker in uninfected people and imputing the time of infection from external sources, it may be possible to improve estimates of progression.

Whether the focus of study is individual progression of HIV infection, community spread of HIV, or effect of intervention programs on spread, modelers need to be able to combine sources of information from many different areas of research. Combining evidence requires detailed knowledge of the methods by which estimates have been produced as well as knowledge above the uncertainty of these estimates. Thus the development of useful epidemic models requires close collaboration between mathematicians concerned with the simulation of complex systems and statisticians concerned with inference from observational studies.

Acknowledgement

This work was supported by grant AI24643 from the National Institute of Allergy and Infectious Diseases, National Institutes of Health. We are grateful to the reviewers for their helpful comments.

References

Auger, I., P. Thomas, V. De Gruttola, D. Morse, D. Moore, R. Williams, B. Truman and C. Lawrence. (1988). Incubation periods for pediatric AIDS patients. Nature **336**:515-517.

Bacchetti P. (1988). Estimating the incubation period of AIDS using population seroprevalence estimates. Annual Meeting of the Western North American Region of the Biometrics Society, June 1988, Honolulu.

Brookmeyer, R. and J. Goedert. (1989). Censoring in an epidemic with an application to hemophilia-associated AIDS. Biometrics **45**:325-335.

Darrow, W., H. Jaffee, A. Hardy, W. Meade Morgan, R. Selik and T. Dondero. (1988). Behavior associated with HIV-1 infection and the development of AIDS. AIDS 1988: AAAS Symposia Papers.

De Gruttola, V. and K. Mayer. (1988). Assessing and modelling heterosexual spread of the human immunodeficiency virus in the United states. Reviews of Infectious Diseases **10(1)**:138-150.

De Gruttola, V. and S. Lagakos. (1989). Analysis of doubly censored survival data, with application to AIDS. Biometrics **45:1-11**.

De Gruttola, V., G. Seage, K. Mayer and R. Horsburgh. (1989). Infectiousness of HIV between Homosexual Partners. Journal of Clinical Epidemiology (in press).

Fischl, M., G. Dickinson, G. Scott, N. Klimas, M.A. Fletcher and W. Parks. (1987). Evaluation of heterosexual partners, children, and household contacts of adults of AIDS. JAMA 257:640-644.

Goedert, J., M. Eyster, J. Biggar and W. Blattner. (1987). Heterosexual transmission of Human Immunodeficiency Virus: Association with severe depletion of T-helper lymphocytes in men with hemophilia. AIDS Research and Human Retroviruses **3(4)**:355-361.

Goedert, J., M. Eyster and M. Ragni. (1988). Rate of heterosexual HIV transmission and associated risk with HIV-antigen. Abstract No. 4019, IVth International Conference on AIDS.

Harris, J. (1988). The incubation period for Human Immunodeficiency Virus. Working Paper of the Department of Economics, Massachusetts Institute of Technology.

Kalbfleisch, J. and J. Lawless. (1988). Inference based on retrospective ascertainment: an analysis of the data on transfusion related AIDS. Department of Statistics and Actuarial Science, University of Waterloo.

Kim, M. and S. Lagakos. (1989). Estimating the per contact risk of HIV transmission. Presented at AAAS Meetings, San Francisco, January, 1989.

Lagakos, S., L.M. Barraj and V. De Gruttola. (1988). Non-parametric analysis of trucated survival data. Biometrika **75(3)**:515-523.

Lagakos, S. and V. De Gruttola. (1989). The conditional latency distribution of AIDS for persons infected by blood transfusion. Journal of AIDS **2**:84-87.

Lui, K., D.N. Lawrence, W.M. Morgan, T.A. Peterman, H.H. Haverkos and D.J. Bregman. (1986). A model-based approach for estimating the mean incubation period of transfusion-associated acquired immunodeficiency sydrome. Proc. Nat. Acad. Sci. **84**, 2913-7.

Medley, G., L. Billard, D. Cox and R. Anderson. (1987). Incubation period of AIDS in patients infected via blood transfusion. Nature **328**:719-21.

Osmond, D., P. Bacchetti, R. Chaisson, T. Kelly, R. Stempel, J. Carlson and A. Moss. (1988). Time of exposure and risk of HIV infection in homosexual partners of men with AIDS. American Journal of Public Health **78(8)**:944-948.

Padian, N., S. Glass, L. Marquis. (1988). Heterosexual transmission of HIV in California: results from a heterosexual partner study. Abstract 4020, IVth International Conference on AIDS.

Peterman, T., R. Stoneburner and J. Allen. (1988). Risk of Human Immunodeficiency Virus transmission from heterosexual adults with transfusion-associated infection. JAMA **259(1)**:55-58.

Seage, G., D. Horsburgh, A. Hardy and K. Mayer. (1988). Increase suppressor T-calls in probable transmitters of the Human Immunodeficiency Virus infection. Technical Report. Boston University School of Medicine, Harrison Avenue, Boston, MA 02114.

Turnbull, B. (1976). The empirical distribution function with arbitrarily grouped, censored, and trucated data. J. Roy. Stat. Soc., Ser. B **38**:290-295.

Wiley, J., S. Hershkorn and N. Padian. (1989). Heterogeneity in the probability of HIV transmission per sexual contact: The case of male-to-female transmission in penile-vaginal intercourse. Stat. in Med., **8(1)**:93-102.

PREDICTING AIDS INCIDENCE BY EXTRAPOLATING FROM RECENT TRENDS

John M. Karon, Owen J. Devine, W. Meade Morgan
AIDS Program (G-29), Centers for Disease Control
Atlanta, Georgia 30333 U.S.A.

Abstract

Projections of future acquired immunodeficiency syndrome (AIDS) cases are important for public health planning. This report provides a detailed description of the extrapolation method that the Centers for Disease Control has used to make 5-year projections. Reported incidence is first adjusted for reporting delays. The prediction model extrapolates recent trends in incidence by fitting a Box-Cox model to adjusted incidence by maximum likelihood. Prediction intervals can be computed from least squares regression prediction intervals conditional on the Box-Cox transformation parameter or from a bootstrap procedure. Projections for subgroups can also be made by modeling the time series of proportions of AIDS cases in the subgroups. Projections made in early 1986 were quite accurate for 1986 and 1987, but improved methods for adjusting for reporting delays could yield better projections. Our experience indicates that the form of the extrapolation model must be chosen carefully, using both statistical criteria and substantive knowledge.

1. Introduction

Projections of future numbers of acquired immunodeficiency syndrome (AIDS) cases indicate the likely magnitude of the problem posed by human immunodeficiency virus (HIV) disease and are useful for estimating the health care and soçial services that will be needed by those who will become ill. For example, in May 1986, about 21,000 AIDS cases diagnosed in the United States had been reported to the Centers for Disease Control (CDC). Extrapolating the trend of AIDS cases diagnosed each month led to a prediction that, under current diagnostic and reporting practices, 270,000 cases diagnosed by the end of 1991 would be reported to CDC (Morgan and Curran, 1986). This suggested that the cases reported at that time represented a public health problem that would become much more severe in the next 5 years.

The primary methods used to predict future numbers of AIDS cases in the United States are extrapolation from recent trends (Morgan and Curran, 1986) and the back-calculation procedure (Brookmeyer and Gail, 1986, 1988; Brookmeyer and Damiano, 1989). The back-calculation method is based explicitly on the latency or incubation time distribution, the distribution of time from HIV infection to a diagnosis of AIDS. Estimates of this distribution in adults (Medley et al., 1987; Lui, Darrow, and Rutherford, 1988; Lui, Peterman et al., 1988; Harris, 1988) show that only a few percent of those infected with HIV are diagnosed as having AIDS within 3 years after infection. The risk of an AIDS diagnosis then rises and is relatively high from perhaps 5 to at least 10 years after infection. As a result, any change in HIV incidence will cause little change in AIDS incidence for at least 3 years, with the effect spread over at least 5 years later on. If diagnostic and reporting practices remain consistent in a large population, therefore, the trend in AIDS incidence will not change rapidly. Thus the long and varied latency period provides a substantive basis for making short-term predictions by extrapolating recent trends in AIDS incidence.

This report contains a detailed description and a discussion of the extrapolation method the CDC has used to predict AIDS incidence. We first describe the data available (Section 2), emphasizing the effect of a change in the case definition made in 1987. We then present the method we use to adjust for reporting delays (Section 3) and our procedure to extrapolate trends in incidence (Section 4). We discuss the important problem of estimating the uncertainty in predictions (Section 5) and outline a method for predicting AIDS incidence within subgroups by modeling a time series of proportions (Section 6). After illustrating these methods using recent data (Section 7), we conclude by discussing our extrapolation procedure, with emphasis on areas in which additional research is needed, and by comparing our procedure to several alternatives (Section 8).

We wish to emphasize that the projections in Section 7 are for illustration only. Because we do not investigate carefully the effect of the change in the case definition, and we do not adjust for diagnosed cases never reported to CDC, the projections in this report do not supercede the 1988 Public Health Service projections (U.S. Public Health Service, 1988).

2. Data available

Since 1981, AIDS cases meeting a surveillance definition have been reported to CDC by state and local health departments. Surveillance for AIDS is conducted by health departments in each state, U.S. territory, and the District of Columbia. In most of these areas, surveillance is both active and passive. In many areas, public health officials not only contact hospital personnel for assistance in detecting and reporting cases, but also use other record systems such as death certificates and tumor registries. In 1985-1986, most diagnosed AIDS cases were being reported: a study of deaths during that year in four cities (Hardy et al., 1987; Starcher et al., 1987) suggested that only about 10% of cases meeting the surveillance definition had not been reported to the appropriate state or local health department.

Reporting to CDC is voluntary and uses a standard format. For each case, the data reported include date and geographic location of diagnosis, diseases present, laboratory results, patient risk information and demographic data. The use of a variety of record systems to detect cases can result in substantial delays in reporting AIDS cases.

The CDC AIDS surveillance definition was revised in September 1987. Before that date, any patient reported as an AIDS case had to have a diagnosis of certain opportunistic diseases, including *Pneumocystis carinii* pneumonia (PCP) or candidiasis, or a cancer, such as Kaposi's sarcoma, confirmed by culture of a tissue specimen or by pathology; for all but a few percent of reported cases, no test for HIV infection was required (World Health Organization, 1986). In September 1987, two types of expanded criteria were added for patients with HIV infection confirmed by laboratory test (Centers for Disease Control, 1987). To reflect a trend in diagnostic practice, presumptive diagnoses (without laboratory confirmation) were allowed for some opportunistic diseases, most notably PCP. To include other life-threatening conditions resulting from HIV infection, a case could be reported based on HIV encephalopathy (dementia), wasting syndrome, or some additional opportunistic infections.

These changes have affected trends in recent AIDS incidence. About 13% of the cases diagnosed in September 1987 - December 1988 were diagnosed only on the basis of these additional conditions. Cases diagnosed before the fall of 1987 meeting only the new definition have been reported to the surveillance system recently as a result of retrospective reviews of records. For example, of all cases diagnosed in the second quarter of 1987 and reported through 1988, 14.8% met the criteria for the new definition only; for cases diagnosed in the first quarter of 1985 and 1986, 2.8% and 8.6% were reportable only under the new definition.

An adjustment for the change in the case definition should be considered in extrapolating from past trends. A correct adjustment would require knowing how the revised case definition affected the reporting of cases. While relevant studies have yet to be done, surveillance data show that AIDS patients reported only under the revised definition are more likely to be black or Hispanic, more likely to be intravenous drug users, and less likely to be homosexual men (U.S. Public Health Service, 1988). Many presumptive diagnoses of the diseases in the pre-1987 case definition may, however, represent a shift in diagnostic practice as physicians became more familiar with treating patients with HIV. Cases with any diagnosis (including a presumptive diagnosis) of a disease in the pre-1987 case definition can be regarded as being consistent with that definition. Even though such cases with only presumptively diagnosed diseases represent 15% of all cases diagnosed since the change in the case definition, there is a smooth trend in the quarterly AIDS incidence of cases consistent (in this sense) with the pre-1987 definition, rather than a shift late in 1987 (see Figure 1).

3. Adjusting for reporting delays

Many AIDS cases that ultimately will be reported to CDC are not reported promptly. Fewer than 10% are reported in the month of diagnosis; about half are reported within two months, about 85% within 1 year of diagnosis, and about 95% within 2 years. Reporting practices vary geographically, resulting in variation in reporting delays (Brookmeyer and Damiano, 1989).

To use recent data in making projections, it is essential to adjust for these reporting delays by estimating the probability that a case will be reported within a given period after diagnosis. Relevant data available are month of diagnosis, month of report to CDC, and location of diagnosis. If a least squares model is used to make predictions, it is also necessary to estimate the variance of the reporting probabilities in

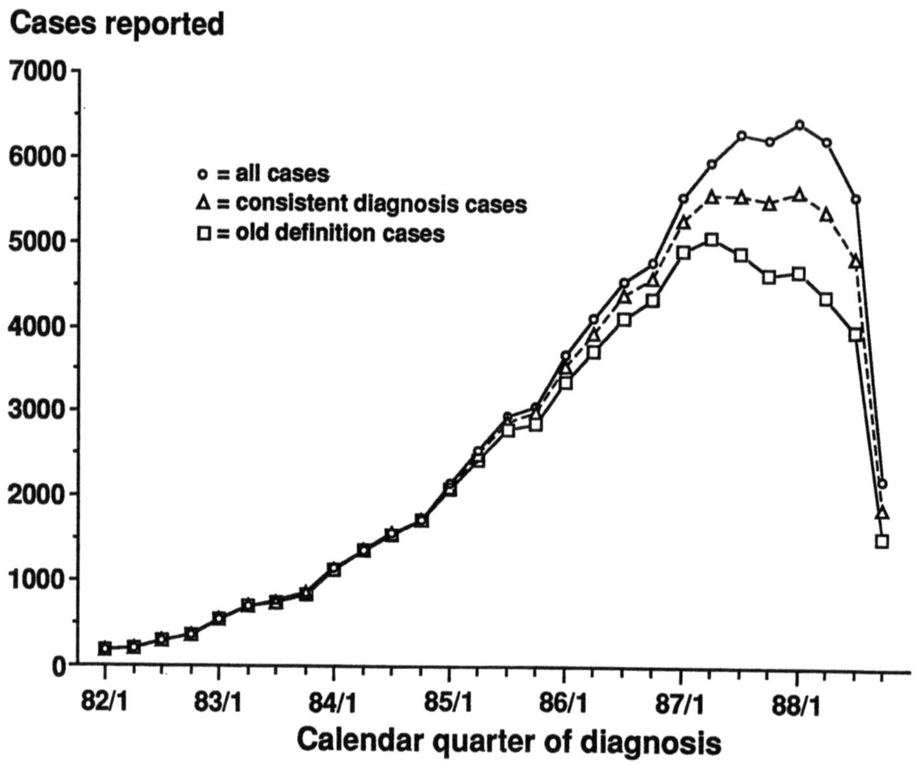

Figure 1. AIDS cases diagnosed in the United States, 1982-1988, and reported to the Centers for Disease Control through December, 1988.

order to estimate inverse variance weights that reflect the uncertainty in adjusted incidence (see Section 4). Several estimation procedures have been proposed.

It is natural to regard data on reporting delays as arising from multinomial distributions. With each period of diagnosis (e.g. calendar month or quarter) defining a population, the problem is to estimate the size of each population (N_t, the number diagnosed with AIDS in period t) from the number of cases diagnosed in period t already reported, I_t. The multinomial probabilities are the probabilities of a case being reported with a delay of 0, 1, 2, ... periods. Harris (1987) obtained maximum likelihood estimates (MLEs) of the population sizes N_t from an iterative procedure by assuming that each N_t has a Poisson distribution. Brookmeyer and Damiano (1989) noted that a conditional MLE (conditional on the number diagnosed in each period who have been reported thus far) can be obtained from a Poisson regression analysis. Their approach facilitates including and testing for geographic and temporal effects. Lui and Rudy (1989) point out that multinomial probabilities can also be modeled by a flexible parametric distribution, incorporating the truncation of each sample in the parameter estimation procedure. They used the Weibull distribution. Geographic and temporal effects can also be incorporated and tested.

We use an adaptation of Harris' procedure, restricting our analysis to those cases that ultimately will be reported and assuming that reporting delays are homogeneous over time. Let t index the periods used to model reporting delays, $t = 1,2,\ldots,T$, where T is the most recent complete period. We assume that, for some fixed $R < T$, the probability of reporting a case with a delay of R or more periods is constant. R is chosen so that nearly all cases are reported within R periods after diagnosis, as indicated by the available data.

We use the following notation. Let n_{tr} be the number of cases diagnosed in period t reported with a delay of r periods, $r = 0,1,\ldots,\min(T-t,R-1)$, with sum $n_{t.}$, and let n_{tR} be the number reported with a delay of at least R periods if $t \le T-R$. For $t = 1,2,\ldots,T$, denote by $\underline{n}_t$ the vector of the number of cases diagnosed in period t reported with delay less than R periods. Let π_r, $r=0,1,\ldots,R-1$, and π_R be the probabilities that a case is reported with delay r periods and at least R periods, respectively; by assumption, the π_r do not depend on time. Let q_t be the probability that a case diagnosed during period t has been reported by the end of period T:

$$q_t = \sum_{r=0}^{T-t} \pi_r, \qquad t > T - R. \tag{1}$$

We assume that N_t is known (the observed value I_t) for $t \le T-R$; by the choice of R, for these values of t, most of the diagnosed cases are believed to have been reported. MLEs of the N_t for $t > T-R$ can be derived conditional on π_R under the assumptions that, for $t > T-R$, the N_t have independent Poisson distributions with means m_t and the vectors $\underline{n}_t$ have independent multinomial distributions.

With the corresponding assumptions (for $R = T$), Harris (1987) observes that, given N_t and q_t, $n_{t.}$ has a binomial distribution. Because N_t is assumed to have a Poisson distribution, the unconditional distribution of $n_{t.}$ is also Poisson. Since the distribution of $\underline{n}_t$ conditional on $n_{t.}$ is multinomial, the likelihood can be written as a product of this multinomial likelihood and the Poisson likelihood for $n_{t.}$.

The MLE of m_t can be computed from the following iterative procedure. Our initial estimate of the reporting distribution is

$$\pi_r^{(0)} = \sum_{t=1}^{T-R} n_{tr} \Big/ \sum_{t=1}^{T-R} N_t, \qquad r = 0,1,\ldots,R-1. \tag{2}$$

We also need an estimate $\hat{\pi}_R$ of π_R. An estimator analogous to (2) is

$$\hat{\pi}_R = \sum_{t=1}^{T-R'} n_{tR} \Big/ \sum_{t=1}^{T-R'} N_t, \tag{3}$$

where $R'>R$; we have typically chosen $R' = R + 2$ in modeling quarterly incidence.

Now let $q_t^{(k)}$ be the estimate of the partial sum q_t at the kth step and $m_t^{(k)}$, the estimate of m_t. The iteration for $k \geq 1$ is obtained from

$$p_r^{(k)} = \sum_{t=1}^{T-r} n_{tr} \Big/ \sum_{t=1}^{T-r} m_t^{(k-1)}, \qquad r = 0,1,\ldots,R-1, \tag{4}$$

$$\pi_r^{(k)} = (1 - \hat{\pi}_R)\, p_r^{(k)} \Big/ \sum_{j=0}^{R-1} p_j^{(k)}, \qquad r = 0,1,\ldots,R-1, \tag{5}$$

$$q_t^{(k)} = \sum_{r=0}^{T-t} \pi_r^{(k)}, \qquad t > T - R, \tag{6}$$

$$m_t^{(k)} = n_{t.} / q_t^{(k)}, \qquad t > T - R. \tag{7}$$

Note that $p_r^{(k)}$ is an estimate of the reporting delay distribution if all cases are reported within R-1 time periods after diagnosis. This algorithm converges very quickly; we have found that all $q_t^{(k)}$ are usually correct to three decimal places after three iterations.

An empirical estimate of the variance of $\hat{q}_t$ can be obtained from the observed n_{tr}, the estimates $\hat{m}_t$ of the N_t, and the estimate $\hat{q}_t$. For

$t' \leq t$, an estimate of the probability that a case will be reported within $r = T-t$ periods, based on cases diagnosed during period t', is $\hat{q}_{t'r} = (n_{t'0} + n_{t'1} + \ldots + n_{t'r}) / \hat{m}_{t'}$. Thus an empirical variance estimate is

$$\mathrm{var}(\hat{q}_t) = \sum_{t'=1}^{t} (\hat{q}_{t',T-t} - \hat{q}_t)^2 / (t-1), \qquad t \geq T - R. \tag{8}$$

4. Fitting the extrapolation model

We model period incidence using an extension of the Box-Cox procedure (Box and Cox, 1964; Atkinson, 1973) for two reasons. This procedure is flexible, so it can model a wide variety of trends in case counts. In addition, because period incidence increases rapidly, we need a transformation such as the Box-Cox to reduce the heteroscedasticity of the model errors. We obtain maximum likelihood estimates (MLEs) of the model parameters by minimizing the -2 log likelihood, calculated from a weighted least squares model fitted to adjusted incidence. The minimization procedure is iterative because the weights depend on the predicted values for adjusted incidence, as in Box and Hill (1974).

First we describe the data fit. Let I_t be the observed incidence for period t, $t = 1,2,\ldots,T_M$, without adjustment for reporting delays. If the period modeled includes periods during which reporting delays were not estimated, we extend the reporting delay and variance estimates derived in Section 3 by setting

$$\begin{aligned} &\hat{q}_t = 1 - \hat{\pi}_R, \\ &\mathrm{Var}(\hat{q}_t) = \mathrm{Var}(\hat{q}_{T-R}), \end{aligned} \qquad t = 1,2,\ldots,T-R-1, \tag{9}$$

where $\hat{\pi}_R$, T, and R are defined in Section 3. The adjusted incidence in period t is $y_t = I_t/\hat{q}_t$.

We will fit models to the Box-Cox transform

$$Z_t = (y_t^{\lambda} - 1) / \lambda \tag{10}$$

with $Z_t = \log y_t$ if $\lambda = 0$. Our models have the form

$$Z_t = p(t) + e_t, \qquad t = 1,2,\ldots,T_M, \tag{11}$$

where p(t) is a polynomial, with changes in level (the intercept term) allowed at suitable times, and e_t is error. To fit the model, we must specify the variance of Z_t. We assume that I_t and $\hat{q}_t$ are independent. Then from (10) and the multivariate delta method (Bishop, Fienberg, and Holland, 1975),

$$\mathrm{Var}(Z_t) \approx y^{2(\lambda-1)}\Big|_{y=\hat{y}_t} \mathrm{Var}(I_t/\hat{q}_t)$$

$$\approx \hat{y}_t^{2(\lambda-1)} [\ \mathrm{Var}(I_t) + y_t^2 \mathrm{Var}(\hat{q}_t)\ ] / \hat{q}_t^2. \tag{12}$$

We described in Section 3 a method for obtaining an empirical estimate of $\mathrm{Var}(\hat{q}_t)$.

We will specify a general form for $\mathrm{Var}(I_t)$. Geographic clustering and variation in reporting mean that the I_t cases diagnosed during period t and reported through period T are not independent counts, so it is unlikely that I_t has a Poisson distribution. We will assume, however, that

$$\mathrm{Var}(I_t) = k\, I_t, \tag{13}$$

where $k \geq 1$ is an overdispersion parameter independent of t. We will conduct a sensitivity analysis to evaluate how the value of k affects our predictions.

We fit the model (11) using weighted least squares with the inverse variance weights

$$w_t(\lambda,\hat{y}_t) = w\ \hat{q}_t^2\ \hat{y}_t^{2(1-\lambda)}\ /\ [kI_t + y_t^2 \mathrm{Var}(\hat{q}_t)], \quad t=1,2,\ldots,T_M; \tag{14}$$

w is a normalizing constant chosen so that the maximum of these weights is 1. Let $\hat{\sigma}^2$ be the mean squared error. Aside from constant terms, the -2 log likelihood is

$$\ell(\lambda) = T_M \log \hat{\sigma}^2 - 2(\lambda - 1) \sum_{t=1}^{T_M} \log y_t - \sum_{t=1}^{T_M} \log w_t \ . \tag{15}$$

We obtain the MLE $\hat{\lambda}$ of λ by minimizing $\ell(\lambda)$, using an iterative procedure. We choose as initial values $\hat{y}_t^{(0)} = y_t$. Step s+1, $s \geq 0$, is:

A. For each λ_i on a grid (i = 1,2,...,g), fit the model (11) using weighted least squares, with the weights $w_t(\lambda, \hat{y}_t^{(s)})$.

B. Choose $\hat{\lambda}^{(s+1)}$ to minimize $\ell(\lambda_i)$, i = 1,2,...,g.

C. Calculate the estimated adjusted incidences $\hat{y}_t^{(s+1)}$ as the predicted values from the model (11) with $\lambda = \hat{\lambda}^{(s+1)}$ and the corresponding coefficients for p(t).

D. If the process has not converged, return to step A.

We make three comments about our experience with this procedure. First, the procedure converges very rapidly. One iteration is usually enough for practical purposes; for most data sets, the second iteration changes at most the third decimal place in $\ell(\hat{\lambda})$ (the sixth significant digit) using a grid spacing of 0.01 in step A. Secondly, the choice of the overdispersion parameter k has little effect on the estimate $\hat{\lambda}$, for k = 1,2,3 and a linear or quadratic polynomial p(t) in the model (11).

Finally, both statistical and substantive considerations should be used in selecting the form of the polynomial p(t) in the model (11). We will discuss substantive issues further in Section 8. Statistical considerations include analysis of the residuals and the significance of additional terms added to the polynomial model. The MLE $\hat{\lambda}$ depends on the model, so the significance of additional terms would ordinarily be assessed from a likelihood ratio test (the difference between the values of $\ell(\hat{\lambda})$ for nested models; see Searle, 1971, sec. 3.7). Because we fit our models using iteratively reweighted least squares, differences between values of $\ell(\hat{\lambda})$ for nested models are not likelihood ratio statistics; in fact, we have observed that $\ell(\hat{\lambda})$ can <u>increase</u> if a term is added to the model p(t). Our experience suggests that we can use a formal likelihood ratio test as part of our model selection procedure, however, as well as to obtain an 100(1-α) percent confidence interval for $\hat{\lambda}$ from those values of λ satisfying

$$\ell(\lambda) \leq \ell(\hat{\lambda}) + X_1^2(1-\alpha). \tag{16}$$

The second term on the right in (16) is the 1-α percentile of a chi-squared random variable with 1 degree of freedom. We will use this confidence interval for $\hat{\lambda}$ to derive prediction intervals for AIDS incidence in the next section.

5. Prediction intervals for the projections

The need to estimate the exponent in the Box-Cox transform makes it hard to calculate prediction intervals for future AIDS incidence. Because we believe that the multivariate delta method (Bishop, Fienberg, and Holland, 1975) might not yield an accurate estimate for the variance of the prediction error, we use a method based on the prediction intervals conditional on the Box-Cox transform exponent. Alternatively, prediction intervals can be calculated from a bootstrap procedure (Efron and Tibshirani, 1986; Stine, 1985).

First we discuss the use of the multivariate delta method. At period t, the predicted value is

$$\hat{y}_t = (1 + \hat{\lambda}\,\hat{p}(t))^{1/\hat{\lambda}}, \tag{17}$$

corresponding to the model (11). Let $\hat{\beta}$ be the MLE of the coefficients of the polynomial p(t) and $\hat{\sigma}^2$ be the mean squared error for that model. Denote by Σ the covariance matrix $Cov(\hat{\lambda},\hat{\beta},\hat{\sigma})$; we estimate Σ as part of the MLE computation using the program BMDPAR (Dixon, 1983). Let $\underline{f}_t$ be the corresponding column vector of the first partial derivatives of the right-hand side of (11) with respect to λ, β, and $-e_t$, evaluated at $\hat{\lambda}$, $\hat{\beta}$, and 0. If $\hat{\lambda}$, $\hat{\beta}$, and $\hat{\sigma}$ have an asymptotic multivariate normal distribution, then the prediction error is asymptotically Gaussian, and from the multivariate delta method its variance is

$$\mathrm{Var}(\hat{y}_t - y_t) \approx \underline{f}_t' \, \Sigma \, \underline{f}_t, \tag{18}$$

from which we can obtain (asymptotically correct) prediction intervals for the prediction error at a set of times.

We have theoretical and computational reservations about this approach. Our theoretical concern is based on a simulation study of the standard deviation of $\hat{\lambda}$ estimated from the inverse of the expected information matrix. Lawrance (1987) found that this estimate may be substantially smaller than the true standard deviation if data are available for 20 or fewer time periods. Our computational concern is based on the large partial derivatives of $\hat{y}_t - y_t$ and on correlations between $\hat{\lambda}$ and $\hat{\beta}$ close to 1 (with correlations between the intercept and slope usually greater than 0.995 in magnitude), resulting in very large terms (as large as the order of 10^7) with both positive and negative signs in the sum $\underline{f}'\Sigma\underline{f}$. Although cancellation results in an estimated variance much smaller than 10^7, relatively small changes in the estimate of Σ would cause large changes in the variance estimate $\underline{f}'\Sigma\underline{f}$.

As an alternative, we compute prediction intervals from a set of prediction intervals conditional on λ (Morgan and Curran, 1986). Let Λ be an $100(1-\alpha)^{1/2}$ percent confidence interval for $\hat{\lambda}$, computed from (16). Given λ in Λ, let $[a(\lambda), b(\lambda)]$ be an $100(1-\alpha)^{1/2}$ prediction interval for the prediction for period t based on the Box-Cox transform with exponent λ. Let (a,b) be the smallest interval containing all the intervals $[a(\lambda), b(\lambda)]$ for λ in Λ, so

$$a = \min_{\lambda \varepsilon \Lambda} a(\lambda) \quad \text{and} \quad b = \max_{\lambda \varepsilon \Lambda} b(\lambda). \tag{19}$$

Assuming that the Box-Cox model is correct, (a,b) is a conservative $100(1-\alpha)$ percent prediction interval for predicted incidence in period t (Appendix).

Prediction intervals can also be obtained from a bootstrap procedure, although at the cost of more computation time. The approach described by Stine (1985) must be modified to incorporate the Box-Cox transform and the use of weighted least squares to fit the model. Our preliminary experience suggests that this method will give prediction intervals close to, but somewhat narrower than, those from the intervals conditional on λ.

6. Predictions for subgroups of cases

For public health purposes, predictions of the numbers of AIDS cases within geographic regions may be even more important than predictions for the United States as a whole. There is also great interest in predictions for other subgroups, such as children, minorities (blacks or Hispanics), and risk groups (e.g. intravenous drug users or heterosexual transmission cases).

An obvious procedure would be to project for each subgroup separately. Since the national HIV epidemic is the sum of epidemics in risk and geographic groups, this might yield an accurate prediction. There are two reasons for not using empirical extrapolation this way. First, this procedure is not additive: in general, the sum of subgroup projections made by our extrapolation procedure will not equal the projection made after combining all the subgroups. Second, for some subgroups period incidences will be small and variable enough that empirical projections will not be reliable. While back-calculation can be implemented to be additive (by using the same incubation and infection distributions for each group), we do not know whether back-calculation is reliable with relatively sparse data.

We propose modeling the time series of the proportions of cases within subgroups. If $\hat{y}(t)$ is the predicted incidence at period t and $\hat{p}_g(t)$ is the predicted proportion of cases diagnosed during period t that are in subgroup g, then the predicted incidence in subgroup g is

$$\hat{y}_g(t) = \hat{p}_g(t)\, \hat{y}(t). \tag{20}$$

We use a generalized logit model to model the proportions $p_g(t)$. Suppose there are G groups, and without loss of generality choose group 1 as the reference group. We use the linear model

$$\log(\, p_g(t) \,/\, p_1(t)\,) = \beta_g\, \underline{t} + e_g, \qquad g = 2,3,\ldots,G, \tag{21}$$

where β_g is a row vector of coefficients, e_g is error, and the column vector $\underline{t}$ may include powers of t and terms allowing for shifts associated with the introduction of the new case definition. Define β_1 to be a vector of zeros. The estimates $\hat{p}_g(t)$ sum to 1 with

$$\hat{p}_g(t) = \exp(\hat{\beta}_g\ \underline{t}) \ / \sum_{j=1}^{G} \exp(\hat{\beta}_j\ \underline{t}), \qquad g = 1,2,\ldots,G. \tag{22}$$

If n_t AIDS cases have been diagnosed durning period t, the variance of the generalized logit in (21) is $(1/p_g(t) + 1/p_1(t))/n_t$. We fit the models (21) using weighted least squares with inverse variance weights.

Prediction intervals may be computed as follows. Obtain maximum likelihood estimates of the coefficients β_g and an estimate of the covariance matrix of the $\hat{\beta}_g$ from a multinomial likelihood incorporating the generalized logit model (22); these MLEs will be nearly identical to the estimates from a weighted regression analysis. Then use the multivariate delta method to obtain an asymptotic prediction interval for each $\hat{p}_g(t)$. An asymptotic prediction interval for $\hat{y}_g(t)$ can be computed by obtaining a set of appropriate prediction intervals for these estimates conditional on the Box-Cox parameter λ, by applying the multi-multivariate delta method to (20) and then using the approach in Section 5.

We have found that the estimated proportions are nearly independent of the group chosen as the reference group in (21), which can be explained intuitively. Let γ_g be the vector of coefficients in the model corresponding to (21) with group k as the reference group. Since $\log(p_g/p_1) = \log(p_g/p_k) + \log(p_k/p_1)$, it follows that $\hat{\beta}_g \simeq \hat{\gamma}_g + \hat{\beta}_k$, and so

$$\hat{p}_g(t) \simeq \exp(\hat{\gamma}_g\underline{t})\ \exp(\hat{\beta}_k\underline{t}) \ / \ \exp(\hat{\beta}_k\underline{t}) \sum_{j=1}^{G} \exp(\hat{\gamma}_j\underline{t}) \tag{23}$$

which reduces to (22) with group k as the reference group.

7. Predictions from current surveillance data

We illustrate our projection methods using AIDS cases reported to CDC through December 1988. We extrapolate the trend in quarterly incidence of all cases, and also of cases consistent with the pre-1987 definition. The latter are cases with a diagnosis (definitive or presumptive: see Section 2) of any disease in the pre-1987 case definition. For our primary results we use cases diagnosed during January 1984 through June 1988; about 75% of the cases diagnosed during

Table 1. AIDS Cases in the United States Reported to CDC Through December 1988, by Quarter of Diagnosis, with Adjustments for Reporting Delays.

Year/ quarter	Reported cases[a]	Reporting probability	Adjusted cases	Regression weight[b]
84/1	1154	0.971	1188	0.92
2	1378	0.971	1419	0.91
3	1575	0.971	1622	0.94
4	1738	0.971	1790	0.92
85/1	2155	0.965	2234	0.83
2	2549	0.958	2660	0.84
3	2975	0.952	3126	0.83
4	3086	0.945	3265	1.00
86/1	3688	0.937	3935	0.95
2	4122	0.930	4431	0.96
3	4568	0.922	4957	0.99
4	4797	0.911	5267	0.84
87/1	5572	0.899	6198	0.69
2	5975	0.884	6758	0.54
3	6309	0.865	7292	0.44
4	6252	0.840	7446	0.32
88/1	6454	0.804	8029	0.24
2	6254	0.751	8326	0.20

[a] Includes all cases diagnosed under the revised case definition.
[b] For a linear model fit to all cases, adjusted for reporting delays, with Box-Cox parameter $\lambda = 0.38$.

the second calendar quarter of 1988 should have been reported by the end of 1988 (Table 1).

First we estimate the reporting delay distribution. To eliminate the effect of delayed reporting caused only by the change in the case definition, we estimate this distribution after deleting those cases diagnosed before September 1987 that are reportable only under the new definition. We model delays of up to 4 years. Our estimates (Table 1) are nearly identical to the corresponding estimates from the Poisson regression procedure mentioned in Section 3. The assumption that reporting delay does not depend on period of diagnosis seems reasonable, as estimates of reporting delays for individual calendar quarters suggest that reporting probabilities representing delays of 6 months or more have remained quite stable since 1984. The adjusted quarterly incidences are also shown in Table 1 and in Figure 2.

We modeled adjusted quarterly incidence using the Box-Cox procedure (Section 4). Quarterly AIDS incidence has increased only slightly from

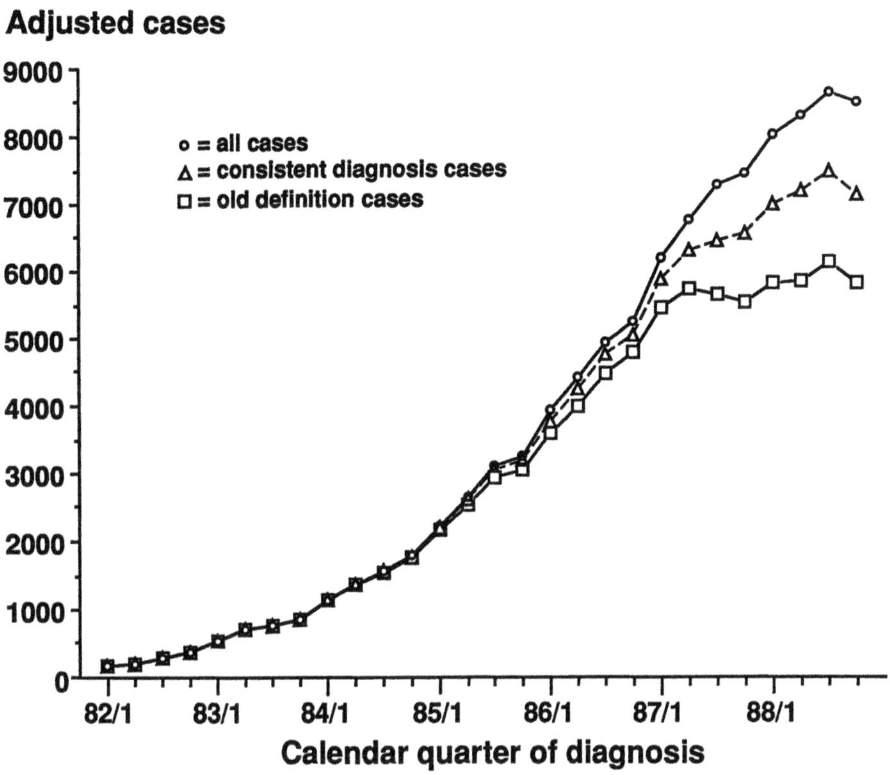

Figure 2. Estimated numbers of AIDS cases diagnosed in the United States, 1982-1988: cases reported through December 1988, adjusted for estimated reporting delays.

the third to the fourth quarter for the last few years (Table 1 and Figure 2), followed by a large increase the next quarter. We assumed that (on the transform scale) each of these annual shifts in incidence is the same and modeled this shift by adding one parameter to the polynomial in the Box-Cox model (11). Because the new case definition took effect in the fourth quarter of 1987, we considered an additional term for a different change in incidence at that time.

We discuss model selection and parameter estimation only for modeling all cases with the dispersion parameter k=1 in (13). Modeling the consistent definition cases or changing the dispersion parameter to k=2 or k=3 gave very similar results. For the linear model, both shift parameters reduce the -2 log likelihood $\ell(\lambda)$, so we included both in the Box-Cox model. For the quadratic model, we need the shift associated

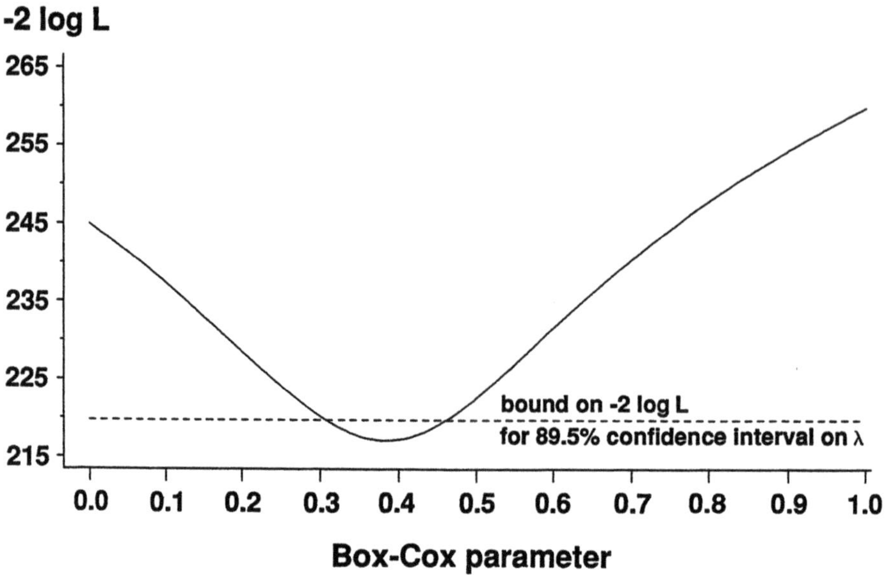

Figure 3. -2 log likelihood curve for a linear prediction model fitted to adjusted quarterly AIDS incidence, January 1984 - June 1988.

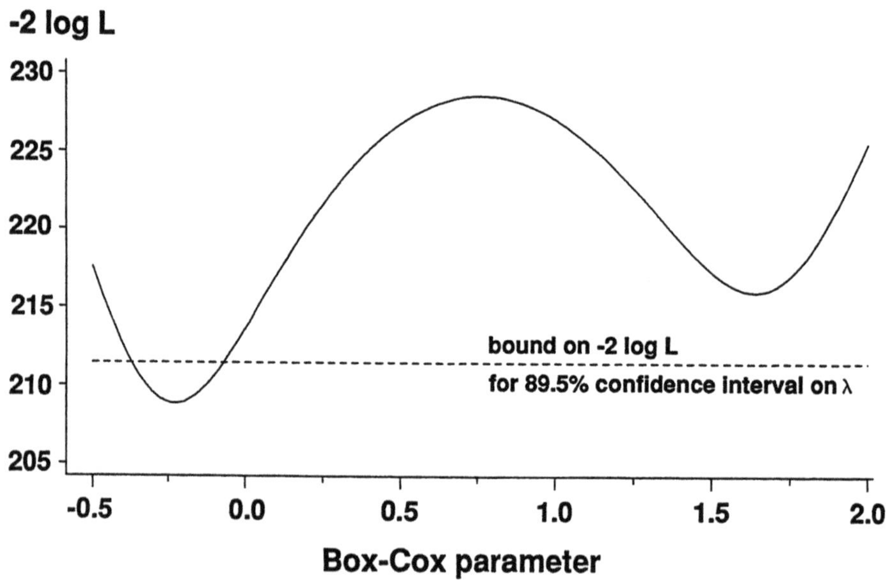

Figure 4. -2 log likelihood curve for a quadratic prediction model fitted to adjusted quarterly AIDS incidence, January 1984 - June 1988.

Table 2. Comparison of AIDS Case Predictions from Models Fit to Adjusted Quarterly Incidence, January 1984 - June 1988.

Model (λ)[a]	-2 log L	Predicted incidence[b] 1988	1990	1992	Total[c]
		Based on all cases			
Linear (0.38)	217.07	37,000	69,000	113,000	425,000
Quadratic (-0.23)	208.83	34,000	28,000	12,000	195,000
Quadratic (log)	213.47	35,000	41,000	29,000	250,000
	Based on cases consistent with the pre-1987 definition[d]				
Linear (0.47)	221.34	34,000	60,000	93,000	375,000
Quadratic (-0.30)	209.78	30,000	19,000	6,000	165,000

[a] Each model includes a term for a change in incidence at each fourth quarter; linear models contain an additional term for a change in incidence in the fourth quarter of 1987. λ is the maximum likelihood estimate of the Box-Cox transformation parameter.

[b] Rounded to the nearest 1,000.

[c] Rounded to the nearest 5,000, and including 84,200 cases estimated to be diagnosed through June 1988.

[d] Based on cases with any disease in the pre-1987 definition, with 7.5% added to the model predictions as an adjustment for the remaining cases.

with each fourth quarter but not the additional shift for 1987. Each model contains five parameters to be estimated.

The -2 log likelihood curves $\ell(\lambda)$ are very different for the linear and quadratic models (Figures 3 and 4). The maximum likelihood estimates $\hat{\lambda}$ are also very different (Table 2). For a linear polynomial, $\hat{\lambda} = 0.38$, with an 89.5% confidence interval of 0.30 to 0.47 (we use 89.5% intervals to obtain 80% prediction intervals $(0.895 = \sqrt{0.80})$, as described in Section 5). For a quadratic polynomial, $\hat{\lambda} = -0.23$ (89.5% confidence interval, -0.37 to -0.06), with a second local minimum at $\lambda \simeq 1.6$. For both models, the residuals show no evident departures from Gaussian distributions and no time trends in magnitude. The residuals also have very small first-order autocorrelations (between -0.05 and 0.05), with Durbin-Watson test statistics between 1.8 and 2.0, in the acceptance region for the hypothesis that the autocorrelation is zero (Neter and Wasserman, 1974). A bootstrap computation (Stine, 1985) for the linear model with 200 bootstrap samples gave a 90% confidence interval for $\hat{\lambda}$ of 0.29 to 0.47. This interval is nearly identical to the interval computed from (16), supporting our proposal to treat differences between $\ell(\hat{\lambda})$ for nested models as likelihood ratio statistics.

As a result of these very different estimates of $\hat{\lambda}$, models with a quadratic polynomial in (11) yield predictions dramatically different from those with a linear polynomial (Table 2). A linear model predicts that annual incidence will continue to increase through 1992, with successively larger annual differences. In contrast, a quadratic model predicts that quarterly incidence will peak in 1988. The -2 log likelihood statistics suggest that the quadratic model gives a better fit to the data than the linear model; we discuss model selection further in Section 8. The predicted incidences for the consistent case definition in Table 2 are obtained by adding 7.5% to the model predictions. This is approximately half of the 13% of cases diagnosed since September 1987 with no disease in the old case definition (7.5% = 1/2 x .13/.87); see Section 2 for further discussion.

In Table 3 we show predicted incidence with 80% prediction intervals, obtained from the data in Table 1 and a linear predictor in the Box-Cox model (11). There is substantial uncertainty in the predictions for later years as indicated by the width of the prediction intervals. Note that the conditional prediction intervals are only slightly wider than those computed from the bootstrap. While our experience is limited to the comparison in Table 3, the bootstrap intervals do require much more computation, so we tentatively recommend using the conditional procedure. The corresponding prediction intervals from the multivariate delta method are very narrow, with half-widths between 500 and 1500 cases for 1988-1992.

Analyses based on adjusted monthly incidence give predicted incidence and prediction intervals very similar to those in Table 3. For monthly data, the MLE $\hat{\lambda}$ is 0.37 (89.5% confidence interval, 0.28 to 0.46). Predicted annual incidences are slightly larger than the corresponding predictions in Table 3 (300 to 2,000 cases, or 1-2% greater); the prediction intervals are slightly narrower.

Our predictions for 3 to 5 years in the future are affected by the time elapsed since the period modeled but do not depend on small changes in that period. This is shown in Table 4, which contains predictions for 1988, 1990, and 1992 from linear polynomials in time based on several reporting periods and on several periods of diagnosis. Because we are making predictions for about 5 years in the future, it is not surprising that increases in adjusted incidence of 1% in late 1987 and early 1988 yield increases of more than 1% in predicted incidence for 1992. For example, more cases diagnosed in 1986 and 1987 were reported between April and December 1988 than had been predicted from the cases reported through March 1988; the increases range from 3% in the first quarter of

1986 to about 6% during the first three quarters of 1987. Using these additional cases in fitting a model to cases diagnosed during July 1983 - September 1987 yields a 1992 predicted incidence 18% higher than the corresponding projections not incorporating cases reported after March 1988. This prediction of 121,000 cases for 1992 in line 3 of Table 4 is just above the 80% prediction interval computed from the model (line 1)

Table 3. Predicted AIDS Incidence and 80% Prediction Intervals[a] from a Linear Model Fit to Adjusted Quarterly Incidence for January 1984-June 1988.

Year	Predicted incidence	Prediction interval Conditional[b]	Prediction interval Bootstrap[c]
1988	37,000	35,000- 38,000	36,000- 38,000
1989	51,000	48,000- 55,000	49,000- 53,000
1990	69,000	63,000- 76,000	64,000- 73,000
1991	89,000	80,000-102,000	80,000- 97,000
1992	113,000	98,000-133,000	98,000-126,000

[a] Computed from a linear function of time fit to the Box-Cox transform (Table 2, footnote a) and rounded to the nearest 1,000.

[b] Computed from intervals conditional on the Box-Cox exponent; see Section 5.

[c] Computed from 200 bootstrap replications using the percentile method (Stine, 1985; Efron and Tibshirani, 1986).

Table 4. Predicted Annual AIDS Incidence from Extrapolation Models[a] Fit to Adjusted Quarterly Incidence for Several Periods.

Period modeled	Predicted AIDS cases 1988	1990	1992
July 1983 - Sept 1987[b]	37,000	65,000	103,000
July 1983 - Sept 1987[c]	39,000	70,000	112,000
July 1983 - Sept 1987[d]	41,000	74,000	121,000
Jan. 1984 - June 1988[d]	37,000	69,000	113,000
Jan. 1984 - Mar. 1988[d]	38,000	70,000	117,000
July 1983 - June 1988[d]	37,000	68,000	111,000

[a] Linear polynomial in time fit to Box-Cox transform (footnote a, Table 2).

[b] Cases reported through March 1988.

[c] Cases reported through June 1988.

[d] Cases reported through December 1988.

fitted to cases reported through March 1988 (upper bound, 116,000 cases).

An additional 9 months to report cases increases the projections because of increases in adjusted incidences and changes in the regression weights. For example, the weight for the third quarter of 1987 increases from 0.17 to 0.42 if the last reporting period changes from the first to the last quarter of 1988. To evaluate the effect of a change in incidence only, we refit a linear Box-Cox model after increasing the adjusted incidences in Table 1 by 1% in the first quarter of 1987, increasing to 10% in the second quarter of 1988. The resulting predictions for 1988, 1990, and 1992 are 9%, 12%, and 16% greater than the predictions in Table 3. The modified predictions for 1988-1990 are slightly above the conditional prediction intervals in Table 3 and just within the corresponding intervals for 1991 and 1992. Projections would be even more sensitive to changes in recent adjusted incidence if the regression weights for recent quarters were larger than those in Table 2. This sensitivity of the projections to the data used emphasizes the importance of computing and reporting prediction intervals.

As an example of our procedure for modeling the proportions of cases within groups, we project trends in incidence for three large metropolitan statistical areas, New York City, San Francisco, and Houston, Texas. Because there are shifts associated with the introduction of the new case definition in September 1987, we use the generalized logit model

$$\log(p_g(t) / p_1(t)) = f_g(t) + \gamma_g(t), \qquad g = 2,3,4, \tag{24}$$

where the remaining U.S. cases constitute the reference group, $f_g(t)$ is a linear polynomial, and $\gamma_g(t)$ is 0 until the fourth quarter of 1987 and a constant thereafter. We fit these models to quarterly data for January 1984 through September 1988, after estimating reporting delays separately within each group. The trends in the logits are quite linear for the New York City and San Francisco areas. The offset term $\gamma_g(t)$ is needed for New York City ($p < .001$) but not for San Francisco ($p = .69$). The logits for Houston show more scatter, and we included the offset term for this analysis even though it was not significant ($p = .22$).

Observed and predicted proportions for these three areas for 1984 through 1990 (Figure 5) show that the observed proportions of cases in the New York City and San Francisco metropolitan areas can be fit very well by linear models in the logits. The observed proportions for Houston are scattered around a prediction that is nearly constant at 3.3% until the change in the case definition in late 1987. Of course, the

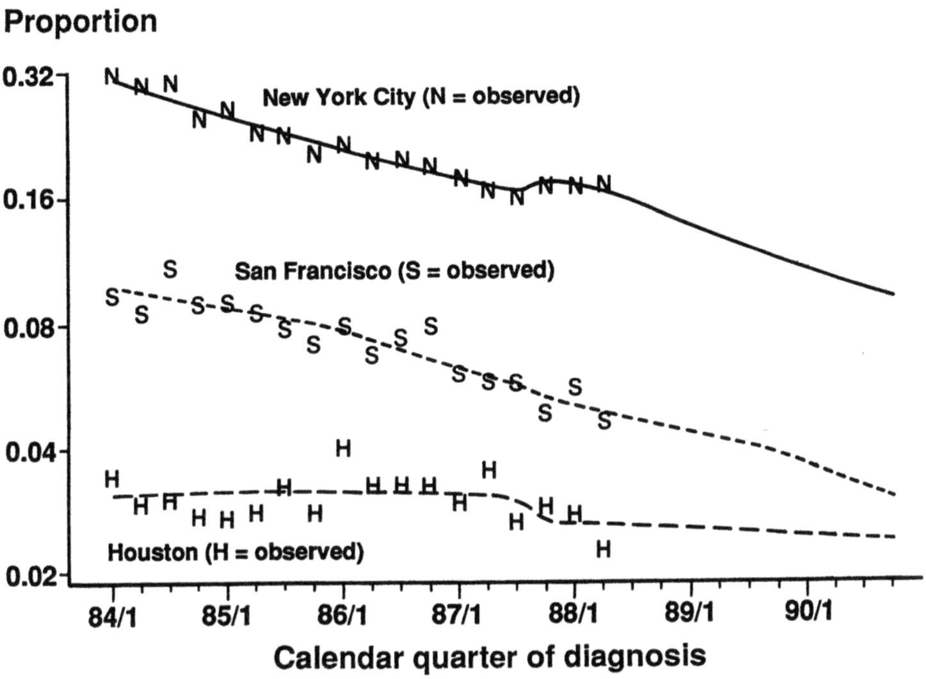

Figure 5. Observed and predicted percent of U.S. AIDS cases diagnosed in three metropolitan statistical areas.

accuracy of the predictions in Figure 5 depends on the assumption that trends in the proportions of cases diagnosed in these areas during the next several years will be the same as for 1984-1987, aside from a shift in level associated with the change in the case definition.

8. Discussion

Although extrapolation makes no explicit use of the natural history of HIV disease, projections of AIDS incidence from recent trends are likely to produce accurate forecasts for the next 3 years if incidence is increasing and if diagnostic and reporting practices remain unchanged. The 1986 projections of 15,800 cases diagnosed in 1986 and 23,000 in 1987 (Morgan and Curran, 1986) are within 13% of current estimates that 17,900 and 25,200 cases (respectively) compatible with the pre-1987 case definition diagnosed during those years will be reported to CDC (Figure

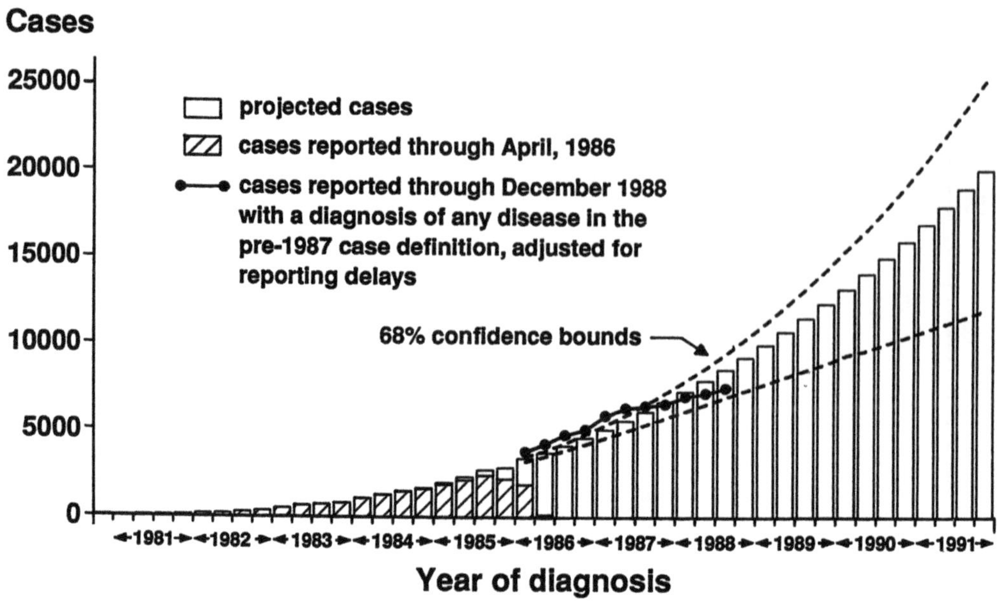

Figure 6. Comparison of estimated quarterly ADIS incidence in the United States, January 1986-September 1988, with predictions made in May, 1986.

6). The accuracy of forecasts from extrapolation depends on the natural history of HIV disease, namely on the long and variable time between infection with HIV and a diagnosis of AIDS (Section 1).

Extrapolation must be used carefully. In this section we discuss our experience with the key issues: choosing the data to be modeled, adjusting for reporting delays, and choosing a model. We conclude with a brief summary of other prediction methods.

The first step is to choose the period to be modeled, the cases diagnosed within this period to be used, and the time unit (e.g. calendar quarter or month). Although recent incidence is important for predicting future incidence, incidence for the last few months should be excluded. If recently diagnosed cases were reported faster or slower than the estimates from historical data, incidence adjusted for estimated reporting delays could differ from true incidence; this could have a substantial effect on predicted incidence, particularly for later years (Section 7). We used only cases diagnosed at least 6 months before the date of our analysis, as about 75% of those cases should have been reported. Our results suggest that the use of monthly instead of quarterly incidence has little effect on the predictions or on the prediction intervals.

Because accurate predictions from extrapolation depend on consistent diagnostic practices, the change in the case definition must be considered. This change undoubtedly resulted in earlier reporting for some cases, causing an apparent temporary increase in AIDS incidence. We suggested one approach to this problem in Section 7: extrapolating from a consistent case definition and adjusting the resulting predictions. Careful study of the effect of the change in the case definition on surveillance data is essential. Data on the progression of disease in patients infected with HIV disease would also be useful.

It is natural to model period incidence instead of cumulative incidence. Modeling period incidence yields direct estimates of future incidence, the quantities of interest for public health planning. In addition, it would be difficult to compute prediction intervals from a model fit to cumulative incidence, as successive cumulative incidences are highly correlated.

There are several problems related to estimating reporting delays. If reporting is homogeneous over time, either Poisson regression or an iterative procedure can be used to estimate delays (Section 3). Empirical data suggest geographic and temporal variation in reporting delays, so it may be desirable to model these effects. Geographic variation can be evaluated from region-specific delay distributions, but choosing an appropriate geographic grouping remains a problem. While recent delays need to be estimated accurately in order to estimate recent incidence accurately, detecting and modeling recent changes in reporting delays may be difficult due to incomplete data, although seasonal terms can be included with Poisson regression (Cox et al., 1988).

We chose the Box-Cox procedure as a flexible modeling strategy. The flexibility offered by the choice of the exponent parameter is essential. For example, while it might be natural to model the logarithm of period incidence, this is too strong a transform: a quadratic polynomial in time is necessary, the quadratic coefficient is negative and relatively large, and consequently AIDS incidence is predicted to peak by 1989 (Table 2) -- in contrast to the recent trend of consistently increasing incidence (Figure 2).

Our analyses of current data show that the degree of the polynomial in the Box-Cox model must be chosen carefully. While a quadratic polynomial yields additional flexibility in modeling trends in incidence, with recent data predicted incidence from this model peaks in 1988 and then falls rapidly. This is consistent neither with the trend in Figure 2 nor with estimates that at least hundreds of thousands of people in the United States are infected with HIV, and consequently, that hundreds of thousands are likely to develop opportunistic infections indicative of AIDS after 1988 (U.S. Public Health Service, 1988).

Another problem with using a quadratic predictor in the Box-Cox model is that the -2 log likelihood curve is unstable. For example, we used a quadratic model to make the U.S. Public Health Service predictions for 1988-1992 (U.S. Public Health Service, 1988; Centers for Disease Control, 1988) in order to gain flexibility in modeling, even though the fit was not significantly better than that from a linear model. We modeled consistent definition cases diagnosed during July 1983 - September 1987; the regression weights were somewhat different from (14). That -2 log likelihood curve has a unique minimum at $\hat{\lambda}$=0.29, although the curve is nearly flat in this region. The annual predicted incidences are somewhat smaller than those in Table 3 but indicate an approximate linear increase in cases, much different from the predictions from quadratic models in Table 2. In contrast, the -2 log likelihood curve for a linear predictor fit to adjusted incidence for July 1983 - September 1987 is very similar to the curve shown in Figure 3. We have also found that quadratic models typically have -2 log likelihood curves with more than one local minimum, and that between the local minima these curves are quite sensitive to changes in the data fit and to changes in the regression weights. This behavior emphasizes that extrapolation cannot be used to forecast AIDS incidence without careful analysis, including a requirement that projections be consistent with recent observed trends.

Prediction intervals for projections are especially important because changes in the incidence modeled can cause marked changes in projections (Section 7). An important unsolved problem with prediction methods (not just extrapolation) is how to compute prediction intervals that incorporate both the uncertainties in the procedure and those in reporting delays. Our conditional procedure will give conservative prediction intervals and the bootstrap (Stine, 1985) should give correct intervals if we use a consistent time series of AIDS incidence, estimate reporting delays correctly, and choose the proper family of models. Because it is impossible to verify these assumptions, we recommend carrying out sensitivity analyses, similar to those summarized in Table 4. It may be worth considering other types of extrapolation models; alternative models are discussed by Cox et al. (1988).

Our extrapolation models seem unreliable for one important situation: when AIDS incidence has leveled. Current examples may be cases attributed to blood transfusions nationwide and to homosexual contact in the San Francisco metropolitan area. A linear predictor in the Box-Cox model does not fit the shift from increasing to constant incidence, while a quadratic predictor tends to forecast a very rapid drop in incidence. This drop certainly seems too fast for transfusion-associated AIDS cases. Modeling the trend in the proportion of AIDS cases may produce more accurate predictions in this situation.

Because extrapolation makes no explicit use of the natural history of HIV disease, our increasing knowledge of this natural history will not lead to more accurate projections. Other prediction methods should also be considered, including back-calculation (Brookmeyer and Gail, 1986, 1988; Gail and Brookmeyer, 1988) and mathematical models of HIV transmission and the natural history of HIV disease (Isham, 1988; Hyman and Stanley, 1988).

Back-calculation is based on the natural history of HIV disease. Historical AIDS incidence and an estimate of the incubation time distribution are used to estimate historical HIV incidence, from which future AIDS incidence can then be predicted from the incubation time distribution. Although we know of no relevant numerical results, it seems likely that projections from this method are not very sensitive to modest changes in recent AIDS incidence, but they are sensitive to the incubation time distribution (Dondero et al., 1987; Gail and Brookmeyer, 1988). This distribution cannot yet be estimated precisely (Kalbfleisch and Lawless, 1988) and will change as therapies are developed to delay the development of opportunistic infections in people infected with HIV. We do not know whether this distribution has changed with time or whether it is the same for other risk groups as for the few specific cohorts (homosexual men [Lui, Darrow, and Rutherford, 1988; Lui, Peterman, et al., 1988], hemophiliacs [Lui, Peterman, et al., 1988; Brookmeyer and Goedert, 1989], and transfusion recipients [Medley et al., 1987; Lui, Peterman, et al., 1988; Harris, 1988]) for which estimates have been made.

Many researchers are developing mathematical models of the transmission of HIV and the natural history of HIV disease (Isham, 1988) While enough is now known to formulate reasonable models, these models are unlikely to yield realistic predictions of national AIDS incidence until estimates are available for such key parameters as the sizes of risk groups, the infectivity during various stages of the infectious period, the frequency of contact between those infected and those at risk, and temporal changes in behavior related to risk. At present, these models are mainly useful in examining the possible effects of alternative intervention strategies (Gail and Brookmeyer, 1988).

We conclude by emphasizing two important research topics that are particularly important for public health planning: AIDS case predictions for local areas and detecting changes in incidence trends. For many areas where predictions are needed, there are too few AIDS cases for extrapolation methods to be used; we have seen no results on how many cases are needed for back-calculation to give accurate short-term projections. Because computational and statistical resources may be limited, methods should be developed that can be implemented easily. Aside from the inherent problems in detecting a change in the form of a model fit to data, very good methods for estimating recent reporting delays are needed to be able to detect promptly a change in the trend in incidence.

9. Summary

Good projections of future AIDS cases will remain important for public health planning for many years to come. HIV incidence and prevalence, while also important for monitoring the current state of the HIV epidemic, are very difficult to estimate (Dondero, Pappaioanou, and Curran, 1988). Currently available projection methods -- extrapolation from recent trends and back-calculation -- are likely to give reasonably accurate predictions (perhaps accurate to within 15%-20%) for perhaps 3 years beyond the data used to make the projections. Additional research is likely to make projections more accurate and reduce uncertainty. The inherent uncertainty in projecting without modeling the biological process, however, as well as incomplete AIDS case reporting make it unlikely that the currently available projection methods will soon yield highly accurate predictions. Because AIDS case projections will continue to be important, better methods are needed for extrapolating trends in reported AIDS incidence.

Acknowledgements

We thank Myron Katzoff and two anonymous referees for helpful comments, and Jane Mulkey for her assistance in preparing the manuscript.

REFERENCES

Atkinson, A.D. (1973). Testing transformations to normality. *J. Royal Statist Soc* B, 35, 473-479.

Bishop, Y.M.M., S.E. Fienberg, and P.W. Holland. (1975). *Discrete Multivariate Analysis*. MIT Press, Cambridge, Massachusetts.

Box, G.E.P. and D.R. Cox. (1964). An analysis of transformations. *J. Royal Stat Soc* B, 26, 211-252.

Box, G.E.P. and W. J. Hill. (1974). Correcting inhomogeneity of variance with power transformation weighting. *Technometrics*, 16, 385-389.

Brookmeyer, R. and A. Damiano. (1989). Statistical methods for short-term projections of AIDS incidence. *Statistics in Medicine*, 8, 23-34.

Brookmeyer, R. and M.H. Gail. (1986). Minimum size of the acquired immunodeficiency syndrome (AIDS) epidemic in the United States. *The Lancet*, 6 December, 1320-1322.

Brookmeyer, R. and M.H. Gail. (1988). A method for obtaining short-term projections and lower bounds on the size of the AIDS epidemic. *J. Amer Statist Assoc*, 83, 301-308.

Brookmeyer, R. and J.J. Goedert. (1989). Censoring in an epidemic with an application to hemophilia-associated AIDS. *Biometrics*, 45, 325-335.

Centers for Disease Control. (1987). Revision of the CDC surveillance case definition for acquired immunodeficiency syndrome. *MMWR*, 36, 3S-15S.

Centers for Disease Control (1988). Quarterly report to the Domestic Policy Council on the prevalence and rate of spread of HIV and AIDS-United States. *MMWR*, 37, 551-554.

Cox, D.R., R.M. Anderson, A.M. Johnson, M.J.R. Healy, V. Isham, A.D. Wilkie, N.E. Day, O.N. Gill, A McCormick. (1988). *Short-term Prediction of HIV Infection and AIDS in England and Wales*. Her Majesty's Stationery Office, London.

Dixon, W.J., ed. (1983). *BMDP Statistical Software*. University of California Press, Berkeley, California.

Dondero, T.J. and the HIV Data Analysis Team. (1987). Human immunodeficiency virus in the United States: a review of current knowledge. *MMWR*, 36, supplement S-6.

Dondero, T.J., M. Pappaioanou, and J.W. Curran. (1988). Monitoring the levels and trends of HIV infection: The Public Health Service's HIV surveillance Program. *Public Health Rep*, 103, 213-220.

Efron, B. and R. Tibshirani. (1986). Bootstrap methods for standard errors, confidence intervals, and other measures of statistical accuracy. *Statistical Science*, 1, 54-77.

Gail, M.H. and R. Brookmeyer. (1988). Methods for projecting course of acquired immunodeficiency syndrome epidemic. *J. Natl. Cancer Institute*, 80, 900-911.

Hardy, A.M., E.T. Starcher, W.M. Morgan, K. Druker, A. Kristal, J.M. Day, C. Kelly, E. Ewing, J.W. Curran. (1987). Review of death certificates to assess completeness of AIDS case reporting. *Public Health Rep*, 102, 386-391.

Harris, J.E. (1987). Delay in reporting Acquired Immune Deficiency Syndrome (AIDS). Working Paper no. 2278, National Bureau of Economic Research, Cambridge, Mass.

Harris, J.E. (1988). The incubation period for HIV-1. In: Kulstad R., ed.; *AIDS 1988: AAAS Symposia Papers*. American Association for the

Hyman, J.M. and E.A. Stanley. (1988). Using mathematical models to understand the AIDS epidemic. *Math Biosciences*, 90, 415-473.

Isham, V. (1988). Mathematical modeling of the transmission dynamics of HIV infection and AIDS: a review. *J. Royal Statist Soc*, A, 151, 5-30.

Kalbfleisch, J.D. and J.F. Lawless. (1988). Estimating the incubation period for AIDS patients (letter). *Nature*, 333, 504-505.

Lawrance, A. J. (1987). A note on the variance of the Box-Cox regression transformation estimate. *Applied Statist*, 36, 221-223.

Lui, K-J., W.W. Darrow, and G.W. Rutherford. (1988). A model-based estimate of the mean incubation period for AIDS in homosexual men. *Science*, 240, 1333-1335.

Lui K-J., T.A. Peterman, D.N. Lawrence, and J.R. Allen. (1988). A model-based approach to characterize the incubation period of paediatric transfusion-associated acquired immunodeficiency syndrome. *Statistics in Medicine*, 7, 395-401.

Lui K-J. and R.K. Rudy. (1989). An application of a mathematical model to adjust for time lag in case reporting. *Statistics in Medicine*, 8, 259-262.

Medley, G.F., R.M. Anderson, D.R. Cox, and L. Billard. (1987). Infection period of AIDS in patients infected via blood transfusion. *Nature*, 328, 719-721.

Morgan, W.M. and J.W. Curran. (1986). Acquired immunodeficiency syndrome: current and future trends. *Public Health Rep*, 101, 459-465.

Neter, J. and W. Wasserman. (1974). *Applied Linear Statistical Models*. Richard D. Irwin, Homewood, Illinois.

Searle, S.R. (1971). *Linear Models*. John Wiley and Sons, New York.

Starcher, E.T., J.K. Biel, R. Rivera Castano, J.M. Day, S.G. Hopkins, J.W. Miller. (1987). The impact of presumptively diagnosed AIDS cases on national reporting of AIDS (abstract). *Abstracts from the Third International Conference on AIDS, 1-5 June 1987, Washington, D.C.*, 125.

Stine, R.A. (1985). Bootstrap prediction intervals for regression. *J. Amer Statist Assoc*, 80, 1026-1031.

U.S. Public Health Service. (1988). Report of the Workgroup on Epidemiology and Surveillance. *Public Health Rep*, 103, Supp. no. 1, 10-18.

World Health Organization. (1986). Acquired immunodeficiency syndrome

(AIDS). WHO/CDC case definition for AIDS. *Wkly Epidemiol Rec*, 61, 69–72.

Appendix: Prediction Intervals for Projections

For a given period modeled and a fixed functional form p(t) in the Box-Cox model (11), let the MLE $\hat{\lambda}$ of the Box-Cox parameter have probability density function $f(\lambda)$. For a fixed time t, let the prediction given λ be $y(\lambda)$. Let $[y_L(\lambda), y_U(\lambda)]$ be an $100(1 - \alpha)^{1/2}$ percent prediction interval for $y(\lambda)$, and let Λ be an $100(1 - \alpha)^{1/2}$ percent confidence interval for $\hat{\lambda}$. Define

$$y_L = \min_{\lambda \varepsilon \Lambda} y_L(\lambda) \quad \text{and} \quad y_U = \max_{\lambda \varepsilon \Lambda} y_U(\lambda). \tag{25}$$

Because $y_L(\lambda)$ and $y_U(\lambda)$ are random variables for each λ, y_L and y_U are also random variables.

Now let y be the (unknown) incidence at time t. By definition,

$$\Pr(y_L \leq y \leq y_U) = \int \Pr(y_L \leq y \leq y_U \mid \lambda=\hat{\lambda})\, f(\lambda)\, d\lambda. \tag{26}$$

From the definition of y_L and y_U, for λ in Λ

$$\Pr(y_L \leq y \leq y_U) \geq \Pr(y_L(\lambda) \leq y \leq y_U(\lambda) \mid \lambda=\hat{\lambda}) = (1 - \alpha)^{1/2}. \tag{27}$$

It follows that

$$\Pr(y_L \leq y \leq y_U) \geq \int_{\Lambda} \Pr(y_L \leq y \leq y_U \mid \lambda=\hat{\lambda})\, f(\lambda)\, d\lambda$$

$$\geq (1 - \alpha)^{1/2} \int_{\Lambda} f(\lambda)\, d\lambda$$

$$= (1 - \alpha)^{1/2} (1 - \alpha)^{1/2} = 1 - \alpha, \tag{28}$$

and so (y_L, y_U) is a conservative $100(1 - \alpha)$ percent prediction interval for incidence at time t.

II. Infectivity and the Human Immunodeficiency Virus (HIV)

MEASURING HIV INFECTIVITY

Scott P. Layne
Theoretical Division
Los Alamos National Laboratory
University of California
Los Alamos, NM 87545

John L. Spouge
Nat. Ctr. for Biotechnology Information
National Library of Medicine
National Institutes of Health
Bethesda, MD 20892

Micah Dembo
Theoretical Division
Los Alamos National Laboratory
University of California
Los Alamos, NM 87545

Abstract

We have developed a mathematical model that quantifies lymphocyte infection by HIV and lymphocyte protection by blocking agents such as soluble CD4. We use this model to suggest standardized parameters for quantifying viral infectivity and to suggest techniques for calculating these parameters from well-mixed infectivity assays. We discuss the implications of the model for our understanding of the infectious process and virulence of HIV *in vivo.*

1. Introduction

Suppose that we give two virologists identical samples of human immunodeficiency virus (HIV) and ask them to independently determine some simple properties of the sample. Questions that we might ask include: How many infectious virions are in the sample? How virulent are the virions? How stable are the virions? How effective are various chemical agents against the virions? How effective are immunoglobulins from infected individuals in neutralizing the virions?

The virologists would set about answering our questions by running a series of viral infectivity assays, where specific conditions would be tailored to tackle each particular problem (Fig. 1). For example, to deal with the question of chemical agents, the virologists would inoculate aliquots of our sample virus into a series of chambers containing target cells plus various concentrations of the agent. The effectiveness of the agent could be judged by the amount required to reduce target cell infection by one half, relative to untreated control. Despite the superficial appearance of scientific objectivity, it would not be surprising to find that the two virologists (with the best of intentions and technique) obtained significantly different activities for the same agent and virus. With further inquiry, we would most likely discover that the virologists used somewhat different assay conditions, i.e., different target cell preparations, cell concentrations, etc. A great deal of detailed and quantitative information would be needed to understand the underlying causes of the discrepancy and allow us to decide which result would be most representative of the agent's activity in clinical situations.

The difficulty of comparing the results of one assay method with those of another is one of the biggest headaches in interpreting viral infectivity assays. For HIV, this problem is particularly important because the screening for potential therapeutic agents and vaccines is frequently based on assay results. To improve the utility of viral infectivity assays, it is useful to study theoretical models of how kinetic processes operate to determine their outcome (Layne et al. 1989).

In this chapter, we present a model for quantifying the infectivity of HIV. We show how the model is used for designing and analyzing viral infectivity assays, and discuss how it answers the kinds of questions posed above. We also use the model to evaluate prospects for blocking therapies, such as soluble forms of CD4 protein (sCD4), and vaccines based on anti-gp120 immunoglobulins.

2. HIV Infection

HIV infects subsets of lymphocytes, monocytes and macrophages exhibiting the CD4 protein on their surface (Fauci 1988). Depending on the particular target cell, infection is manifested by a spectrum of outcomes ranging from prolonged latency to syncytia formation and cell death. Sometimes replication is so explosive that target cell membranes lyse as newborn virions emerge. Unfortunately, $CD4^+$ cells are at the helm of the immune system's response to invasion. Thus HIV infection not only harms individual target cells, it also perturbs the entire communication network for the body's defenses. This results in a catastrophic susceptibility to opportunistic infections.

In a viral infectivity assay, only a single population of target cells is present, for example $CD4^+$ lymphocytes, and only the direct consequences of target cell infection are measured. Although this simplification does not support some mechanisms of infection (e.g., via MHC-restricted interactions, direct cell-to-cell contact, etc.), it does permit investigation of the initial events in HIV infection by a cell-free inoculum. For infectivity assays, three overall steps have been suggested for the infective process. First, HIV diffuses to the cell surface; second, gp120 on the virus' surface and CD4 on the target cell's surface form a bimolecular complex; third, interactions involving CD4, gp120 and gp41 promote fusion of HIV envelope with target cell membrane, resulting in entry of the viral core.

3. The Model

Consider a stock solution prepared from the supernatant of a cell culture infected with a particular strain of HIV. Such a stock solution can be regarded as a mixture of "homogeneous cohorts" of virions (i.e., populations of virions that were born simultaneously and that have been treated identically ever since). At birth, all members of a homogeneous cohort are assumed to be identical. A virion is said to remain "live" at time T, if it has neither participated in an infective event nor been non-specifically killed. As time progresses, some cohort members will die and the "infectivity" of those remaining "live" will diverge due to random processes.

Now suppose that V_0 random members of a homogeneous cohort are selected at birth. These virions are allowed to pre-incubate for a time T_p and are then inoculated at $T = 0$ into a chamber containing a large excess of CD4+ target cells (Fig. 1). The objective of this procedure is to count the number of virions that successfully infect, I, which subsequently yields the probability that a single virion will successfully infect, $i \equiv I/V_0$. Considering each homogeneous cohort separately involves no loss of generality, since the behavior of a mixture of cohorts is obtained by taking a weighted average.

Fig. 2 illustrates the random processes acting on a cohort. Of these, blocking, shedding and infection depend on gp120; non-specific killing does not. Despite the large number of viral states implied by the figure, an old trick from polymer chemistry, the "equivalent site approximation," gives a manageable formulation with a minimal loss of detail. According to this approximation, each gp120 molecule on the surface of a "live" virion has the same chance of being shed, of binding to CD4 on a target cell, or of binding to sCD4 in solution. Furthermore, non-specific killing operates independently on each "live" virion.

Let N be the initial number of gp120 molecules on each virion at birth and let g be the probability that a particular gp120 remains at a later time. Since gp120s can be either free or complexed with sCD4, $g \equiv (F+C)/NV$, where F and C are the numbers of free and complexed gp120 molecules on "live" virions and V is the number of "live" virions. Because of the equivalent site approximation, the probability that a "live" virion's surface will present exactly J gp120s is always given by a binomial distribution:

$$P(J) = \binom{N}{J} g^{J} (1-g)^{N-J} \quad . \tag{1}$$

After applying probabilistic identities, it follows that each infective event causes the loss (on average) of $[1+(N-1)F/NV]$ free gp120 molecules and $[(N-1)C/NV]$ complexed gp120 molecules.

Now let L and B be the respective concentrations of target cells and sCD4 in the reaction chamber. Because the viral inoculum is small, both L and B remain unperturbed and the kinetics in the reaction chamber are governed by:

$$\frac{dI}{dT} = k_l LF \quad , \tag{2}$$

$$\frac{dV}{dT} = -k_l LF - k_n V \quad , \tag{3}$$

$$\frac{dF}{dT} = -k_f BF + k_r C - (k_s + k_n)F - k_l LF \left[1 + (N-1)\frac{F}{NV}\right] \quad , \tag{4}$$

$$\frac{dC}{dT} = k_f BF - k_r C - (k_s + k_n)C - k_l LF \left[(N-1)\frac{C}{NV}\right] \quad . \tag{5}$$

Fig. 2 defines the five rate constants: k_l , k_n , k_s , k_f , and k_r . The terms k_lLF and k_nV are the rates of loss of "live" virions due to target cell infection and non-specific killing, respectively. The terms k_fBF and k_rC are the rates of formation and disassociation of gp120-sCD4 complexes, respectively. The terms $(k_s+k_n)F$ and $(k_s+k_n)C$ are the respective rates of loss of free and complexed gp120 from "live" virions due to the combined effects of spontaneous shedding and non-specific killing of virus. Finally, the terms $k_lLF[1+(N-1)F/NV]$ and $k_lLF[(N-1)C/NV]$ are the respective rates of loss of free and complexed gp120 from "live" virions due to infective events (see Fig. 3).

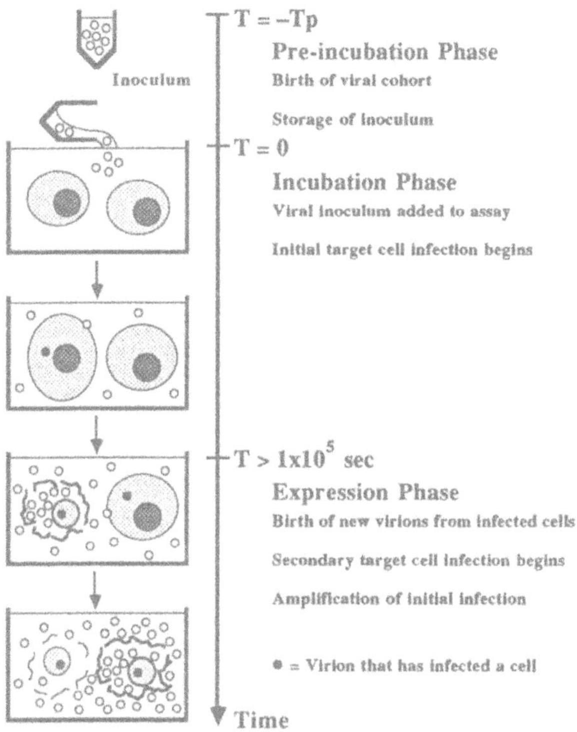

Fig. 1. Schematic diagram of the three phases in a viral infectivity assay. The inoculum is prepared by growing HIV in cell cultures, centrifuging the supernatant to separate virions from cellular debris, and storing the isolated virions. For simplicity, we assume that the inoculum consists of a "homogenous cohort" of virions that was born at $T=-T_p$. During the "pre-incubation" phase, $-T_p \leq T \leq 0$, virions lose activity by shedding gp120 and non-specific killing but target cell infection does not occur. To begin the initial cycle of infection, the reaction chamber is inoculated with a calibrated number of virions at $T=0$. During the "incubation" phase, $0 \leq T \leq 1\times10^5$ sec, all three processes of gp120 shedding, non-specific killing and target cell infection occur. Ordinarily, HIV replicates within 24 – 48 hours (~10^5 sec) after entering a target cell. During the "expression" phase, $T > 1\times10^5$ sec, new virions emerge from initially infected cells and secondary infections occur. A viral infectivity assay is said to be "linear" if the additional cycles of infection manufacture virions (or viral proteins) in proportion to the number of initial infections.

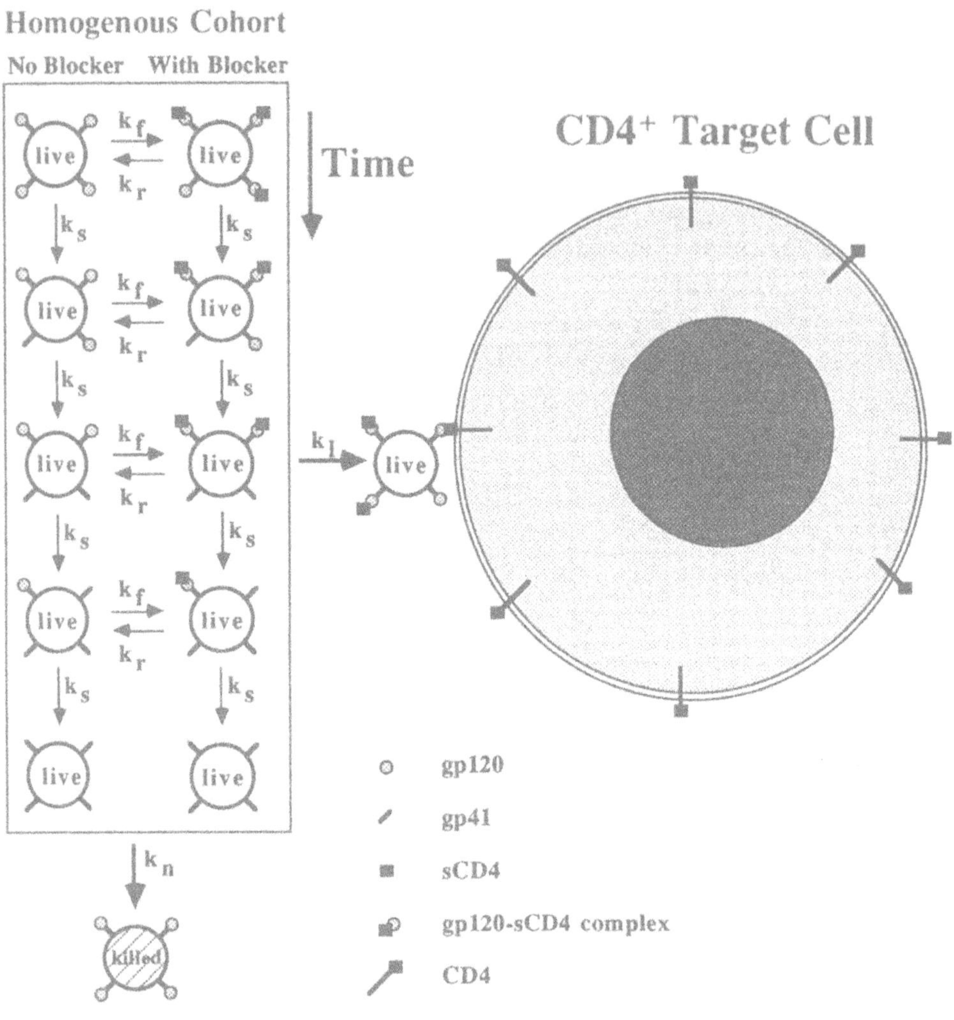

Fig. 2 Schematic diagram of the kinetic processes in a viral infectivity assay. k_l is the rate constant for successful infective contact between viral gp120 and CD4 on a target cell, defined on a per gp120 basis. Hence, a virion with four free gp120s infects at the rate $4k_lL$, with three free gp120s at the rate $3k_lL$, etc. When a virion sheds all of its gp120, it is considered "live" but not infectious. k_n is the rate constant for non-specific killing of virions, which includes mechanisms such as enzymatic degradation and dissolution by soaps (e.g., nonoxynol-9). The processes of infection and non-specific killing both result in the disappearance of virions together with their associated free and complexed gp120s. k_s is the rate constant for spontaneous disassociation of gp120 from gp41. Although gp120 "shedding" causes progressive inactivation of virions, it does not cause the actual disappearance of virions. k_f and k_r are the forward and reverse rate constants for gp120-sCD4 complex formation respectively. These processes result in the masking and unmasking of gp120s, but do not result in the net loss of gp120 nor in the disappearance of virions.

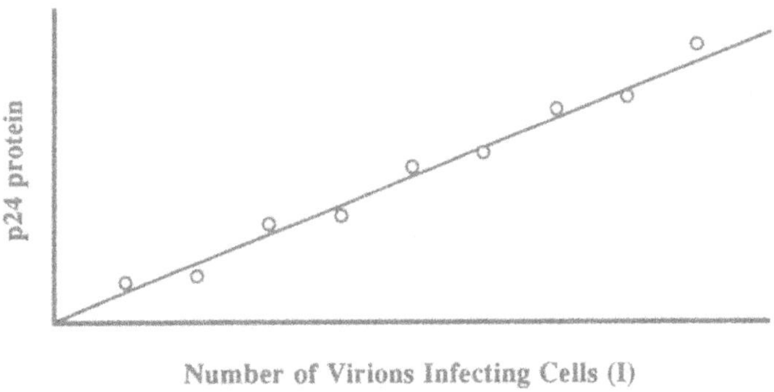

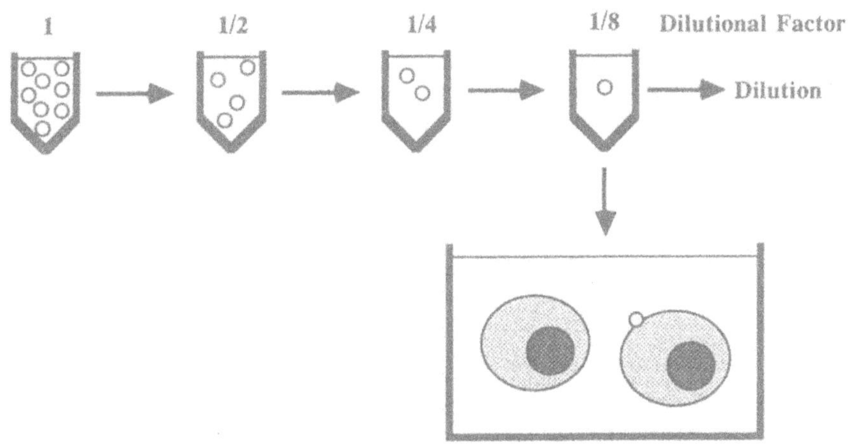

Fig. 3 There are two common methods for measuring I experimentally. First, if there is a linear relationship between I and subsequent expression of an HIV product (e.g., p24 protein) then measurement of the product yields I directly. Second, the probability of exactly k infections in a reaction chamber is Poisson distributed: $p_k = \exp\{-I\} I^k / k!$. In this case, I is determined by serial dilution of viral stock until only 50% of inocula produce one or more infections (i.e., until $p_0 = 0.5$). The reciprocal of the dilution factor required to achieve this result, $I / \ln(2)$, is the "infectious dose" or ID-50. Since $I \equiv i V_0$, the size of a particular inoculum, V_0, can be quantified by measuring the ID-50 with conditions ensuring that $i \approx 1$. Such conditions are favored by $T_p \rightarrow 0$ and $L \rightarrow \infty$.

The initial conditions at inoculation ($T = 0$) depend on circumstances during the pre-incubation phase. In many infectivity assays, for example, virions have no opportunity to infect target cells and are not exposed to sCD4 during pre-incubation. Solving Eqs. 2–5 with $L = 0$ and $B = 0$ for $-T_p \leq T \leq 0$ yields exponential loss of live virions and gp120 due to non-specific killing and shedding processes, respectively. The initial conditions for the incubation phase of the assay are then: $I = 0$, $V = V_0 \exp\{-k_n T_p\}$, $F = NV_0 \exp\{-(k_n+k_s)T_p\}$, and $C = 0$.

To facilitate analysis of Eqs. 2–5, introduce non-dimensional variables $i \equiv I/V_0$, $v \equiv V/V_0$, $f \equiv F/NV$, $c \equiv C/NV$ and $g \equiv (F+C)/NV$. Also introduce non-dimensional time, $t \equiv (k_s+k_n)T$, and non-dimensional parameters $\sigma \equiv k_s/(k_s+k_n)$, $\lambda \equiv k_l L/(k_s+k_n)$, $\gamma \equiv k_r/(k_s+k_n)$ and $\beta \equiv k_f B/k_r$. Then Eqs. 2–5 take the form:

$$\frac{di}{dt} = N\lambda f v \quad , \tag{6}$$

$$\frac{dv}{dt} = -[N\lambda f + 1 - \sigma]\, v \quad , \tag{7}$$

$$\frac{df}{dt} = -\gamma(\beta f - c) - \sigma f - \lambda f(1-f) \quad , \tag{8}$$

$$\frac{dc}{dt} = \gamma\, (\beta f - c) - \sigma c + \lambda f c \quad . \tag{9}$$

To gain insight into the kinetic model's behavior, we will solve Eqs. 6–9 with the aid of a computer. We will use these numerical results to help us obtain analytical solutions to the model. Before doing this, we must estimate the values of the rate constants and parameters.

4. Parameter Estimation

Upper limits for both k_l and k_f are derived from diffusion-limited reaction theory, i.e., the rate of collision between two diffusing spheres. We assume diffusion occurs in water at 37°C.

The rate of collision between HIV (radius $\approx 5\times10^{-6}$ cm) and a CD4$^+$ lymphocyte (radius $\approx 4\times10^{-4}$ cm) is about 1×10^{-10} cm^3 sec^{-1}. CD4$^+$ lymphocytes typically express $\sim2\times10^4$ receptors on their surface, implying that up to ~80% of collisions may result in reaction. In addition, electron micrographs show that a single gp120 complex covers 1/100 of a virion's surface (Özel et al. 1988). Therefore, the rate constant for successful infective contact is $k_l \leq (0.8)(0.01)(1\times10^{-10}) = 8\times10^{-13}$ cm^3 sec^{-1}.

The rate of collision between sCD4 (radius $\approx 2.5\times10^{-7}$ cm) and viral gp120 (radius $\approx 3.3\times10^{-7}$ cm) yields the forward rate constant for blocking: $k_f \leq 3\times10^{-12}$ cm^3 sec^{-1}. Experiments with other viruses indicate that both k_l and k_f are unlikely to be less that 10^4 times smaller than these upper limits.

According to equilibrium binding experiments, the association constant between sCD4 and gp120 ranges from 0.25×10^9 to 1.4×10^9 M^{-1} (Lasky et al. 1987 and Smith et al. 1987). Therefore, we take $k_{assoc} = k_f/k_r \approx 1.2\times10^9$ M^{-1} $= 2.0\times10^{-12}$ cm^3 molecule^{-1}. Given the fixed ratio k_{assoc}, the reverse rate constant for the blocking reaction is $k_r = k_f/k_{assoc} \leq 1.5$ sec^{-1}.

Electron microscope studies on the structure of HIV estimate that 70–80 gp120 complexes completely cover the surface of a mature virion. Therefore, we take $N = 80$.

Nara et al. (1987) have shown that HIV strains HTLV-IIIB and HTLV-IIIRF$_{II}$ lose half of their syncitial forming units within 4-6 hours when incubated in their growth media at 37° C (P. L. Nara and J. Kessler, unpublished data, April 12, 1988, using protocol cited in Nara et al. 1987). This gives $(k_s+k_n) \approx 10^{-4}$ sec^{-1} to within a factor of two.

5. Numerical Solutions

Numerical solutions of the model for typical parameters are illustrated in Fig. 4 – (a) shows a case with no blocker, (b) shows the effect of adding a low concentration of blocker, (c) shows the effect of adding a higher concentration of blocker, and (d) shows the effect of a high concentration of blocker in conjunction with non-specific killing agent (e.g., nonoxynol–9). These four solutions are useful for gaining insight into the temporal behavior of the model.

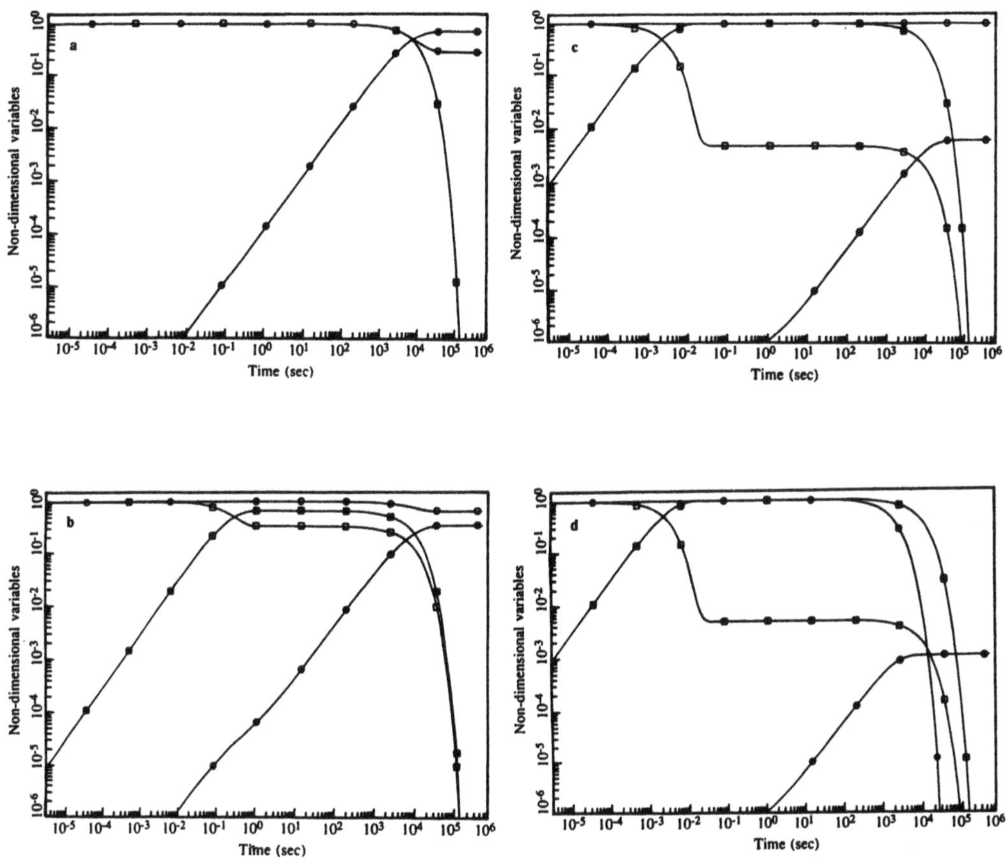

Fig. 4 Four numerical solutions of the model illustrating the progress of an untreated infection, an infection treated with two different concentrations of sCD4, and an infection treated with sCD4 plus an agent that enhances non-specific killing. The corresponding parameters are (a) $B = 0$ and $k_n = 0$, (b) $B = 1\times10^{12}$ molecules cm^{-3} and $k_n = 0$, (c) $B = 1\times10^{14}$ molecules cm^{-3} and $k_n = 0$, (d) $B = 1\times10^{14}$ molecules cm^{-3} and $k_n = 5\times10^{-4}$ sec^{-1}. Plots are labeled by (■) $c \equiv C/NV$, (□) $f \equiv F/NV$, (●) $i \equiv I/V_0$ and (○) $v \equiv V/V_0$. For all solutions $T_p = 0$ and $L = 2\times10^6$ cells cm^{-3}, which is a typical lymphocyte concentration for infectivity assays. See the parameter estimation section for other values.

In Fig. 4(a), the number of infected target cells (●) rises linearly until $T \approx 1\times10^3$ sec. Subsequently, at the characteristic shedding-time $k_s^{-1} \approx 1\times10^4$ sec, there is a drop in the number of gp120 molecules on the surface of virions and the rate of target cell infection diminishes. The obvious decline in the number of virions at $T \approx 1\times10^2$ sec (○) is due to target cell infection. When target cell infection stops, $T \approx 1\times10^5$ sec, 72% of initial virions have infected target cells (●); the remaining 28%, now completely lacking gp120 molecules and hence non-infectious, remain in the media (○). In this computation there is no non-specific killing, therefore, at least in theory these "live" but non-infectious particles remain in solution indefinitely.

Fig. 4(b) shows the effects of adding a small concentration of sCD4 to the culture medium. The initial rate of target cell infection (●) is unchanged from Fig. 4(a) until viral gp120 and sCD4 begin to equilibrate at $T \approx 1\times10^{-1}$ sec, (□) and (■). Immediately following this, the rate of target cell infection declines by a factor of 2–3 and because of this decline, only 35% of the initial virions ultimately find target lymphocytes (●), a decline comparable to the blocking ratio.

In Fig. 4(c), the concentration of sCD4 is 100 fold higher than in Fig. 4(b). Consequently, equilibration of the blocker with gp120 occurs in only 3×10^{-3} sec and 199 out of 200 gp120 molecules are blocked, (□) and (■). The rate of infectious events (●) declines by the same proportion but the gp120 shedding is unchanged. Therefore, the final proportion of infecting virions (●) is only 0.6%.

Fig. 4(d) shows the synergy of a high concentration of sCD4 with non-specific killing of virus. The rate-constant for non-specific killing, $k_n = 5\times10^{-4}$ sec^{-1}, is fivefold faster than the rate constant for gp120 shedding, $k_s = 1\times10^{-4}$ sec^{-1}. As in Fig. 4(c), binding of sCD4 to viral gp120 and the shedding of viral gp120 are independent of non-specific killing and occur on a "per live virion" basis. Non-specific killing causes the disappearance of virions (○) and so infection stops before virions shed all of their gp120 molecules, (□) and (■). As a result, the number of infective events per virion is diminished by six fold relative to Fig. 4(c) (●).

6. Analytical Solutions

Because $\gamma \equiv k_r/(k_s+k_n) \approx 10^4$ is large for physically relevant parameters, perturbation expansions of the form $f = f_0 + \gamma^{-1} f_1 + \gamma^{-2} f_2 + \ldots$ and $c = c_0 + \gamma^{-1} c_1 + \gamma^{-2} c_2 + \ldots$ lead to solutions of Eqs. 6–9. The zeroth order truncation, $f = f_0$ and $c = c_0$, is equivalent to the usual quasi steady-state approximation, $k_f BF \approx k_r C$, which holds for time-scales longer than the gp120-sCD4 equilibration time (Spouge et al. 1989). This approximation gives $c \approx \beta g/(1+\beta)$ and $f \approx g/(1+\beta)$.

For convenience, define the non-dimensional parameter $\rho \equiv \lambda/(1+\beta)$. Adding Eqs. 8 and 9 and applying the steady state approximation yields the Bernoulli equation, which is solvable by separation of variables:

$$\frac{dg}{dt} = -\sigma g - \rho g(1-g) \quad . \tag{10}$$

Eqs. 6 and 7 non-dimensionalize to

$$\frac{dv}{dt} = -(N\rho\, g + 1 - \sigma)\, v \quad , \tag{11}$$

$$\frac{di}{dt} = N\rho\, gv \quad . \tag{12}$$

Applying the product rule to Eqs. 10 and 11 gives:

$$\frac{d(gv)}{dt} = -\,\{\,[(N-1)g + 1]\rho + 1\,\}\; gv \quad . \tag{13}$$

Now consider Eqs. 10–13 for fixed initial conditions but for two different shedding rates, σ_1 and σ_2. Because viral infectivity assays requires g, i and v to be non-negative, the right hand sides of Eqs. 10–13 are monotonic in σ and other variables. If ρ are fixed non-negative functions of time, at any fixed time t,

$$\sigma_1 < \sigma_2 \;\Rightarrow\; g_{\sigma_1} > g_{\sigma_2} \;\Rightarrow\; g_{\sigma_1} v_{\sigma_1} < g_{\sigma_2} v_{\sigma_2} \;\Rightarrow\; i_{\sigma_1} < i_{\sigma_2} \quad . \tag{14}$$

The subscript on g, i and v indicates a solution for a particular value of σ. The implications in Eq. 14 are consequences of an elementary theorem (Hartman 1964). The theorem yields the first implication because the right-hand side of Eq. 10 is monotonic in σ. The other implications follow similarly from Eqs. 13 and 12 respectively. Therefore, at any time t, infection rates i for extreme values of σ ($\sigma = 0$ and $\sigma = 1$) bracket infection rates for all other values of σ. We use this property below.

Eqs. 10–12 can be solved explicitly for all σ. Substituting $g(t)$ into Eq. 11 gives $v(t)$. Next, substituting $g(t)$ and $v(t)$ into Eq. 12 gives $i(t)$. Define initial conditions as $g(t_0) = g_0$, $v(t_0) = v_0$ and $i(t_0) = i_0$. Also for convenience, define the auxiliary quantity

$$m(t) = g_0 \int_{t_0}^{t} \rho \;\; e^{-\int_{t_0}^{u} (\rho + \sigma)\, dw}\, du \quad . \tag{15}$$

The solutions to Eqs. 10–12, written as implicit functions of t, are:

$$g = g_0\, (1-m)^{-1}\, e^{-\int_{t_0}^{t} (\rho + \sigma)\, du} = \rho^{-1}(1-m)^{-1}\frac{dm}{dt} \quad , \tag{16}$$

$$v = v_0\, e^{-\int_{t_0}^{t} (1-\sigma)\, du}\, (1-m)^{N} \quad , \tag{17}$$

$$i = i_0 + v_0 \int_{t_0}^{t} e^{-\int_{t_0}^{u} (1-\sigma)\, dw}\, N\, (1-m)^{N-1} \frac{dm}{du}\, du \quad . \tag{18}$$

In Eqs. 16–18, u and w are dummy variables. m is a function of either u or t, depending on whether m appears in an integrand or not. In Eq. 16, the second equality is valid when $\rho \neq 0$.

When there are no target cells, $\rho = 0$. Therefore, during the pre-incubation phase ($-t_p \le t < 0$) Eqs. 10–12 describe constant functions and exponential decays. Solving Eqs. 10–12 with $\rho = 0$ and the initial conditions $g(-t_p) = 1$, $v(-t_p) = 1$ and $i(-t_p) = 0$ yields the initial conditions for the subsequent incubation phase ($t \ge 0$):

$$g(0) = e^{-\int_{-t_p}^{0} \sigma\, du}\ , \quad v(0) = e^{-\int_{-t_p}^{0} (1-\sigma)\, du} \quad \text{and } i(0) = 0.$$

If there is no shedding of gp120 ($\sigma = 0$), then $g(0) = 1$, $v(0) = \exp\{-t_p\}$ and $i(0) = 0$. The solutions to Eqs. 15 and 18 are

$$m = 1 - e^{-\int_0^t \rho\, du}\ , \tag{19a}$$

$$i = e^{-t_p} \int_0^t e^{-(u + N\int_0^u \rho\, dw)}\, N\rho\, du\ . \tag{19b}$$

If viral inactivation occurs entirely by shedding of gp120 ($\sigma = 1$), then $g(0) = \exp\{-t_p\}$, $v(0) = 1$ and $i(0) = 0$. The solutions to Eqs. 15 and 18 are

$$m = e^{-t_p} \int_0^t \rho\, e^{-(u + \int_0^u \rho\, dw)}\, du\ , \tag{20a}$$

$$i = 1 - (1-m)^N\ . \tag{20b}$$

Next, assume that the non-dimensional parameters λ, β, σ and ρ are constant with time, which is reasonable for viral infectivity assays. Both Eqs. 19 and 20 (which bracket all solutions for $i(t)$ by the monotonicity property) become:

$$m(t) = e^{-\sigma t_p} \frac{\rho}{\rho+\sigma} \left[1 - e^{-(\rho+\sigma)t}\right]\ , \tag{21a}$$

$$i = e^{-t_p} N\rho \int_0^t e^{-(\rho+1)u}\, (1-m)^{N-1}\, du\ . \tag{21b}$$

Setting $t = \infty$ in Eqs. 21 and using $(1-m)^N \approx \exp\{-m N\}$ gives an approximation that is uniformly valid to order $1/N$,

$$i_\infty \approx \left(\frac{N}{N-1}\right) e^{-(1-\sigma)t_p} \frac{\zeta}{\delta} \int_0^\infty \exp\left[-(u/\delta) - (\zeta/\delta)(1 - e^{-u})\right] du\ , \tag{22}$$

where $\zeta \equiv \exp\{-\sigma t_p\}(N-1)\lambda / (\lambda+1+\beta)$ and $\delta \equiv [\lambda + \sigma(1+\beta)] / (\lambda+1+\beta)$.

A change of variables from u to $z = -(\zeta/\delta)\exp\{-u\}$ relates the integral in Eq. 22 to the incomplete gamma function (formulas 6.5.1 and 6.5.4 in Abramowitz and Stegun 1972):

$$i_\infty \approx \left(\frac{N}{N-1}\right) e^{-(1-\sigma)t_p} (\zeta/\delta)\, e^{-(\zeta/\delta)}\, \Gamma(1/\delta)\, \gamma^*(1/\delta, -\zeta/\delta)\ . \tag{23}$$

The incomplete gamma function has an expansion (formula 6.5.29 in Abramowitz and Stegun 1972):

$$i_\infty \approx e^{-(1-\sigma)t_p} \frac{\zeta N}{N-1}\, e^{-\zeta/\delta} \sum_{j=0}^{\infty} \frac{(\zeta/\delta)^j}{(1+\delta j)\, j!}\ . \tag{24}$$

Notice that $\zeta \leq N-1$ and $\delta \leq 1$. The parameter ζ is a measure of the degree to which assay conditions promote target cell infection. Expressing ζ in dimensional variables gives:

$$\zeta \equiv e^{-(k_s+k_n)T_p} \frac{(N-1)\, k_l\, L}{k_l\, L + (1+k_{assoc}\, B)\, (k_s+k_n)} \quad . \tag{25}$$

Target cell infection is less probable as $\zeta \to 0$, i.e., $T_p \to \infty$, $L \to 0$, $B \to \infty$ or $(k_s+k_n) \to \infty$. Conversely, target cell infection is more probable as $\zeta \to N-1$, i.e., $T_p \to 0$, $L \to \infty$, $B \to 0$ or $(k_s+k_n) \to 0$. The expansions of Eq. 24 for both $\zeta \to 0$ and $\zeta \to N-1$ lead to the expressions

$$I_\infty \approx \frac{N\, V_0\;\, k_l\, L\;\, e^{-(k_s+k_n)\,T_p}}{k_l\, L + (k_s+k_n\,)\,(1 + B\; k_{assoc})}\left[1 - \frac{\zeta}{1+\delta} + \cdots\right] \tag{26}$$

and

$$I_\infty \approx \frac{V_0\, N\, e^{-k_n T_p}}{N-1}\left[1 - \frac{1-\delta}{\zeta} + \cdots\right] , \tag{27}$$

respectively. For both of these limiting cases, notice that δ appears only in the higher order terms.

Eqs. 26 and 27 are for designing and analyzing experiments to measure the characteristic viral parameters k_{assoc} , k_s , k_n, k_l and NV_0 . Fig. 5 shows some characteristics of the transition from the regime of Eq. 26 (small ζ) to the regime of Eq. 27 (large ζ).

7. Experimental Techniques

A primary motivation for developing our model is measuring the range of HIV's characteristic parameters – k_{assoc} , k_s , k_n, k_l , NV_0 – from viral infectivity assays. For example, separate HIV isolates may shed gp120 at differing rates and separate target cell lines may differ in their susceptibility to infection. Also an equally important motivation is measuring a parameter's change as a function of assay conditions. For example, increases in k_n after adding nonoxynol-9 to the assay media. Quantifying experiments is the key to answering our opening questions.

Consider an experiment to determine k_{assoc} . In such an experiment, I_∞ would be measured at various values of the blocker concentration, B, with all other variables held constant. When target cell concentration L is moderate, Eq. 26 implies that a plot of $I_\infty\,(B = 0)\; / \;I_\infty\,(B \geq 0)$ versus B will be linear with slope = $k_{assoc}/[1+ k_l L\; /(k_s+k_n\,)]$ and intercept = 1. Fig. 6 shows five plots generated by numerical solutions of Eqs. 2–5, simulating such an experiment at different lymphocyte concentrations, L . Although the plots for all values of L appear linear, the slopes seriously underestimate k_{assoc} except at the lowest cell concentrations. Hence, when determining k_{assoc} from the inhibition of viral infectivity, the experiment must be performed within the regime where the results are independent of cell concentration, i.e., $k_l L\; /(k_s+k_n\,) << 1$.

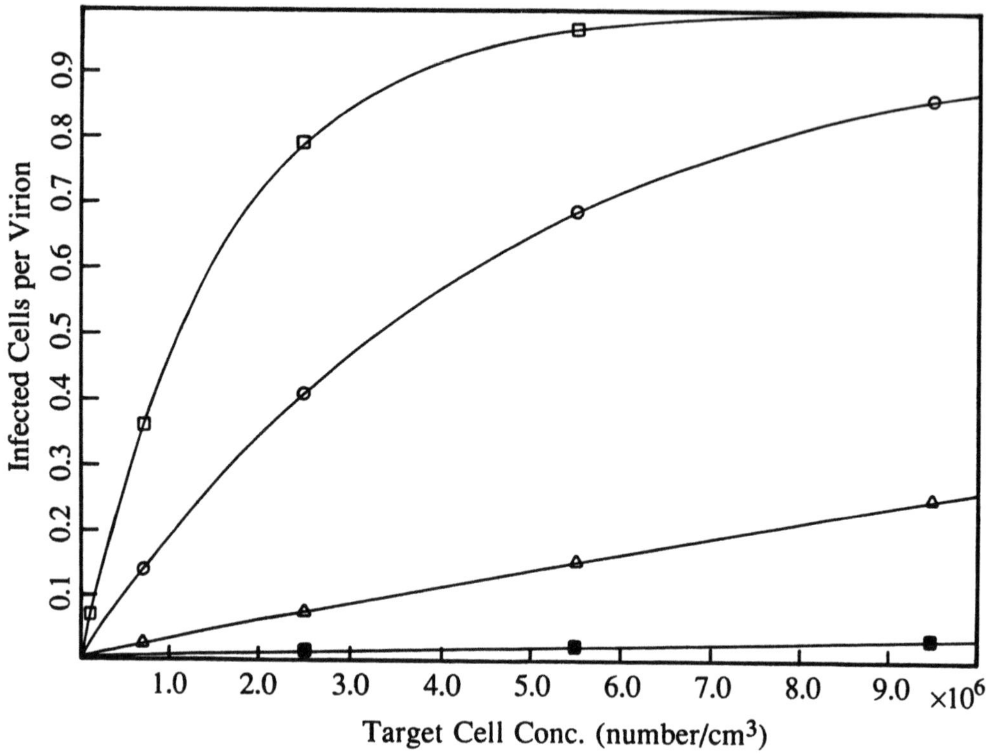

Fig. 5 Numerical solutions of the model illustrating a progression from small to large ζ (see Eqs. 26 and 27). The four solutions in each graph correspond to different sCD4 concentrations: (□) $B = 0$, (○) 1×10^{12}, (△) 1×10^{13} and (■) 1×10^{14} molecules cm^{-3}. The life of a virion consists of a race between finding a target cell and inactivation. Small values of ζ reflect a situation in which a given virion is likely to have only one chance to infect a target cell in its lifetime. Conversely, large values of ζ reflect a situation in which a given virion has multiple chances to infect a target cell. Since there is no pre-incubation, $T_p = 0$, small values of ζ occur only when $k_l\, L \,/\, [(k_s+k_n)(1+B\, k_{assoc})] \ll 1$, i.e., if $L \rightarrow 0$ or $B \rightarrow \infty$. In both instances, Eq. 26 implies that $I_\infty \propto L$. The breakdown of this proportionality occurs as $\zeta \rightarrow N-1$, i.e., $L \rightarrow \infty$. The figure also shows the effects of adding various concentrations of sCD4. Notice that the region of transition between linear and nonlinear behavior depends strongly on the blocker concentration. For all solutions $k_n = 0$, $k_s = 1\times10^{-4}$ sec^{-1} and the incubation time $T = 6.48\times10^4$ sec. See the parameter estimation section for other values.

Measuring the decay of viral infectivity with increasing pre-incubation times allows estimation of k_n and k_s. Fig. 7 shows five curves generated by numerical solution of Eqs. 2–5 simulating such experiments at different choices of non-specific killing, k_n. Target cell concentration is made as large as possible ($L \rightarrow$ maximum of $\sim10^8$ cells cm^{-3} for lymphocytes) and no blocker is added ($B = 0$). Under these conditions, it can be shown (see Eq. 27) that the initial decay rate gives k_n and that the final decay rate gives k_s+k_n (see Eq 26). The increase in decay rate with pre-incubation is a consequence of a fundamental kinetic difference between non-specific killing and shedding. The former is a so-called "single-hit" processes, whereas the later is a "multi-hit" process that inactivates the virus via many incremental steps. In other words, loosing a few gp120s makes little difference to the initial infection rate. The lumped quantity, k_s+k_n, is a direct measure of the ability of a viral strain to survive until it finds a target cell. A change in either k_n or k_s+k_n provides an objective measure of the potencies of viracidal agents.

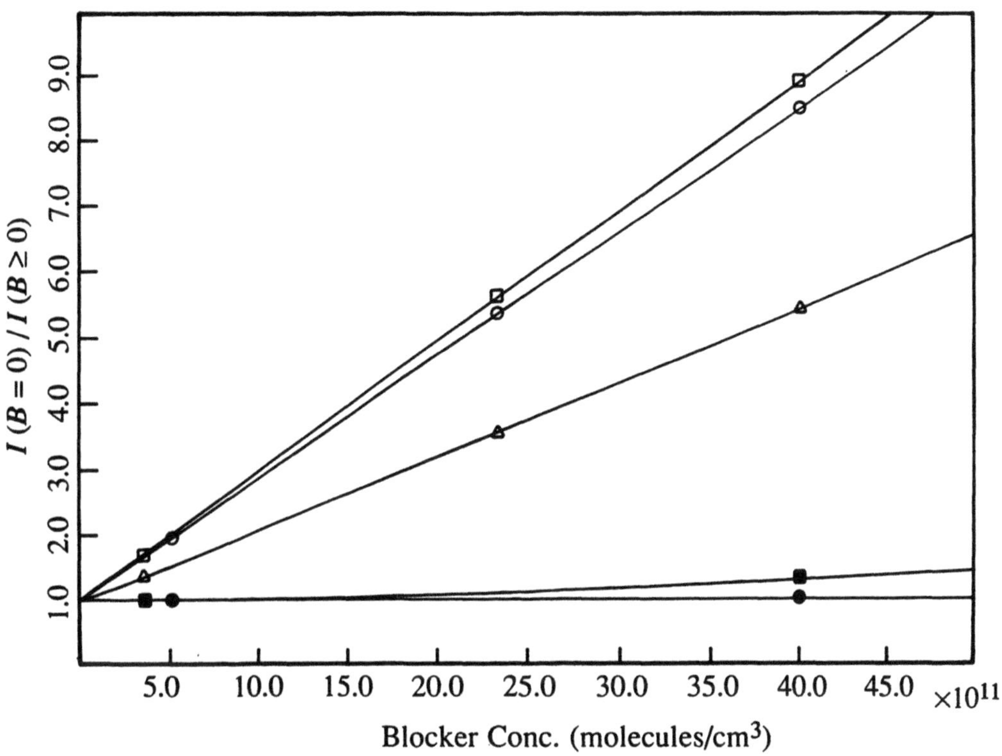

Fig. 6 Numerical solutions simulating a series of infectivity assays for quantifying blocker affinity (k_{assoc}). Activity is measured by comparing an assay without blocker to an assay with blocker, holding other conditions identical. This "control" to "experiment" ratio is expressed by $I(B = 0) / I(B > 0)$. The five straight lines correspond to increasing concentrations of target cells: (□) $L = 2\times10^4$, (○) 2×10^5, (△) 2×10^6, (■) 2×10^7 and (●) 2×10^8 cells cm^{-3}. The corresponding slopes for these solutions are 2.0×10^{-12}, 1.9×10^{-12}, 1.1×10^{-12}, 8.0×10^{-14} and zero cm^3 $molecule^{-1}$, respectively. According to Eq. 26, these slopes provide estimates of the quantity $k_{assoc} / [1+ k_l L /(k_s+k_n)]$, which is the "apparent" association constant between blocker and gp120. The decline of the slopes with increasing target cell concentration occurs because $k_l L /(k_s+k_n)$ increases. For all solutions $T_p = 0$, $k_n = 0$, $k_s = 1\times10^{-4}$ sec^{-1} and the incubation time $T = 6.48\times10^4$ sec. See the parameter estimation section for other values.

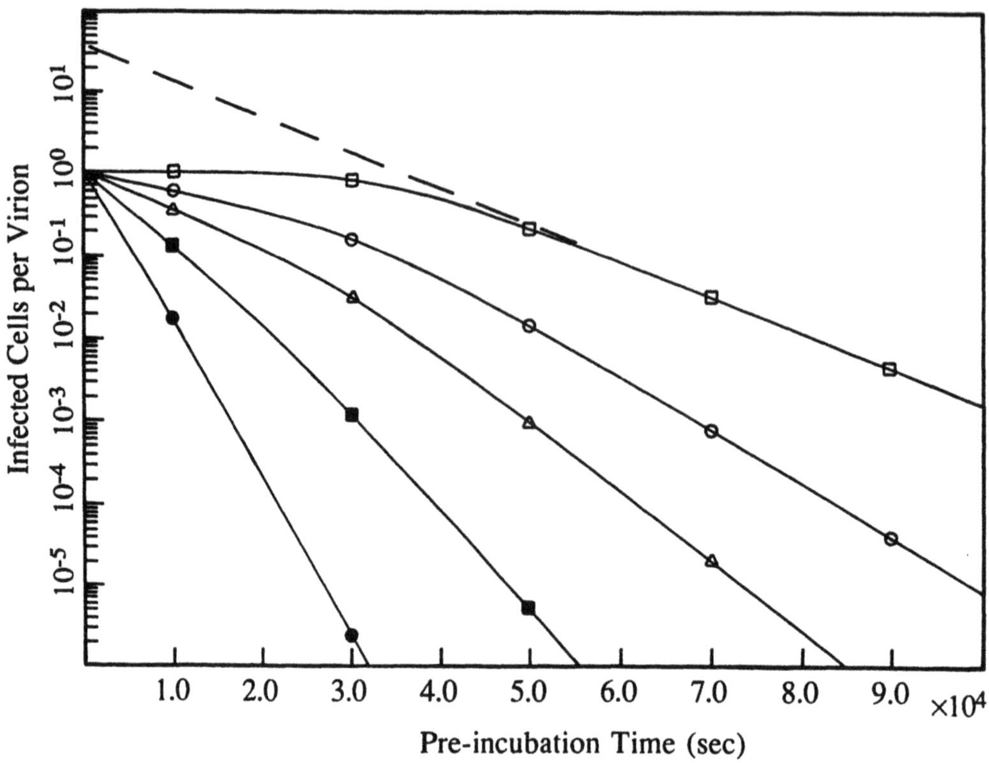

Fig. 7 Five numerical solutions of the model simulating a series of experiments to determine k_s and k_n. In all five simulations, virions are allowed to pre-incubate for various times T_p and are then inoculated into a reaction chamber. The five plots correspond to increasing amounts of non-specific killing: (□) $k_n = 0$, (○) 0.5×10^{-4}, (△) 1×10^{-4}, (■) 2×10^{-4}, and (●) 4×10^{-4} sec^{-1}. The abscissa is normalized by the initial number of virions, a procedure equivalent to taking $V_0 = 1$ in Eqs. 26 and 27. Initially, the slope of each plot is k_n but at longer pre-incubation times, the slope increases and approaches k_s+k_n. The transition to the final slope occurs when T_p satisfies $\zeta \ll 1$. Based on Eq. 25, extrapolating the final slope to $T_p = 0$ (shown for top curve) gives the intercept $NV_0\, k_lL\,/(k_lL + k_s+k_n)$. For all solutions $k_s = 1\times10^{-4}$ sec^{-1}, $B = 0$, $L = 1\times10^{8}$ cm^{-3} and the incubation time $T = 6.48\times10^{4}$ sec. See the parameter estimation section for other values.

Conducting two "pre-incubation assays" as above with different target cell concentrations yields estimates of both NV_0 and k_l (Fig. 8). The quantity NV_0 is useful for estimating the number of "infectious" virions in the inoculum. The rate constant k_l is important because it quantifies the susceptibility of a particular target cell type to infection by a particular HIV strain. A decrease in k_l can be caused by a number of independent factors, e.g., a decrease in the surface density of CD4, an increase in the viral uncoating and penetration time, or an increase in the abortive disassociation of the initial virus-target cell complex.

Fisher et al. (1988) report HIV isolates from infected individuals displaying markedly varying capacities to propagate *in vitro*. As HIV infection progresses, Cheng-Mayer et al. (1988) also report more virulent strains of HIV emerging that propagate in a wider variety of target cells. A numerical ranking of virus–target cell "tropism" according to the value of k_l would help to clarify whether such increased virulence is due to increased transmission or increased reproduction of virus.

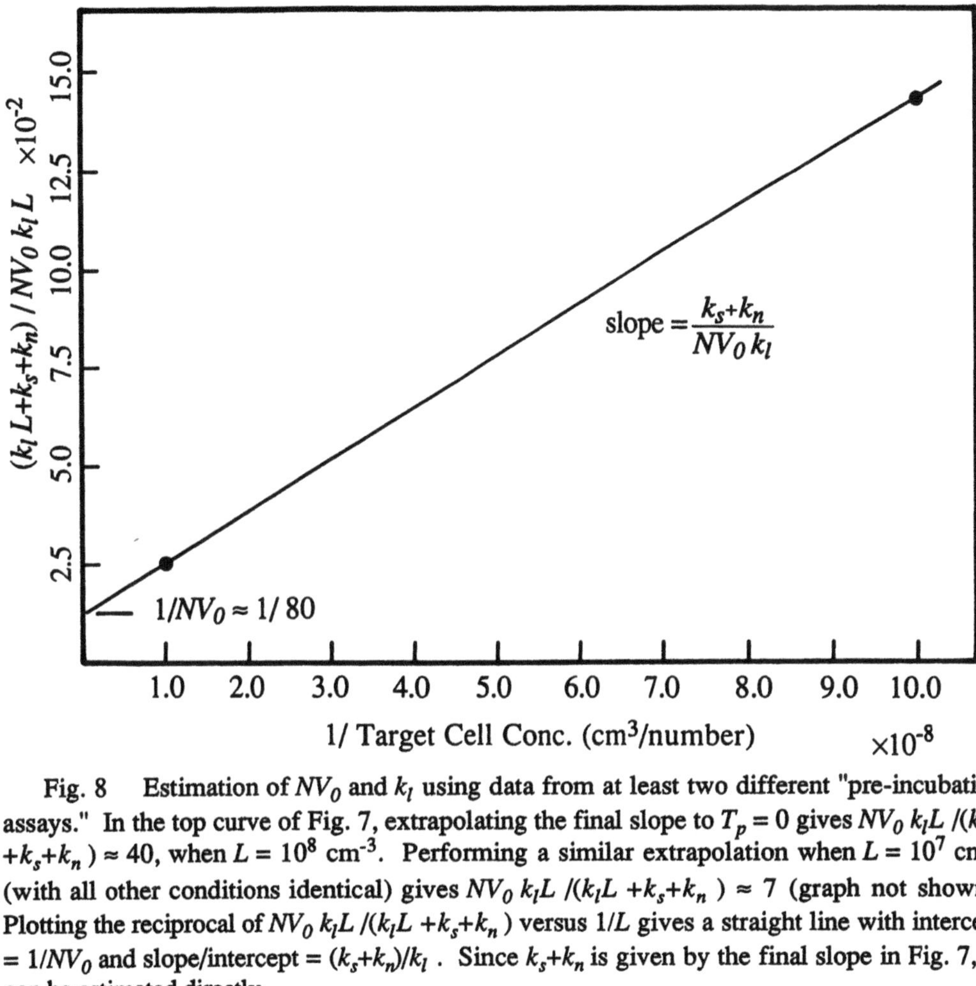

Fig. 8 Estimation of NV_0 and k_l using data from at least two different "pre-incubation assays." In the top curve of Fig. 7, extrapolating the final slope to $T_p = 0$ gives $NV_0\, k_l L\,/(k_l L + k_s + k_n) \approx 40$, when $L = 10^8$ cm^{-3}. Performing a similar extrapolation when $L = 10^7$ cm^{-3} (with all other conditions identical) gives $NV_0\, k_l L\,/(k_l L + k_s + k_n) \approx 7$ (graph not shown). Plotting the reciprocal of $NV_0\, k_l L\,/(k_l L + k_s + k_n)$ versus $1/L$ gives a straight line with intercept $= 1/NV_0$ and slope/intercept $= (k_s+k_n)/k_l$. Since k_s+k_n is given by the final slope in Fig. 7, k_l can be estimated directly.

8. Comparison to Experiments

A number of publications report that sCD4 blocks HIV infection of $CD4^+$ lymphocytes, but of these, only two provide sufficient information for measuring k_{assoc} by our analytical techniques (Fig. 6). From Deen et al. (1988), we calculate $k_{assoc} \approx 3.4\times10^{-12}$ cm^3 molecule^{-1}. From Hussey et al. (1988), we calculate $k_{assoc} \approx 3.8\times10^{-12}$ cm^3 molecule^{-1} for both of their sCD4 derivatives.

These "biological" results should be compared to measurements of k_{assoc} by direct "physical" methods: $0.42\times10^{-12} \leq k_{assoc} \leq 2.3\times10^{-12}$ cm^3 molecule^{-1} for various analogs of sCD4. The close agreement between "biological" and "physical" methods strongly supports the fundamental assumption that infection proceeds at a rate proportional to the number of free gp120s on a virion's surface (equivalent site approximation). This agreement would not ensue if there were significant mechanisms of infection not requiring gp120, nor if blocking essentially all gp120s were necessary to diminish infection. The fact that sCD4 blocks target cell infection despite long incubation times also verifies the existence of non-specific killing or shedding processes, k_n+k_s , and points out that such processes ultimately limit target cell infection.

9. *In Vitro* Versus *In Vivo*

HIV is transmitted from infected to susceptible individuals via cell-free virions and whole infected cells (e.g., infected CD4$^+$ lymphocytes). The relative contributions of these two mechanisms of infection have not been determined and could well depend on the circumstances surrounding transmission.

Once HIV invades the body, there are a number of distinct mechanisms for protecting against initial and sustained infection, such as neutralizing antibodies, antibody-dependent cellular cytotoxicity, natural killer cells, and HLA-restricted cytotoxic cells.

The relative importance and temporal evolution of these immune responses have not been elucidated for HIV. Paradoxically, these protective responses may also contribute to the immune system's decline. For example, Siciliano et al. (1988) have shown that HLA-restricted cytotoxic cells kill CD4$^+$ lymphocytes displaying gp120 fragments on their surface This killing occurs regardless of whether the cells are infected with HIV or merely exposed to gp120 before adding cytotoxic cells.

Our model deals primarily with quantifying the initial events of infection by a cell-free inoculum *in vitro*. It may also apply to the initial HIV infection *in vivo* and to protection by blocking agents and immunoglobulins during this initial phase of spread. It does not apply, however, to three of the protective mechanisms mentioned above nor to the longer-term dynamics of immune decline. Below we discuss the model's application *in vivo*.

10. Branching Process

The expression phase of an infectivity assay can be likened to a branching process (Fig. 9). In this process, each primary infection generates (on average) V_n secondary virions that enter the culture medium without pre-incubation ($T_p = 0$). These secondary virions, in turn, infect new target cells with probability i_∞. A growing infection develops if the branching number (the average number of successfully infecting secondary virions) is $V_n i_\infty > 1$.

Blocking secondary infection with sCD4 allows estimation of the branching number for an unblocked infection. Define B_{min} as the minimum sCD4 concentration extinguishing the branching process. Under many circumstances (see Eq. 26), it can be shown that $V_n i_\infty \approx NV_n k_l L / (k_s + k_n) \approx (1 + B_{min} k_{assoc})$. Estimating $B_{min} > 10\ \mu g\ cm^{-3} \approx 1\times10^{14}$ molecules cm^{-3} from Deen *et al.* (1988), and using $k_{assoc} \approx 3\times10^{-12}\ cm^3$ molecule^{-1} yields $1 + B_{min} k_{assoc} > 300$, which is surprisingly large.

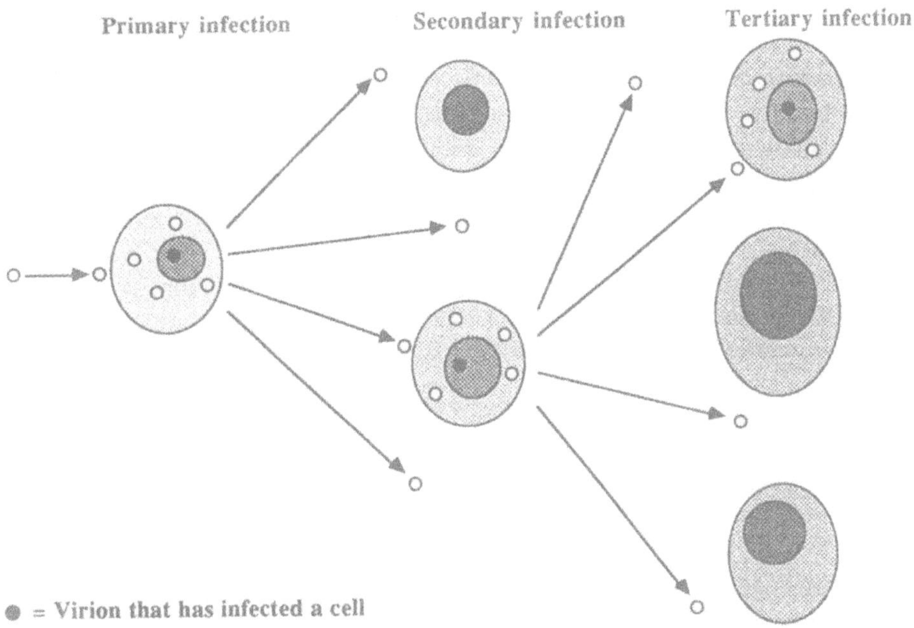

Fig. 9 The spread of HIV infection from cell to cell can be viewed as a branching process. In the figure, the expected number of progeny virions from an infected cell is $V_n = 4$ and the probability that a given progeny virions will find a target is $i_\infty = 1/4$. Since the branching number is equal to $V_n i_\infty = 1$, the process is just self-sustaining.

We note, however, that Deen et al. (1988) stimulated the CD4$^+$ lymphocytes in their assay with phytohemagglutinin (PHA). Recent work by Gowda et al. (1989) suggests that immune stimulation by mitogens significantly increases the rate of human CD4$^+$ lymphocyte infection. Based on this, it is conceivable that PHA stimulation significantly increased the probability of target cell infection, i_∞, and the number of secondary virions, V_n. Therefore, additional experiments to determine the branching number of both resting and stimulated lymphocytes are needed.

Since the branching number, $NV_n k_l L / (k_s + k_n)$, is proportional to target cell concentration, we can extrapolate from the conditions of Deen et al. (1988) ($L \approx 10^6$ cells cm^{-3} and $B_{min} > 10$ μg cm^{-3}) to the conditions in human blood ($L \approx 10^6$ cells cm^{-3}) and lymph node ($L \approx 10^8$ cells cm^{-3}). Such extrapolation indicates a minimum therapeutic dose of ~1000 μg cm^{-3} of sCD4 to treat established infections *in vivo*. Even more pessimistically, target cell infection from direct cell-to-cell contacts is probably less easily blocked than infection from the fluid medium. Experiments examining this situation are also required.

These results hold if the primary mechanism of action of sCD4 is simply to block the infective process as occurs in viral infectivity assays. As mentioned above, Siciliano et al. (1988) and Lanzavecchia et al. (1988) have suggested that sCD4 may also act to protect CD4$^+$ lymphocytes from indirect or autoimmune effects of gp120. If this is the case, then much lower concentrations of sCD4 may be of therapeutic use.

The branching process can also be used for estimating the immune response that an anti-gp120 vaccine must induce to protect against HIV infection. In this instance, k_{assoc} is the association constant between gp120 and neutralizing immunoglobulin (Ig), and B_{min} is the minimum concentration of Ig required to extinguish the spread of infection. Assuming that neutralizing Ig has a k_{assoc} identical to sCD4's (a rather high affinity Ig), a molecular weight ≈ 150,000, and $V_n i_\infty \approx 300$ yields $B_{min} \approx 0.03$ mg cm^{-3} for blood. For lymph node, we calculate that ~3 mg cm^{-3} will be required to prevent growth of infection. Normally, serum contains ~20 mg cm^{-3} of all classes of Ig. Thus an anti-gp120 vaccine must induce and maintain an extremely high titer of antibody.

11. Summary of Variables and Parameters

L ≡ concentration of target cells
B ≡ concentration of blocker
V ≡ number of live virions
I ≡ number of virions that successfully infect a target cell
F ≡ number of free gp120 molecules on live virions
C ≡ number of complexed gp120 molecules on live virions
N ≡ initial number of gp120 molecules on each live virion at birth
T ≡ time
T_p ≡ pre-incubation time
V_0 ≡ number of live virions from a homogenous cohort that are selected at birth
V_n ≡ expected number of progeny virions from an infected
B_{min} ≡ minimum blocker concentration extinguishing the branching process.
k_l ≡ rate constant for successful infective contact between viral gp120 and target cell CD4
k_n ≡ rate constant for non-specific killing of virions
k_s ≡ rate constant for spontaneous disassociation of gp120 from gp41
k_f ≡ forward rate constant for gp120-sCD4 complex formation
k_r ≡ reverse rate constant for gp120-sCD4 complex formation

$$i \equiv I/V_0$$

$$v \equiv V/V_0$$

$$f \equiv F/NV$$

$$c \equiv C/NV$$

$$g \equiv (F+C)/NV$$

$$t \equiv (k_s+k_n)T$$

$$\sigma \equiv k_s/(k_s+k_n)$$

$$\lambda \equiv k_l L/(k_s+k_n)$$

$$\gamma \equiv k_r/(k_s+k_n)$$

$$\beta \equiv k_f B/k_r$$

$$\rho \equiv \lambda/(1+\beta)$$

$$\zeta \equiv \exp\{-\sigma t_p\}(N-1)\lambda/(\lambda+1+\beta)$$

$$\delta \equiv [\lambda+\sigma(1+\beta)]/(\lambda+1+\beta)$$

REFERENCES

Abramowitz, A. and I. Stegun. (1972). *Handbook of Mathematical Functions with Formulas, Graphs, and Mathematical Tables*. Dover, New York.

Cheng-Mayer, C., D. Seto, M. Tateno and J.A. Levy. (1988). Biologic Features of HIV-1 That Correlate with Virulence in the Host. *Science*, **240**, 80-82.

Deen, K.C., J.S. McDougal, R. Inacker, G. Folena-Wasserman, J. Arthos, J. Rosenberg, P.J. Maddon, R. Axel and R.W. Sweet. (1988). A soluble form of CD4 (T4) protein inhibits AIDS virus infection. *Nature*, **331**, 82-84.

Fauci, A.S. (1988). The Human Immunodeficiency Virus: Infectivity and Mechanisms of Pathogenesis. *Science*, **239**, 617-622.

Fisher, A.G., B. Ensoli, D. Looney, A. Rose, R.C. Gallo, M.S. Saag, G.M. Shaw, B.H. Hahn and F. Wong-Staal. (1988). Biologically diverse molecular variants within a single HIV isolate. *Nature*, **334**, 444-447.

Gowda, S.D., B.S. Stein, N. Mohagheghpour, C.J. Benike and E.G. Engleman. (1989). Evidence that T Cell Activation Is Required for HIV-1 Entry in $CD4^+$ Lymphocytes. *J. Immun.*, **142**, 773-780.

Hartman, P. (1964). *Ordinary Differential Equations*. John Wiley and Sons, New York. p. 27.

Hussey, R.E., N.E. Richardson, M. Kowalski, N.R. Brown, H.-C. Chang, R.F. Siliciano, T. Dorfman, B. Walker, J. Sodroski and E.L. Reinherz. (1988). A soluble CD4 protein selectively inhibits HIV replication and syncytium formation. *Nature*, **331**, 78-81.

Layne, S.P., J.L. Spouge and M. Dembo. (1989). Quantifying the Infectivity of HIV. *Proc. Natl. Acad. Sci. USA*, **86**, 4644-4648.

Lanzavecchia, A., E. Roosnek, T. Gregory, P. Berman and S. Abrignani. (1988). T cells can present antigens such as HIV gp120 targeted to their own surface molecules. *Nature*, **334**, 530-532.

Lasky, L.A., G. Nakamura, D.H. Smith, C. Fennie, C. Shimasaki, E. Patzer, P. Berman, T. Gregory and D.J. Capon. (1987). Delineation of a Region of the Human Immunodeficiency Virus Type 1 gp120 Glycoprotein Critical for Interaction with the CD4 Receptor. *Cell*, **50**, 975-985.

Nara, P.L., W.C. Hatch, N.M. Dunlop, W.G. Robey, L.O. Arthur, M.A. Gonda and P.J. Fischinger. (1987). Simple, Rapid, Quantitative, Syncytium-Forming Microassay for the Detection of Human Immunodeficiency Virus Neutralizing Antibody. *AIDS Res. and Hum. Retroviruses*, **3**, 283-302.

Özel, M., G. Pauli and H.R. Gelderblom. (1988). The organization of the envelope projections on the surface of HIV. *Arch. Vir.*, **100**, 255-266.

Siciliano, R., T. Lawton, C. Knall, R. Karr, P. Berman, T. Gregory and E. Reinherz. (1988). Analysis of Host–Virus Interactions in AIDS with Anti-gp120 T Cell Clones: Effect of HIV Sequence Variation and a Mechanism for $CD4^+$ Cell Depletion. *Cell*, **54**, 561-575.

Smith, D.H., R.A. Byrn, S.A. Marsters, T. Gregory, J.E. Groopman and D.J. Capon. (1987). Blocking of HIV–1 Infectivity by a Soluble, Secreted Form of the CD4 Antigen. *Science*, **238**, 1704-1707.

Spouge, J.L., S.P. Layne and M. Dembo. (1989). Analytic Results for Quantifying HIV Infectivity. *Bull. Math. Biol.* In press.

THE STAGES OF HIV INFECTION: WAITING TIMES AND INFECTION TRANSMISSION PROBABILITIES

Ira M. Longini, Jr. W. Scott Clark, Michael Haber
Dept. of Epidemiology and Biostatistics
Emory University
Atlanta, GA 30322

Robert Horsburgh, Jr.
AIDS Program, Centers
for Disease Control
Atlanta, GA 30333

Abstract

We use stochastic models to estimate the waiting time distributions for progressive stages of HIV infection and to estimate stage-specific infection transmission probabilities between exposed and infected persons. We partition the infection period into four progressive stages: 1. infected but antibody negative; 2. antibody positive but asymptomatic; 3. pre-AIDS symptoms and/or abnormal hematologic indicator; and 4. clinical AIDS. We also define a fifth stage, death due to AIDS. A time-dependent Markov model is fitted to data on 45 persons with known time of HIV exposure to estimate the waiting time in stage 1, i.e., the pre-HIV-antibody period. The mean pre-HIV-antibody period is estimated to be 2.6 ± 0.2 months. A time-homogeneous Markov model was previously used to estimate the waiting time distributions for stages 2-3 from data on a sample of 513 homosexual and bisexual men from San Francisco. By combining this model with the model for stage 1, we estimate the mean AIDS incubation period, i.e., the waiting time in stages 1-3, as 9.8 ± 0.7 years. The estimated mean HIV infectious period, i.e., the waiting time in stages 1-4, is 11.8 ± 0.8 years. The estimated AIDS incubation period distribution is combined with a stochastic transmission model to estimate the stage-specific infection transmission rates from a sample of 45 heterosexual sex partners of persons with AIDS. The probability that an exposed person will be infected by a single sexual contact with an

infected person in stage 4 is estimated to be 0.0057 ± 0.0016. For stage 3, this probability is estimated to be 0.0007 ± 0.0002, and it is estimated to be very near to 0 for stage 2. Thus, an exposed person is about eight times more likely to be infected by a person who has AIDS than by one who has pre-AIDS symptoms
($p < 0.001$). The stochastic models that we developed can be extended to assess the risk of HIV transmission for different levels of important risk factors when more detailed data become available.

1. Introduction

The natural history of HIV in the human host can be visualized as a progression of stages from initial infection to death. In addition, the infectiousness of infected persons may vary considerably with respect to the stage of infection. These two important characteristics of HIV, coupled with the complicated social patterns of human contacts, largely determine the spread of HIV. The staging process and infectious contact patterns have been incorporated into dynamic mathematical models of HIV transmission to better understand HIV epidemiology and control (Jacquez et al. 1988; Koopman et al. 1988; Hethcote 1988). This paper presents some of the progress that has been made by using stochastic models of the staging process to estimate key parameters that govern the natural history and transmissibility of HIV.

Using the work of Longini et al. (1989), we model the natural history of HIV as a five-stage Markov process. The period of infection is partitioned into four transient states (stages) which are as follows:
1) infected but antibody negative; 2) antibody positive but asymptomatic;
3) pre-AIDS symptoms and/or abnormal hematologic indicator; and
4) clinical AIDS. The fifth stage is the absorbing state, death.
Infected persons are modeled to flow irreversibly through the stages as shown in Figure 1. There are several waiting time distributions embedded in Figure 1 which are epidemiologically important. The waiting time in stage 1 is the pre-HIV-antibody period, which will be referred to as the pre-antibody period in this paper. The sum of the waiting times in stages 1-3 is the AIDS incubation period while the sum of the waiting times in stages 1-4 is the HIV infectious period as well as the time from initial

infection to death (i.e., HIV survival time). The AIDS survival time is the waiting time in stage 4.

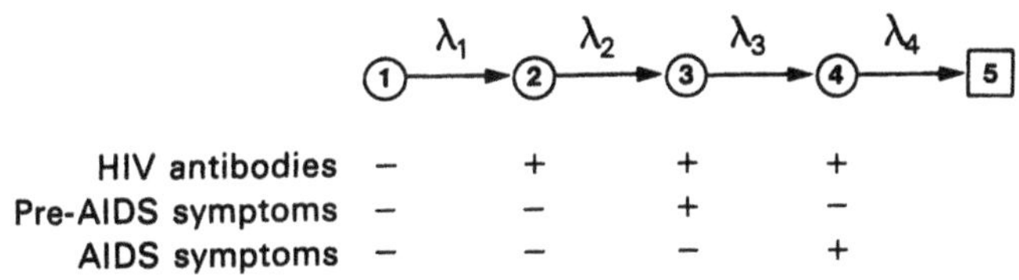

Figure 1: Flow diagram for the modeled natural history of HIV.

Section 2 of this paper deals with fitting a time-dependent, two-stage Markov model to data on newly infected persons in order to estimate the distribution of the pre-antibody period. In Section 3, this work is integrated with previous results of Longini et al. (1989) to provide estimates of the distributions of the AIDS incubation and HIV infectious periods. In Section 4, the estimated distribution of the AIDS incubation period is coupled with a stochastic model for estimating the stage-specific infectious transmission rates. We then apply the model to data collected by Fischl et al. (1987) on the sexual transmission of HIV between heterosexual partners. Finally, a discussion is given in Section 5.

2. The pre-antibody period

The pre-antibody period, i.e., waiting time in stage 1, was estimated from data on 45 persons who were infected with a known time of exposure to HIV (Horsburgh et al. 1989). The data, including the most likely route of exposure, are given below in Table 1. However, the route of exposure is not a factor in the analysis. Some of the persons were tested for infection just after the time of exposure and then again within six months. All persons were tested within six months of the time of exposure, and were followed for a relatively short period of time. Thus, they provide reliable information only about stage 1.

Table 1: Data used to estimate pre-antibody period

Person	Time sequence			States			Route of exposure
j		τ_j months			y_j		
1	0	2.53		1	2		Factor VIII
2	0	2.17		1	2		Factor VIII
3	0	3.52	7.50	1	1	2	Factor VIII
4	0	2.80	4.18	1	1	2	Factor VIII
5	0	0.79	2.86	1	1	2	Factor VIII
6	0	3.45	4.93	1	1	2	Factor VIII
7	0	2.96		1	2		Factor VIII
8	0	2.50		1	1		Factor VIII
9	0	5.10	6.91	1	1	2	Factor VIII
10	0	0.99	1.18	1	1	2	Factor VIII
11	0	0.89	3.85	1	1	2	Factor VIII
12	0	2.80		1	2		Factor VIII
13	0	0.66	2.20	1	1	2	Factor VIII
14	0	0.46	6.51	1	1	2	Factor VIII
15	0	2.73		1	2		Factor VIII
16	0	1.15	2.80	1	1	2	Factor VIII
17	0	1.22	1.45	1	1	2	Factor VIII
18	0	1.22	1.45	1	1	2	Factor VIII
19	0	0.76	1.15	1	1	2	Blood Transfusion
20	0	0.86	1.32	1	1	2	Blood Transfusion
21	0	0.29	1.48	1	1	2	Blood Transfusion
22	0	0.59	1.51	1	1	2	Blood Transfusion
23	0	0.43	3.82	1	1	2	Blood Transfusion
24	0	0.92	3.22	1	1	2	Blood Transfusion
25	0	2.37	3.45	1	1	2	Blood Transfusion
26	0	0.30	6.05	1	1	2	Needlestick
27	0	1.22	3.82	1	1	2	Needlestick
28	0	0.03	3.98	1	1	2	Needlestick
29	0	0.89	1.61	1	1	2	Needlestick
30	0	1.91	5.92	1	1	2	Needlestick
31	0	0.43	2.24	1	1	2	Needlestick
32	0	2.96	5.92	1	1	2	Needlestick
33	0	1.64	2.47	1	1	2	Organ Transplant
34	0	0.99	2.63	1	1	2	Organ Transplant
35	0	1.32	1.84	1	1	2	Organ Transplant
36	0	1.64		1	2		Organ Transplant
37	0	1.38		1	2		Organ Transplant
38	0	1.32	7.99	1	1	2	Organ Transplant
39	0	1.32	7.99	1	1	2	Organ Transplant
40	0	1.84	9.05	1	-1	2	Cutaneous
41	0	1.38	4.01	1	1	2	Cutaneous
42	0	0.69	1.41	1	1	2	Cutaneous
43	0	0.53	1.55	1	1	2	Sexual
44	0	1.61	2.07	1	1	2	Sexual
45	0	1.05	2.96	1	1	2	IV drug use

Because the time of exposure is known for these 45 persons, the transition intensity (i.e., hazard function) for stage 1, $h_1(t)$ can be modeled as a time-dependent function, where $h_1(t)\Delta t + o(\Delta t)$ is the probability that a person who has been in stage 1 for t units of time will make the transition to stage 2 during the time interval $[t, t+\Delta t]$, and where $\lim o(\Delta t)/\Delta t = 0$ as $\Delta t \longrightarrow 0$.

We selected a three-parameter Weibull distribution to model the waiting time in stage 1. This distribution can have an increasing, decreasing, or constant hazard function depending upon the value of the shape parameter. Thus, the Weibull distribution should be sufficiently flexible to model the waiting time distribution in stage 1. In addition, the exponential distribution, which we previously used to model the waiting time distribution for stage 1 (see Longini et al. 1989), is a special case of the Weibull distribution. The probability density function (pdf) and the transition intensity (hazard) function, respectively, of the three-parameter Weibull distribution are

$$f_1(t) = \begin{cases} 0 & \text{if } t \le \delta \ , \\ \lambda_1^{\alpha}\, \alpha[(t-\delta)^{\alpha-1}] \exp\{-[\lambda_1(t-\delta)]^{\alpha}\} & \text{if } t > \delta \ , \end{cases} \tag{1}$$

$$h_1(t) = \begin{cases} 0 & \text{if } t \le \delta \ , \\ \lambda_1^{\alpha}\, \alpha(t-\delta)^{\alpha-1} & \text{if } t > \delta \ , \end{cases}$$

where $\lambda_1 > 0$, $\alpha > 0$ and $\delta \ge 0$. The time delay δ is needed since a finite amount of time is required for a primary antibody response (i.e., it is biologically impossible for a person to seroconvert immediately after infection). When $\alpha = 1$, then (1) reduces to a two-parameter exponential distribution.

Let j ($j = 1,2,\ldots,45$) be the index for each of the persons in the cohort, and let m_j be the number of times person j was observed. Then the array $\boldsymbol{\tau}_j = (\tau_{j0}, \tau_{j1}, \ldots, \tau_{jm_j})$ represents the times at which person j was observed to be in the stages given by the array $\mathbf{y}_j = (y_{j0}, y_{j1}, \ldots, y_{jm_j})$, where $\tau_{j0} = 0$ and $y_{j0} = 1$ for all j. Since the mean waiting time in stage 1 (about 2.5 months) is much shorter than that in stage 2 (about 53 months--see Section 3), and the period of observation for each person is short, we modeled the system as simply two stages with stage 2 being closed. Given the above assumptions, we are interested in the probability, $p_j(\boldsymbol{\tau}_j;\mathbf{y}_j)$, of observing the array $\mathbf{y}_j$ at times $\boldsymbol{\tau}_j$. Table 1 presents the data for the arrays $(\boldsymbol{\tau}_j,\mathbf{y}_j)$, where the time units are months.

The following array patterns were observed in the data: $(0,\tau_{j1};1,1)$, $(0,\tau_{j1};1,2)$ and $(0,\tau_{j1},\tau_{j2};1,1,2)$. The probabilities of these patterns are given below in terms of $h_1(t)$ which is defined in (1):

$$p_j(0,\tau_{j1};1,1) = \begin{cases} 1 , & \text{if } \tau_{j1} \leq \delta, \\ \exp[-h_1(\tau_{j1}-\delta)], & \text{if } \tau_{j1} > \delta, \end{cases} \tag{2}$$

$$p_j(0,\tau_{j1};1,2) = 1 - p_j(0,\tau_{j1};1,1) , \tag{3}$$

$$p_j(0,\tau_{j1},\tau_{j2};1,1,2) = \begin{cases} 0 , & \text{if } \tau_{j1}\leq \delta,\ \tau_{j2} \leq \delta, \\ 1-\exp[-h_1(\tau_{j2}-\delta)], & \text{if } \tau_{j1}\leq \delta,\ \tau_{j2} > \delta, \\ \exp[-h_1(\tau_{j1}-\delta)] - \exp[-h_1(\tau_{j2}-\delta)] , & \\ & \text{if } \tau_{j1}> \delta,\ \tau_{j2} > \delta. \end{cases} \tag{4}$$

The likelihood function for estimating the parameters $\boldsymbol{\theta} = (\delta,\lambda,\alpha)$ was found by taking the product of the functions (2-4) for all 45 persons. It is

$$L(\boldsymbol{\theta}) = \prod_{j=1}^{45} p_j(\boldsymbol{\tau}_j; \mathbf{y}_j) . \tag{5}$$

Maximum likelihood estimates (MLEs) of the parameters, $\boldsymbol{\theta}$, were found by numerically maximizing the natural logarithm of (5) for λ_1 and α at fixed values of δ. This was accomplished with the derivative-free pseudo-Gauss-Newton algorithm in the BMDP statistical package (Ralston 1985). This algorithm also provided the asymptotic variance-covariance matrix of the conditional MLE's $\hat{\lambda}_1$ and $\hat{\alpha}$. Hypothesis tests were conducted using the likelihood ratio test (see Chapter 10 of Hogg and Craig, 1970).

The log-likelihood function was maximized at preset values of δ in the interval [0.00,1.14] using a step size of 0.01. Selected results are given in Table 2. When no delay is modeled, i.e., δ = 0.00, the Weibull distribution provides a significantly better fit to the data than does the exponential distribution (i.e., $\chi^2_{(1)} \cong 23$, $p < 0.001$, by the likelihood ratio test). However, from Table 2, the likelihood function is greatest for both the Weibull and exponential distributions at $\delta = 0.99$, but the log-likelihood functions were relatively flat around $\delta = 1$. Thus, we will use this value as our estimate. At this value of δ, the Weibull does not provide a significantly better fit to the data than does the exponential distribution (i.e., $\chi^2_{(1)} \cong 0.6$, $p \cong 0.55$, by the likelihood ratio test). The estimated value of α when $\delta = 1$ is 0.876 ± 0.152, which provides another check on the conjecture that the waiting-time distribution in stage 1 is a two-parameter exponential distribution. Thus, we select the two-parameter exponential distribution as the most parsimonious model for the data.

Table 2: Estimating the pre-antibody period: Maximized log-likelihood function values at preset values of δ

Delay δ Months	Maximized value of $\ell n\,[L(\boldsymbol{\theta})]$ Exponential $\alpha = 1$	Weibull $\alpha \neq 1$
0.00	-74.73	-63.16
0.40	-65.94	-60.79
0.80	-57.90	-57.54
0.90	-56.67	-56.67
0.98	-56.29	-56.10
0.99	-56.27	-55.99
1.00	-56.33	-55.99
1.01	-56.39	-55.99
1.02	-56.47	-56.00
1.10	-57.85	-56.33
1.14*	-60.15	-57.31

*For $\delta \geq \min\{\tau_{j2}\} = 1.15$ the value of $\ell n\,[L(\boldsymbol{\theta})] \longrightarrow -\infty$.

The estimate of λ_1 is 0.625 ± 0.081, conditional on $\delta = 1$. The mean waiting time in stage 1, i.e., pre-antibody period, is estimated to be $\hat{\mu}_1 = 1 + 1/\hat{\lambda}_1 = 2.6$ months. The estimated standard error of $\hat{\mu}_1$ is obtained using the method of statistical differentials (see pages 69–72 in Elandt-Johnson and Johnson, 1980). It is $\widehat{\text{s.e.}}(\hat{\mu}_1) \cong \widehat{\text{s.e.}}(\hat{\lambda}_1)/\hat{\lambda}_1^2 = 0.2$ months when δ is assumed constant. Thus, an approximate 95% confidence interval on the mean pre-antibody period, μ_1, is [2.2,3.0] months. The median length of the pre-antibody period is estimated to be $\hat{\tilde{\mu}}_1 = 1 + (\ell n\ 2)/\hat{\lambda}_1 = 2.1$ months. The approximate 95% confidence interval on $\tilde{\mu}_1$ is [1.8,2.4] months. The estimated time at which 95% of the infected persons could be expected to seroconvert is $\hat{\tau}_{.95} = 1 - \ell n(.05)/\hat{\lambda}_1 = 5.8$ months, with an approximate standard error of 0.6 months. Then the approximate 95% confidence interval on $\tau_{.95}$ is [4.6,7.0] months.

3. The AIDS incubation period

The AIDS incubation period, i.e., waiting time in stages 1-3, was estimated by combining the results from Section 2 with data on a sample of 513 seropositive men who were from a larger cohort of homosexual and bisexual men from San Francisco (Jaffe et al. 1985). These men were periodically bled for serostatus and examined for pre-AIDS and AIDS indicators and symptoms. While the men in this study were presumably infected by sexual contact, the time of exposure was unknown. The time of seroconversion was observed to an interval for 90% of the men, while the remaining 10% entered the sample as seropositive for HIV. Thus, this cohort yielded information about the waiting times in stages 2-4, but not about stage 1. Of the 513 men included in the analysis, 130 (25%) had developed AIDS and 76 of these 130 (58%) had died, during the seven to eight years of follow-up.

A time-homogeneous, staged Markov model was fitted to these data by Longini et al. (1989) to estimate the waiting times in stages 1-4. In that analysis, they estimated the mean pre-antibody period to be 2.2 ± 0.7 months from a cohort of 90 persons with transfusion and factor VIII-associated infections. We now propose to use the model described in Section 2 to model stage 1 with the somewhat improved data given in table 1. For this model, the mean pre-antibody period is estimated to be 2.6 ± 0.2 months, as described above.

The progression of an infected person through the stages of infection and ultimately to death is modeled as a time-homogeneous Markov process with a time delay δ in the first stage. The transition intensities for stages 2-4 are the constants $\lambda_i > 0$, $i = 2,3,4$, and the transition intensity for stage 1 is zero, if $t \leq \delta$, and it is $\lambda_1 > 0$, if $t > \delta$. The probability that a person who is in stage i at time τ will be in stage $k \geq$

i at time $t > \tau$ is defined as $p_{ik}(\tau,t)$. Explicit formulae for this probability are easily found using standard methods for Markov processes (see Chapter 11.7 in Chiang 1980). If all the transition intensities are distinct, i.e., $\lambda_i \neq \lambda_j$ for all $i \neq j$, then the transition probabilities from stage 1, starting at time 0, to the other states are

$$p_{1k}(0,t) = \begin{cases} 0 & , \text{ if } t \leq \delta, \\ (-1)^{k-1}\lambda_1 \cdots \lambda_{k-1} \sum_{j=1}^{k} \exp[-\lambda_j\,(t-\delta)] \Big/ \prod_{\substack{\ell=1 \\ \ell\neq j}}^{k} (\lambda_j-\lambda_\ell) & , \text{ if } t>\delta, \end{cases} \tag{6}$$

k = 1,2,3,4,

$$p_{15}(0,t) = \begin{cases} 0 & , \text{ if } t \leq \delta \\ -\lambda_1 \cdots \lambda_4 \sum_{j=1}^{4} \{1-\exp[-\lambda_j\,(t-\delta)]\}/[\lambda_j \prod_{\substack{\ell=1 \\ \ell\neq j}}^{4} (\lambda_j-\lambda_\ell)], & \text{if } t>\delta. \end{cases} \tag{7}$$

Since the transitions among stages 2–4 are assumed to be time homogeneous, the transition probabilities among these stages for all $\tau > \delta$ and $t > \tau$ are

$$p_{ik}(\tau,t) = (-1)^{k-i}\,\lambda_i \cdots \lambda_{k-1} \sum_{j=i}^{k} \exp[-\,\lambda_j\,(t-\tau)] \Big/ \prod_{\substack{\ell=i \\ \ell\neq j}} (\lambda_j-\lambda_\ell), \tag{8}$$

$i = 2,3,4;\ i \leq k \leq 4,$

$$p_{i5}(\tau,t) = (-1)^{4-i}\,\lambda_i \cdots \lambda_4 \sum_{j=i}^{4} \{1-\exp[-\lambda_j(t-\tau)]\}/[\lambda_j \prod_{\substack{\ell=i \\ \ell\neq j}}^{4} (\lambda_j-\lambda_\ell)], \tag{9}$$

$i = 2,3,4.$

We define T_I as the random variable for the AIDS incubation period, i.e., the waiting time in stages 1–3. The probability that a person who was infected at time 0 is in stage 3 at time t, and then makes the transition to stage 4 at time t + dt is $\lambda_3 p_{13}(0,t)dt$, where $p_{13}(0,t)$ is given in (6). Thus, the pdf for T_I is $f_I(t) = \lambda_3 p_{13}(0,t)$. Note that $f_I(t)$ is a special case of the three-parameter general gamma distribution (see page 222 in Johnson and Kotz 1970). The hazard function, $h_I(t)$, for the AIDS incubation period is

$$h_I(t) = f_I(t)/[1 - F_I(t)], \tag{10}$$

where $F_I(t) = \int_0^t f_I(\omega)d\omega$ is the cumulative distribution function (cdf) of T_I.

It follows from the modeling assumptions that the mean waiting time in stage 1 is $\mu_1 = \delta + 1/\lambda_1$, and the mean waiting time in the other stages is $\mu_i = 1/\lambda_i$; i = 2,3,4. The median waiting time in stage 1 is $\tilde{\mu}_1 = \delta + \mu_1 \ell n2$, while it is $\tilde{\mu}_i = \mu_i \ell n2$ for i = 2,3,4. Then the expected length of the AIDS incubation period is

$$E(T_I) = \int_0^\infty \omega \, f_I(\omega) \, d\omega = \mu_1 + \mu_2 + \mu_3 \, , \tag{11}$$

and the variance of T_I is

$$Var(T_I) = 1/\lambda_1^2 + 1/\lambda_2^2 + 1/\lambda_3^2 \, . \tag{12}$$

We define T as the random variable for the length of the HIV infectious period, i.e., the waiting time in stages 1-4. (Note that T is also the time from infection to death.) If we use the same argument as the one above, then the pdf of T is $\lambda_4 p_{14}(0,t)$. This is a special case of the four-parameter general gamma distribution. The cdf of T is

$$F(t) = \int_0^t \lambda_4 p_{14}(0,\omega) \, d\omega, \tag{13}$$

and the expected length of the HIV infectious period is

$$E(T) = \mu_1 + \mu_2 + \mu_3 + \mu_4. \tag{14}$$

The parameters λ_i, i = 2,3,4, were estimated by Longini et al. (1989) by ML methods for Markov processes using the data on the 513 homosexual and bisexual men from the San Francisco study. The parameters δ and λ_1 were estimated as described in Section 2. The estimated parameters and mean and median waiting times are given in Table 3. The estimated mean

AIDS incubation period from (11) and Table 3 is 9.8 years (117.7 months) with a 95% confidence interval of [8.4, 11.2] years. The asymptotic standard error of the estimated AIDS incubation period was obtained by the use of the method of statistical differentials (Elandt-Johnson and Johnson, 1980). Based on the model, the estimated median AIDS incubation period is 8.3 years (99.4 months). The estimated hazard function for progression to AIDS is monotonically increasing in t (see Fig. 2), which agrees with the form of the hazard functions used to model the AIDS incubation period by other investigators (see Longini et al. 1989 for a discussion of this point). Based on the estimated density function, the probability that a newly infected person will have developed AIDS within five years of infection is 0.26.

Table 3: Estimated parameters, mean and median waiting times in each stage of infection based on the staged Markov model with $\delta = 1$

Stage	Parameter estimate	Waiting time	
		Mean	Median
i	$\hat{\lambda}_i \pm$ one s.e.	$\hat{\mu}_i$	$\hat{\tilde{\mu}}_i$
	mos.$^{-1}$	mos. (yrs.)	mos. (yrs.)
1	0.625 ± 0.081	2.6 (0.2)	2.1 (0.2)
2	0.019 ± 0.002	52.6 (4.4)	36.5 (3.0)
3	0.016 ± 0.002	62.5 (5.2)	43.3 (3.6)
4	0.042 ± 0.004	23.8 (2.0)	16.5 (1.4)

The estimated parameters for stages 2, 3, and 4 are from Longini et al. (1989).

If we assume that persons remain infectious up to their time of death, the estimated mean HIV infectious period from (14) and Table 3 is 11.8 years (141.5 months) with a 95% confidence interval of [10.3, 13.3] years. Based on the model, the estimated median HIV infectious period is 10.3 years (124.0 months). The estimated probability density and hazard functions have the same shape as those shown in Fig. 2. As mentioned above, the HIV infectious period is also the time to death from the beginning of stage 1, i.e., time of initial infection. Statistics concerning the survival time from each stage of infection are easily derived from the staged Markov process and the parameter estimates (see

Longini et al. 1989 for detailed estimates).

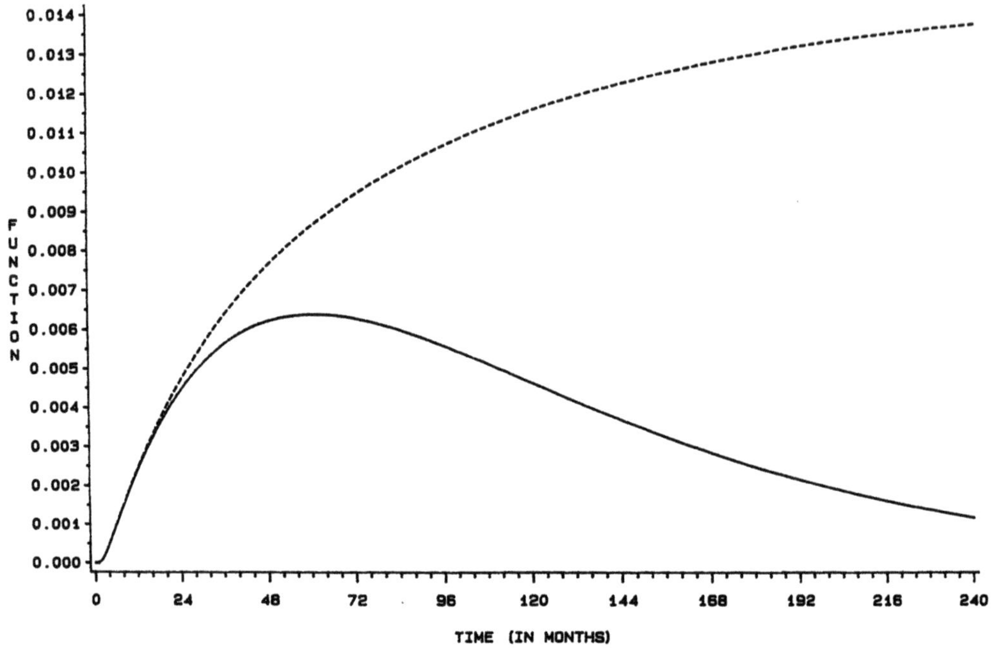

Figure 2: The estimated pdf $\hat{f}_I(t) = \hat{\lambda}_3\hat{p}_{13}(0,t)$, solid line, and hazard function $\hat{h}_I(t)$ (see (10)), dashed line, of the AIDS incubation period, where the estimated parameters come from Table 3.

4. Stage-specific infection transmission probabilities

As shown in the above sections, HIV has a long, variable infectious period, and the level of infectiousness is thought to vary considerably as the disease progresses (Lange et al. 1986; Hyman and Stanley 1988; and Anderson and May 1988). A number of host factors may affect HIV transmissibility, including concomitant venereal infections and T-helper cell numbers. However, it has been proposed that infectiousness increases with the stage of infection, i.e., progression (Burke and Redfield 1988; Goedert et al. 1987; Laga et al. 1988). With regard to the four stages of infection described above, it is possible that persons are highly infectious, on the average, during stages 1 and 4, not very infectious during stage 2, and infectious at an intermediate level, on the average, during stage 3 (Seage et al. 1989). In this section, we test this hypothesis by developing a statistical model for estimating the probability that a susceptible person is infected given that the susceptible is exposed to an infected person who is in a particular stage of infection. Such probabilities can best be estimated from prospective cohort studies where susceptibles are exposed to known infectives for specified lengths of time.

We will develop the model for the following study design which was employed by Fischl et al. (1987) to study the heterosexual transmission of HIV from persons diagnosed with AIDS to their sex partners. "Monogamous" sexual partners are ascertained when one partner (the index case) is diagnosed with AIDS. We will label this time of diagnosis as time 0. The exposed partner (to the index case) is then bled periodically at times $0, t_1, \ldots, t_k$, and the samples are examined for HIV. (We assume that the intervals $[t_j, t_{j+1}]$, and $j = 0, \ldots, k-1$ are wide enough so that if a person is infected during an interval, then seroconversion will probably occur during that same interval.) In addition, the amount of time that the partners had sexual contact prior to diagnosis of the index case is known and labeled as variable $u \geq 0$. Then, the period of exposure prior to AIDS diagnosis of the index is $\min\{T_I, u\}$, where T_I is the random variable for the length of the AIDS incubation period, with pdf $f_I(t)$ given in Section 3. In addition, the amount of time that the partners continue to have sexual relations after time 0 is known and labeled as w. Then the total period of exposure to the index case, when the infection status of the exposed person is known, is $\min\{T_I, u\} + w$. Fischl et al. (1987) assumed that the exposed sex partner in the pair did not have exposure to infected persons outside of the relationship, although there was evidence of limited outside exposure for some exposed partners. We use this assumption in our analysis, although the statistical model can be easily modified to incorporate exposure from outside of the relationship (see Longini et al, 1988).

The infection transmission rate is modeled to vary over the length of the infectious period. For exposure prior to time 0, the infectious transmission rate is $\beta(\tau,x)$, so that $\beta(\tau,x)d\tau + o(d\tau)$ is the probability that a susceptible will be infected during the interval of time $(\tau,\tau+d\tau)$, where τ is measured backwards from time 0, given exposure to an infected person who has an AIDS incubation period of length $T_I = x$. Since T_I is a random variable, it is unlikely that we would know precisely when the index was infected. Thus, we need to incorporate the distribution of T_I into our analysis. Then the cumulative infection transmission rate for exposure prior to time 0 is

$$\beta(\tau) = \int_0^{\infty} \beta(\tau,x)\, f_I(x)dx, \quad 0 \leq \tau \leq u. \tag{15}$$

For exposure after time 0, we let $\gamma(\tau)$ be the infection transmission rate for exposure τ time units after time 0. Then, the cumulative hazard function (for being infected) for an exposed person who has been exposed to the index for u time units before time 0 and w time units afterwards is

$$\Lambda(u,w) = \int_0^{u} \beta(\tau)d\tau + \int_0^{w} \gamma(\tau)d\tau. \tag{16}$$

It follows directly that the probability that an exposed person is still not infected at time w is $\exp[-\Lambda(u,w)]$. Additional risk due to exposure to infectives outside the relationship could be modeled by adding the appropriate terms to the cumulative hazard function (16).

The functions $\beta(\tau,x)$ and $\gamma(\tau)$ are assumed to have particular parametric forms, with parameters $\boldsymbol{\beta}$ and $\boldsymbol{\gamma}$, respectively. These parameters, $\boldsymbol{\theta} = (\boldsymbol{\beta},\boldsymbol{\gamma})$, can be estimated using ML methods as long as they are identifiable. With the study design described above, three types of observations can be seen in the data. Each type is listed below with the appropriate contribution to the likelihood function:

1. If the exposed person is positive (for infection) at time 0, then the contribution is
$$L_1(\boldsymbol{\theta}) = 1 - \exp[-\Lambda(u,0)]. \tag{17}$$
2. If the exposed person is not positive at time $t_{k-1} < w$ and is positive at time t_k, then the contribution is
$$L_2(\boldsymbol{\theta}) = \exp[-\Lambda(u,t_{k-1})] - \exp[-\Lambda(u,s_k)], \tag{18}$$

where $s_k = \min(w, t_k)$.

3. If the exposed person is negative at the time of the last observation, t_k, then the contribution is

$$L_3(\theta) = \exp[-\Lambda(u, s_k)]. \tag{19}$$

The total likelihood function is the product of the appropriate contributions (17-19) for all the exposed persons in the data set. The total likelihood function is maximized using standard methods as described in Section 2.

Since the infectiousness of a person is thought to vary approximately with respect to the stages of infection described in Section 3, the function $\beta(\tau,x)$ is modeled as a step function with each step corresponding roughly to a stage of infection. The function is

$$\beta(\tau,x) = \begin{cases} \beta_3, & \text{if } \quad 0 \leq \tau \leq x(1-\delta_2), \\ \beta_2, & \text{if } \quad x(1-\delta_2) < \tau \leq x(1-\delta_1), \\ \beta_1, & \text{if } \quad x(1-\delta_1) < \tau \leq x, \\ 0, & \text{if } \quad \tau > x, \end{cases} \tag{20}$$

$\beta_1 \geq 0,\ \beta_2 \geq 0,\ \beta_3 \geq 0,$

where δ_1 is the fraction of the mean waiting time in stage 1 relative to the mean AIDS incubation period. Similarly, δ_2 is the fraction corresponding to the mean waiting times in stages 1 plus 2. We make no *a priori* assumptions about the ordering of the β_i's. From the data in Table 3, we estimate $\delta_1 = 2.6/117.7 = 0.022$ and $\delta_2 = (2.6 + 52.6)/117.7 = 0.469$. Thus, β_1, β_2, and β_3 correspond to the infection transmission rates with an infected person who is in stages 1, 2, and 3 of infection respectively. Since a person is in stage 4 of infection after AIDS diagnosis by definition, then the function $\gamma(\tau)$ is

$$\gamma(\tau) = \beta_4, \quad \beta_4 \geq 0, \text{ for } \tau \geq 0. \tag{21}$$

Thus, β_4 is the transmission rate for a person in stage 4 of infection.

Once the above parameters are estimated, two infection transmission probabilities of epidemiologic interest can be calculated. The first is the probability that a susceptible will be infected given t time units of exposure to an infective who is in stage 1 of infection, which is

$$P_i(t) = 1 - \exp(-\beta_i t), \qquad i = 1,2,3,4. \tag{22}$$

The second alternative is the probability that a susceptible will be infected in a single sex act with an infective who is in stage i of infection. In order to calculate this probability, we will assume that all couples have an average rate of r sexual contacts per unit of time. This probability is

$$p_i = 1 - \exp(-\beta_i/r), \qquad i = 1,2,3,4. \tag{23}$$

The model described by equations (15-19) was fitted to data on 45 heterosexual couples that were followed by Fischl et al.(1987), where the index case had AIDS. The exposed person was bled every six months up to 18 months after the AIDS diagnosis of the index case. Infection was identified by seropositivity to HIV. The complete data set is given in Table 1 of Fischl et al. (1987) and will not be given here. Of the 45 exposed persons, 13 were seropositive at time 0 (i.e., the time of AIDS diagnosis of the index case). Their contribution to the likelihood function is modeled by (17). In addition, 13 persons seroconverted after time 0, and their contribution to the likelihood function is modeled by (18). Finally, 19 exposed persons remained seronegative, and their contribution to the likelihood function is modeled by (19). Thus, 58% of the exposed persons were infected. Because stage 1 represents such a small proportion of the AIDS incubation period, 2.2%, we were unable to estimate β_1. Three different distributions were used to model the AIDS incubation period: 1) The three-parameter general gamma distribution used in Section 3, i.e., $f_I(t) = \lambda_3 p_{13}(0,t)$, 2) the two-parameter Weibull distribution, which has been used by a number of other researchers (see Longini et al. 1989), and 3) the degenerate (i.e., constant) distribution for the sake of comparison. The parameters were set so that the mean was the same for all three distributions, $E(T_I) = 118$ months. The parameter estimates were similar for all three distributions. Thus, only the results when the general gamma distribution is used are presented in Table 4.

The first row of Table 4 shows the results for a model that ignores the stages of infection and assumes a uniform transmission rate, β, through the entire infectious period. In this case, the probability of infection per sexual contact would be 0.0010. This probability was calculated using a constant rate of r = 11 (mostly) unprotected sexual contacts per month, the average of the rate reported by Fischl et al. (1987). The value of the maximized log-likelihood function is -73.5. The next three rows in table 4 show the estimated parameters for the model with stage-specific transmission rates (20). The value of the maximized log-likelihood function for this model is -56.6. Thus, we reject the null hypothesis that $\beta_1 = \beta_2 = \beta_3 = \beta_4 = \beta$ ($p < 0.001$) when we use the likelihood ratio test (with 3 degrees of freedom), and we conclude that there is a significant difference in the infectiousness of an infected person in stages 2, 3, and 4. From Table 4, the infection transmission rate for exposure to an infected person in stage 2, i.e., the asymptomatic state, is estimated to be 0. However, this occurs because the estimate of β_2 hit the lower bound of 0 at the maximum of the likelihood function. Thus, the standard error for β_2 cannot be computed. We can only state that the transmission rate for stage 2 is probably close to 0 for this particular data set.

Table 4: Estimated infection transmission rates and probabilities

Stage	Transmission rate	Transmisson probability	
	mo.^{-1}	Per 12 mos.	Per sexual contact
i	$\hat{\beta}_i$	$\hat{P}_i(12)^{*}$	$\hat{p}_i^{**}$
no stages†	0.011 ± 0.002	0.124 ± 0.021	0.0010 ± 0.0002
2	0††	0††	0††
3	0.008 ± 0.002	0.093 ± 0.024	0.0007 ± 0.0002
4	0.061 ± 0.017	0.518 ± 0.101	0.0057 ± 0.0016

*Calculated from (22). **Calculated from (23) based on a constant rate of 11 sexual contacts per month (Fischl et al. 1987). †Fitted model with $\beta_1 = \beta_2 = \beta_3 = \beta_4 = \beta$. ††Standard error not available.

From Table 4, the risk ratio per sexual contact for a susceptible when comparing exposure to an infected person in stage 4 with that in stage 3 is estimated to be $\hat{p}_4/\hat{p}_3 = 0.0057/0.0007 = 8.1$, which is significantly different from 1 ($p < 0.001$). Therefore, a person who has a single sexual contact with an infected person who has AIDS is eight times more likely to be infected than if he or she has a single sexual contact with an infected person who has pre-AIDS symptoms. Table 4 also gives the risk of infection to a susceptible who has sex with an infected person over the period of one year. Note that the probability that a person would be infected after a year of sexual contact with a partner who has AIDS (stage 4) is estimated to be 0.518--a rather high probability. The average period of sexual contact following AIDS diagnosis was 11.2 months for the 45 couples in the data set.

5. Discussion

In this paper, we have used a staged Markov model to describe the transitions of infected persons from infection to AIDS diagnosis and ultimately, to death. The estimated transition intensity rates provide statistical estimates of the length of the pre-antibody period, AIDS incubation period, HIV infectious period, and the time to death (i.e., survival time) for infected persons. In addition, by combining the staging distribution with a non-homogeneous Poisson process for the risk of infection, we were able to estimate the stage-specific infection transmission rates for exposed susceptible persons. Thus, we were able to use the general concept of staging for HIV infection to construct a relatively complete statistical picture of the progression to disease for infected persons and the risk that such persons may pose to others through heterosexual contact.

The estimates of the transition intensities, $\lambda_1,\ldots,\lambda_4$, given in Table 3 and those of the infection transmission rates, β_3 and β_4, given in Table 4, have been used by Koopman et al. (1988) and Hethcote et al. (1988) in dynamic models of HIV transmission. These models have been used to investigate questions of HIV epidemiology and control as well as to make long-term projections for the course of the HIV epidemic in specific populations.

As pointed out in Section 1, the pre-antibody period (i.e., waiting time in stage 1) is important because persons can have infective virus in their blood during this period (Ward et al. 1988). Thus, they may be highly infectious to others at a time when they are antibody negative and difficult to detect as infected. Our estimate of 2.1 months for the median of the pre-antibody period is close to that estimated by Horsburgh, et al. (1989) of 2.4 months from experimental data. That analysis used a staged Markov model for estimation similar to the model described in Section 2, and was based on data from pre- and post-seroconversion blood samples from 39 infected persons whose infection status was also assessed by detection of HIV DNA using the polymerase chain reaction technique. Both the above estimates are in general agreement with direct observations on newly infected persons (see Horsburgh et al. 1989 for details). Our estimate that 95% of infected persons would seroconvert within 5.7 months of exposure is consistent with the observations of Nekwei et al. (1988). They reported that 96% of the newly infected persons that they studied seroverted within six months.

A potential bias exists in the data in Table 1 because subjects in which HIV infection has persisted for several years without the detection of antibody may not yet have been reported. However, this is unlikely since infection without antibody detection has not been reported to persist for longer than 14 months, and no delays in the recognition of infection have been reported from prospective studies of exposed persons who have been followed for at least 24 months (see Horsburgh et al. 1989 for details).

With respect to the estimation procedure used in Section 2, there is no MLE for the time delay, δ, for right interval-censored data. In the case of no interval censoring, the MLE for δ is the minimum observed waiting time from infection to seroconversion (see page 245 in Kalbfleisch and Prentice 1980). Thus, it was necessary to find the MLEs for λ and α, conditioned on the preset values of δ. The estimated standard errors of $\hat{\lambda}$ and $\hat{\alpha}$ are probably underestimated since they do not reflect variation in the estimate of δ.

The interval censoring causes some inflation in the estimated standard error of $\hat{\lambda}_1$. In the case of no interval censoring, then we have $\text{var}(\hat{\lambda}_1) \cong \lambda_1 / \sum_{j=1}^{n} W_j$, where W_j is the time spent by person j in stage 1 (see chapter 11 in Chiang, 1980). The estimates of λ_1 and W_j from the interval-censored data in Table 1 are $\hat{\lambda}_1 = 0.625$ and $\hat{W}_j \cong 2.6$, $j = 1, \ldots, 45$. If we assume that the data were not interval-censored, then $\widehat{\text{var}}(\hat{\lambda}_1) \cong (0.625)/[(45)(2.6)] = 0.0053$, and we have $\widehat{\text{s.e.}}(\hat{\lambda}_1) \cong \sqrt{0.0053} = 0.073$. This estimatated standard error is only slightly smaller than the estimate of 0.081 that was found for the interval-censored data.

The most parsimonious model for the pre-antibody period is the two-parameter exponential distribution, which is time homogeneous except for the time delay, δ. This distribution provides as good an explanation of the data as the time-dependent, three-parameter Weibull distribution. The implication is that the hazard rate of transition from the antibody-negative to the antibody-positive stage of infection is probably constant over time following an initial time delay of about one month (i.e., $\delta = 1$). We also used a nonparametric method (see Turnbull 1976) to estimate the cdf of the waiting-time distribution in stage 1 from the data in Table 1. However, the censoring pattern in the data resulted in a number of gaps in the empirical cdf, and it is difficult to compare the two curves. The nonparametric estimate of the time delay is the shortest observed seropositive time from Table 1, which is $\delta = 1.15$. It is clear that the actual time delay must be somewhat less than 1.15 months, and our estimate of $\delta = 1$ seems reasonable.

Our estimate of the mean AIDS incubation period of 9.8 years is consistent with estimates obtained by others using different statistical methods and data sets (see the discussion in Longini et al. 1989). Because 75% of the observations used to estimate the distribution of the AIDS incubation period were right-censored for the development of AIDS, our estimates of the mean and median AIDS incubation periods are highly distribution dependent. These estimates are extrapolations based on limited data and the selected model. Another possible approach to data analysis would be to use a semi-Markov model (Lagakos et al. 1978). This approach relies on nonparametric estimation of the waiting-time distribution in each stage. Unfortunately, the interval-censoring in our data is too severe for us to employ this approach. Nonetheless, we believe that our analysis provides the most efficient use of the available data.

Brookmeyer et al. (1987) have identified several sources of bias that can arise in the analysis of cohort data of HIV infected persons. The estimate of the AIDS incubation period can be affected by length-biased sampling if persons were selected because they developed AIDS. Such a bias results in an underestimate of the mean and median AIDS incubation period. Our data are not subject to this source of bias because persons in our samples were selected only because they were known to be infected. In addition, Brookmeyer et al. (1987) have described other forms of bias that arise in prevalent HIV cohorts (i.e., cohorts with some or all of the persons being seropositive upon entry into the cohort) if the hazard function of the AIDS incubation period distribution is time dependent. Since the hazard function of the general gamma distribution that we employ is monotonically increasing, there is potential for such biasing. However, this problem is minimized in our analysis because the staged Markov model that we use partitions the AIDS incubation period into three stages, each with a constant hazard function.

A final caveat with respect to our estimate of the AIDS incubation period concerns how the data were combined. The waiting-time distribution for stage 1 was estimated largely from persons with nonsexual sources of infection (see Table 1), while the distributions for stages 2 and 3 were estimated from persons who probably were sexually infected. Thus, we make the assumption that the waiting-time-distribution for stage 1 does not vary with the source of infection.

Our estimates of the stage-specific infectious transmission rates appear to be the first such estimates made. Anderson and May (1988) review 23 published reports where the probability of transmission per sexual partnership was estimated. None of these reports considered stage-specific infection rates and the general trend was to calculate the probability of transmission per partnership rather than per sexual contact. Transmission probabilities that are calculated in the former fashion are difficult to compare since the duration of partnerships and rate of sexual contact per partnership may vary considerably. For male-to-female transmission (16 reports), the calculated probability ranged from 0.03 to 0.73 per sexual partnership. For female-to-male transmission (5 reports) it ranged from 0.08 to 0.71, while for male-to-male (2 reports) it varied from 0.10 to 0.60. The above reports included that of Fischl et al. (1987), which involved both male-to-female and female-to-male transmission, although Fischl et al. report no significant difference in the probability of infection by sex of the index case. As pointed out in Section 4, the overall probability of infection per partnership was 0.58 for that study.

Recently, Wiley et al. (1989) estimated the average probability of infection per male-to-female sexual contact (unprotected penile-vaginal intercourse) to be 0.001 from two cohorts of heterosexual partners where the man was the index infected person (see Padian et al. 1987 and Peterman et al. 1988). Their mean estimate is equal to ours when we assume that the transmission rate is a constant across the stages of infection (see Table 4). However, they note that there is considerable heterogeneity in the per-contact infection transmission probability, and they speculate that this is due to considerable variation in infectiousness and/or susceptibility. DeGruttola et al. (1989) have estimated the transmission probability to be in the range of 0.005 to 0.010 per unprotected receptive anal contact for homosexually active men. They also report substantial heterogeneity in the transmission probability. Our results strongly support the hypothesis that the infection transmission rate exhibits considerable variation over the HIV infectious period. This is evident since the model with a constant transmission rate was rejected when compared to one with variation.

We found that the estimated probability of infection per sexual contact is eight times as high with an infected person with AIDS (stage 4) as with a person with pre-AIDS symptoms. Thus, it appears that persons with AIDS are much more infectious than those with pre-AIDS symptoms. This finding is supported by the study of Osmond et al. (1988) where 117 homosexual men, who were regular sexual partners of men with AIDS, were tested for HIV antibody. They found that receptive anal intercourse was a strong risk factor for infection for those men who had such contact beyond the date of AIDS diagnosis in the index case, but not if receptive anal intercourse ceased before the date of AIDS diagnosis.

There are several important points that need to be addressed when interpreting the estimated transmission rates and probabilities in table 4. First, we used a constant rate of 11 sexual contacts per month to calculate the probability of infection per sexual contact, p_i, because Fischl et al. (1987) did not report the number of sexual contacts per couple per month. If such data had been available, they could have been included in (15) to provide a direct estimate of p_i.

Second, for those couples in which both persons were found to be seropositive at the time of AIDS diagnosis of the "index" case, it may not be clear who was infected by whom. In fact, the person labeled "exposed" may have infected the "index," or both could have been infected from outside of the relationship (see Longini et al. 1982). If the former is true, our estimates would not be affected since the two persons are indistinguishable in terms of risk factors, and they are exposed to one another for the same period of time. If the latter is true, then information on exposure outside of the relationship would have to be incorporated into the analysis to provide accurate estimates of the parameters (see Longini et al. 1982; Longini et al. 1988; and Haber et al. 1988).

Third, nine of the index cases were IV drug users. If their partners were also IV drug users, then they may have shared needles, and there would be an additional route of transmission among these couples. This would lead to an additional risk of transmission, which should be modeled and included in the analysis.

Fourth, all the index cases under study had AIDS. This could be a source of bias since our estimates of the infectious contact rates for the pre-AIDS stages are conditioned on exposure to persons who developed AIDS in a relatively short period of time. Such estimates could be different for exposure to persons who may take a very long period of time to develop AIDS.

Fifth, our estimate of the infectious contact rate during stage 2 turned out to be 0. This is because the parameter β_2 hit the lower bound of 0 at the maximized value of the likelihood function. This is a particular result from the data and the mean length of the AIDS incubation period that we used. When we used a mean AIDS incubation period of shorter length, the estimate for β_2 was a very small number, but not 0. We feel that this result indicates that the risk of infection given exposure to an asymptomatic, antibody-positive person is low in general, but such a person could be quite infectious if the right cofactors were present.

Finally, we were unable to obtain any estimate for the infectious contact rate in stage 1, β_1. This is because of the retrospective nature of the data prior to AIDS diagnosis of the index case and the extremely short duration of stage 1 with respect to the rest of the AIDS incubation period. The parameter β_1 could be estimated from a study that followed couples prospectively from the time of early detection of infection (or at least seroconversion) of the index case. However, such a study would be difficult to perform.

The transmission model presented here (15-21) was used to examine the risk of transmission by stage of infection. The data of Fischl et al. (1987) contained risk factor information that could have been examined, such as the type of index case (e.g., IV drug user, bisexual), the use of barrier contraceptives, the presence of concomitant venereal infections, and the direction of sexual transmission (i.e., male-to-female or female-to-male); but numbers in each risk category were small. The effect of these risk factors on the infectious contact rates could be examined by formulating risk-specific rates. Longini et al. (1988) and Haber et al. (1988) have formulated such models for the transmission of viral diseases such as influenza. In the case of HIV, the infectious contact rate may be β_{ri}, which is the contact rate between a susceptible of risk category r with an infective who is in stage i of infection. Then the parameters could be estimated and the appropriate risk ratios examined. For example, let $r = 1$ if the susceptible has genital ulcers and $r = 0$ if not. Then the risk ratio $RR_i = \beta_{1i}/\beta_{0i}$ would measure the increased risk due to genital ulcers given exposure to an infected person in the i-th stage of infection. In addition, the index i could indicate additional categories for infectiousness such as use of condoms by infected males. Longini et al. (1988) have shown that risk ratios based on infectious contact rates provide a more accurate and less confounded measure of risk than do those based on infection attack rates. Such analyses should become feasible as more data become available.

Acknowledgements

This research was partially supported by contracts 200-07-0515 and 88060702 from the CDC and by NIH Grant 1-R01-AI22877.

References

Anderson, R.M. and R.M. May. (1988). Epidemiological parameters of HIV transmission. *Nature* London 333, 514-519.

Burke, D.S. and R.R. Redfield. (1988). Letter to the editor, *New England Med.* 318, 1202-1203.

Brookmeyer, R., M.H. Gail, and B.F. Polk. (1987). The prevalent cohort study and the acquired immunodeficiency syndrome. *Am. J. Epidemiol.* 126, 14-24.

Chiang, C.L. (1980). *An Introduction to Stochastic Processes and Their Applications*, 2nd ed. Krieger, New York.

DeGruttola, V., G.R. Seage, K.H. Mayer, and C.R. Horsburgh. (1989). Infectiousness of HIV between male homosexual partners, *J. Clin.*

Epidemiol. (In Print).
Elandt-Johnson, R.C. and N.L. Johnson. (1980). *Survival Models and Data Analysis.* Wiley, New York.
Fischl, M.A., G.M. Dickinson, G.B. Scott, N. Klimas, M.A. Fletcher, and W. Parks. (1987). Evaluation of heterosexual partners, children, and household contacts of adults with AIDS. *JAMA* 257, 640-644.
Goedert, J.J., M.E. Eyster, R.J. Biggar, and W.A. Blattner. (1987). Heterosexual transmission of human immunodeficiency virus: association with severe depletion of T-helper lymphocytes in men with hemophilia. *AIDS Res. Hum. Retrov.* 3, 355-361.
Haber, M., I.M. Longini and G.A. Cotsonis. (1988). Statistical analysis of infectious disease data. *Biometrics*, 44, 163-173.
Hethcote, H.W. (1988). Mathematical and computer models for the prediction of AIDS incidence: HIV prevalence and AIDS in San Francisco, Unpublished report to the CDC.
Hogg, R.V. and A.T. Craig. (1970). *Introduction to Mathematical Statistics*, 3rd ed. Macmillan, London.
Horsburgh, C.R., Y.O. Chin, J. Jason, S.D. Holmberg, I.M. Longini, C. Schable, K.H. Mayer, A.R. Lifson, G. Schochetman, J.W. Ward, G.W. Rutherford, G.R.Seage, and H.W. Jaffe. (1989). Defining the interval between human immunodeficiency virus infection and detection of antibody to the virus. Submitted, *Ann. Int. Med.*
Hyman, J.M. and E.A. Stanley. (1988). Using mathematical models to understand the AIDS epidemic. *Math. Biosci.* 90, 415-473.
Jacquez, J.A., C.D. Simon, J.S. Koopman, L. Sattenspiel, and T. Perry (1988). Modeling and analyzing HIV transmission: the effect of contact patterns. *Math. Biosci.* 92, 119-199.
Jaffe, H.W., W.W. Darrow, D.F. Echenberg, D.F., P.M. O'Malley, J.P. Getchell, V.S. Kalyanaraman, R.H. Byers, D.P. Drennan, E.H. Braff, J.W. Curran, and D.P. Francis. (1985). The acquired immunodeficiency syndrome in a cohort of homosexual men: a six-year follow-up study. *Ann. Int. Med.* 103, 210-214.
Johnson, N.L. and S. Kotz. (1970). *Continuous Univariate Distributions - 1.*Wiley, New York. Kalbfleisch, J.D. and R.L. Prentice. (1980). *The Statistical Analysis of Failure Time Data.* Wiley, New York.
Koopman, J.S., C. Simon, J. Jacquez, J. Joseph, L. Sattenspiel., and Park, T. (1988). Sexual partner selectiveness effects on homosexual HIV transmission dynamics. *J. AIDS* 1, 486-504.

Laga, M., H. Taeman, L. Bonneux, P. Cornet, G. Vercauterent, and P. Piot. (1988). Risk factors for HIV infection in heterosexual partners of HIV infected Africans and Europeans. *IV Int. Conf. AIDS, Stockholm* (Abstr.) I, 260.

Lagakos, S.W., C.J. Summer, and M. Zelen. (1978). Semi-Markov models for partially censored data. *Biometrika* 65, 311-317.

Lange, J.M.A., D.A. Paul, H.G. Huisman, deWolf, F., Van Den Berg, H., Coutinho, R.A., Danner, S.A., Van Der Noordaa, J. and Goudsmit, J. (1986). Persistent HIV antigenaemia and decline of HIV core antibodies associated with transition to AIDS. *Brit. Med. J.* 293, 1459-1462.

Longini, I.M., W.S. Clark, R.H. Byers, G.F. Lemp, J.W. Ward, W.W. Darrow, and H.W. Hethcote. (1989). Statistical analysis of the stages of HIV infection using a Markov model. *Statist. Med.* 8, 831-843.

Longini, I.M., J.S. Koopman, M. Haber, and G.A. Cotsonis. (1988). Statistical inference on risk-specific household and community transmission parameters of infectious diseases. *Am. J. Epidemiol.* 128, 845-859.

Longini, I.M., J.S. Koopman, A.S. Monto, and J.P Fox. (1982). Estimating household and community transmission parameters for influenza. *Am J. Epidemiol.* 115, 736-751.

Nekwei, W., R.L. Colebunders, Y. Bahwe, I. Leburghe, H. Francis, and R. Ryder. (1988). Acute manifestations of HIV infection following blood transfusion. *IV Int. Conf. AIDS, Stockholm* (Abstr.) II, 350.

Osmond, D., P. Bacchetti, R.E. Chaisson, T. Kelly, R. Stempel, J. Carlson, and A.R. Moss. (1988). Time of exposure and risk of HIV infection in homosexual partners of men with AIDS. *Am. J. Pub. Health* 78, 944-948.

Padian, N., J. Wiley, and W. Winkelstein. (1987). Male-to-female transmission of human immunodeficiency virus (HIV): current results, infectivity estimates, and San Francisco population seroprevalence estimates. *III Int. Conf. AIDS, Stockholm* (Abstr.) THP. 3-48, 171.

Peterman, T.A., R.L. Stonebrunner, J.R. Allen, H.W. Jaffe, and J.W. Curran. (1988). Risk of human immunodediciency virus transmission for heterosexual adults with transfusion-associated infections. *JAMA* 259, 55-58.

Ralston, M. (1985). Derivative-free nonlinear regression, in *BMDP Stat. Software Manual*. U. Cal. Press, Berkeley, 302-329.

Seage, G.R., C.R. Horsburgh, A.M. Hardy, K.H. Mayer, M.A. Barry, J.E. Groopman, H.W. Jaffe, and G.A. Lemp (1989). Increased suppressor T cells in probable transmitters of human immunodeficiency virus infection, submitted. *Am. J. Pub. Health.*

Turnbull, B.W., (1976). The empirical distribution function with arbitrary grouped, censored, and truncated data. *J. Roy. Statist. Soc., Series B* 38, 290-295.

Ward, J.W., S.D. Holmberg, J.R. Allen, J.R., Cohn, D.O., Kritchley, S.E., Cleinman, S.H., Lenes, B.A., Ravenholt, O., Davis, J.R., Quinn, M.G. and Jaffe, H.W. (1988). Transmission of human deficiency virus (HIV) by blood transfusions screened as negative for HIV antibody. *New England Med.* 318, 473-478.

Wiley, J.A., S.J. Herschkorn, and N.S. Padian. (1989). Heterogeneity in the probability of HIV transmission per sexual contact: the case of male-to-female transmission in penile-vaginal intercourse. *Statist. Med.* 8, 93-102.

MODELING HETEROGENEITY IN SUSCEPTIBILITY AND INFECTIVITY FOR HIV INFECTION

N. Scott Cardell
Washington State University
Pullman, WA 99164

David E. Kanouse
The RAND Corporation
Santa Monica, CA 90406

Abstract

Models of the spread of human immunodeficiency virus (HIV) infection must deal with substantial heterogeneity in the populations at risk. The virus is spread by behaviors that are far from uniformly distributed in the population, and substantial variations in biological aspects of susceptibility and infectivity are also likely. How adequately a model represents this heterogeneity will substantially determine its accuracy and usefulness for capturing the dynamics of the epidemic, for making forecasts of future spread, and for answering questions of policy interest.

There are two main ways in which a model may handle heterogeneity: by partitioning the population into discrete risk groups that are in some respect homogeneous within group but heterogeneous between groups, and by introducing model parameters to capture the effects of heterogeneity in a group or in the population as a whole. This paper discusses the dynamics of heterogeneity in HIV spread and develops a theory of heterogeneity in susceptibility and infectivity within a population that allows a simple representation of key phenomena within an epidemic model. It is suggested that the effects of heterogeneity-related phenomena can be captured by letting two key parameters, the mean susceptibility over time of the uninfected and the mean infectivity of the infected, depend upon $\frac{X}{P}$, the proportion of the population that is uninfected. (The mean infectivity may also depend on the cumulative proportion of the population that is removed through death or other causes). Because $\frac{X}{P}$, as we define it, is monotonic over time, this approach is general, and it allows considerable flexibility in the choice of functional form to fit available data.

1. Introduction

Models of the spread of human immunodeficiency virus (HIV) infection must deal with substantial heterogeneity in the populations at risk. The virus is spread within and between populations that differ in both type and frequency of behaviors that are epidemiologically linked to HIV transmission, as well as in other ways that may be relevant to the goals underlying development of a model. How adequately a model represents this heterogeneity will substantially determine its accuracy and usefulness for capturing the dynamics of the epidemic, for making forecasts of future spread, and for answering questions of policy interest.

The heterogeneity dealt with in this paper concerns the extent of variation within a population in individuals' susceptibility to infection or infectivity to others. We define susceptibility as proportional to the probability per unit time that an uninfected individual will become infected, holding factors external to the individual constant. Susceptibility has both biological and behavioral components; that is, it will depend both on the nature and frequency of epidemiologically risky behaviors that the individual engages in and on biological resistance to becoming infected. This definition is broader than the usual definition, which is restricted to the biological component.[1] We define infectivity similarly, as proportional to the probability per unit time that an infected individual will infect another (uninfected) person, again holding factors external to the individual constant. Like susceptibility, infectivity has both biological and behavioral components.

Within a population, the extent of variation in susceptibility and infectivity will reflect the extent of variation in relevant biological and behavioral factors. If all individuals behave in the same way and all have the same biological propensity to infect or acquire infection, then individual susceptibility and infectivity at any given time will reflect only the individual's current status (infected or uninfected) and the population mean for individuals with that status. If behavioral or biological factors vary, however, that variation introduces selection dynamics that alter the course of an epidemic over time. Those dynamics should be taken into account in epidemiological modeling.

The effects of population heterogeneity on the spread of an infectious agent are greatest when modes of transmission are relatively inefficient, as is the case with HIV (Friedman and Klein, 1987; Wiley, 1987). In these circumstances, the effects of variability in the probability of transmission per exposure or in the frequency of exposure are much greater than when transmission is relatively efficient. Growth is expected to occur at a constant exponential rate in the early phases of an epidemic. As we shall show, however, heterogeneity may first substantially accelerate and then moderate the rate of growth that would occur in the absence of heterogeneity.

Although the HIV epidemic is in some ways quite complex, its essential features are those of a relatively simple class of epidemics that may be described by an SI model, in which a constant-sized population consists entirely of those susceptible and those infected; no one is immune and no one recovers (Hethcote, 1976). The early growth of such an epidemic within a homogeneous population is at a constant exponential rate, gradually slowing to half this initial rate when the proportion infected reaches 50 percent. Manifestly, the HIV epidemic has not followed this pattern but has instead exhibited a steady increase in the doubling time (Curran et al., 1988). The existence of biological or behavioral heterogeneity in the populations in which HIV is spreading is one possible explanation.

---

[1] We have adopted this broader definition of susceptibility because it offers distinctive advantages over the more usual definition. In particular, it allows unitary representation of the effects of sources of individual variation that are functionally equivalent. For instance, the effects of biological resistance may be difficult to distinguish from the effects of using condoms.

Because of the important role that heterogeneity may play in the dynamics of the HIV epidemic, an AIDS epidemiological model needs to account for its effects. A model may handle heterogeneity in either or both of two ways: by partitioning the population into discrete risk groups that are in some respect homogeneous within group but heterogeneous between groups (e.g., Jacquez et al., 1988; Sattenspiel and Simon, 1988), and/or by introducing model parameters to capture the effects of heterogeneity in a group or in the population as a whole. In Section 2 of this paper, we discuss the qualitative effects of within-group heterogeneity on the course of an epidemic. In Section 3, we develop a theory of heterogeneity in susceptibility and infectivity that allows a simple representation of the key phenomena associated with this heterogeneity in the spread of HIV. In Section 4, we illustrate the dynamics involved using a simple one-population simulation, and show how these dynamics may be represented in a model using an approach to parameterization adopted in our own deterministic simulation model of the spread of HIV infection in the United States (Cardell et al., 1987).

2. Effects of Heterogeneity

In the standard epidemiological model, all individuals are equally susceptible to infection and equally infectious once infected. If we allow for individual variation in susceptibility, the most susceptible individuals become infected first. As a result, the average susceptibility of those who remain uninfected declines over time and is greatest when no one is infected. Because the epidemic growth rate is a function of the average susceptibility of those who remain uninfected, variation in susceptibility results in slower growth for the same average susceptibility for the total population.

Individual variation in susceptibility can occur without individual variation in infectivity. If infectivity varies as well, the consequences depend on the relationship between infectivity and susceptibility. If infectivity varies independently of susceptibility, infectivity variation will have no effect on the epidemic, because there will be no reason for the most infectious to become infected first and therefore the mean infectivity of those who are infected at any given time will remain at the population average. If, however, both susceptibility and infectivity vary and are positively correlated (e.g., if both represent a tendency to engage in behaviors that are epidemiologically linked to HIV infection), then the most infectious, being more susceptible on average, will tend to become infected first. As a result, the mean infectivity of the infected will exceed the mean infectivity that the population would have if all its members were infected.

When susceptibility and infectivity are positively correlated, the mean infectivity of the infected will be greatest when the smallest fraction is infected. When this fraction is very small, the mean susceptibility of those uninfected will also be near its maximum value (the mean value for the total population). Therefore, introducing both susceptibility variation and a correlated infectivity variation will increase the rate at which the epidemic spreads in its earliest stages. As the epidemic progresses, however, both the mean susceptibility of the uninfected and the mean infectivity of the infected will decline, and the rate of spread will fall to a lower level than would prevail at the same level of infection if there were no variation. In fact, it can be shown that the growth rate will fall below the "no variation" rate before one half the population is infected.

Although our larger model (Cardell et al., 1987) includes many additional factors, our focus in this paper is on heterogeneity among individuals in susceptibility and infectivity. We do not deal with stages of HIV infection or with variation in infectivity over the course of the disease (Blythe and Anderson, 1988; Hyman and Stanley, 1988). We treat the population as constant in size, ignoring vital dynamics. We also ignore behavioral change over time and heterogeneity of other types than that considered here, such as in mixing.

Susceptibility when uninfected and infectivity when infected are constants associated with an individual. Since there is no recruitment, and we assume that no one recovers, we continue to include those removed through death in our definition of the population. An important consequence of this is that the proportion uninfected can only be monotonically nonincreasing. These assumptions can reasonably be applied to cohorts over time, but would require modification to apply to fixed age groups.

3. Accounting for Heterogeneity in Epidemiologic Models

Given that variations in susceptibility and infectivity can potentially have important effects, what can be done to deal with these effects in epidemiological models? In the discussion that follows, we will begin with the simplified one-population SI model but will extend the model to consider some of the particulars of the HIV epidemic and what heterogeneity entails in that context.

Consider a simplified case where we have only one population and include only subgroups for uninfected, infected, and dead from HIV-related causes. Further let the latency between infection and death be a fixed time period, τ. (For discussions of models in which the latency between infection and death is not fixed, see for example, Cardell et al., 1987 and Castillo-Chavez et al., 1989.) Let $X(t)$ denote the uninfected population, $Y(t)$ the infected and living population, and $Z(t)$ those dead of HIV-related causes. To allow for individual variation in susceptibility and infectivity, characterize each individual by what his susceptibility to infection is when uninfected and what his infectivity to others is when infected. Denote susceptibility by s and infectivity by h. Let $x(s,h,t,)$, $y(s,h,t)$, $z(s,h,t)$ denote the distribution of individuals over s and h at time t for the uninfected, infected and dead groups, respectively. Thus $X(t) = \int_0^\infty \int_0^\infty x(s,h,t)dsdh$, $Y(t) = \int_0^\infty \int_0^\infty y(s,h,t)dsdh$, and $Z(t) = \int_0^\infty \int_0^\infty z(s,h,t)dsdh$. Let $P = X(t) + Y(t) + Z(t)$, and $p(s,h) = x(s,h,t) + y(s,h,t) + z(s,h,t)$. (Note that $Z(t) = P - X(t-\tau)$, $Y(t) = X(t-\tau) - X(t)$). In this simplified model the only processes are infection and death. Because these processes move individuals between the above categories, P and $p(s,h)$ *do not depend on time*. Assuming random contact (or proportionate mixing; see Hethcote and Van Ark, 1987), we can write the probability per unit time (or hazard) that an infected individual characterized by s_1 and h_1 will infect an uninfected individual characterized by s_2 and h_2 as:

$$\alpha s_2 h_1.$$

That is, if person 2 is uninfected at time 0, the probability that infected person 1 will *not* have infected person 2 by time t is (ignoring all other sources of infection):

$$e^{-\alpha s_2 h_1 t}.$$

The constant α is chosen to allow the convenient normalizations

$$\bar{s} \equiv \frac{1}{P}\int_0^\infty \int_0^\infty s \cdot p(s,h) ds dh = 1, \quad \bar{h} \equiv \frac{1}{P}\int_0^\infty \int_0^\infty h \cdot p(s,h) ds dh = 1.$$

Note that the size of α depends on the units of time and that α may exceed one.

We assume that the population groups are large enough to treat without loss of generality all functions as continuous, and hence we can use deterministic equations. (In practice, this means we can only apply these equations after a significant number of people are infected.)

$$\frac{dx(s,h,t)}{dt} = -\alpha s \left(\int_0^\infty \int_0^\infty r \cdot y(q,r,t) dq dr \right) x(s,h,t) \tag{1}$$

Given as initial conditions x, y, z specified for $t \in [\tau, 0]$.

$$\begin{aligned} z(s,h,t) &= y(s,h,t-\tau) + z(s,h,t-\tau) \\ &= p(s,h) - x(s,h,t-\tau) \end{aligned} \tag{2}$$

$$\begin{aligned} y(s,h,t) &= p(s,h) - x(s,h,t) - z(s,h,t) \\ &= x(s,h,t-\tau) - x(s,h,t). \end{aligned} \tag{3}$$

Let $b(t) = \alpha \int_0^t \left(\int_0^\infty \int_0^\infty r \cdot y(q,r,u) dq dr \right) du$; then the solution to equation 1 above is $x(s,h,t) = x(s,h,0)e^{-b(t)\cdot s}$. If we assume that the same infection process held before $t=0$, $x(s,h,0) = p(s,h)e^{-ks}$. Let $a(t) = b(t) + k$; then:

$$x(s,h,t) = p(s,h)e^{-a(t)\cdot s}, \tag{4}$$

substituting into equation (2)

$$\begin{aligned} z(s,h,t) &= p(s,h) - p(s,h)e^{-a(t-\tau)\cdot s} \\ &= p(s,h) \cdot \left(1 - e^{-a(t-\tau)\cdot s}\right), \end{aligned} \tag{5}$$

substituting into equation (3)

$$\begin{aligned} y(s,h,t) &= p(s,h) - p(s,h)e^{-a(t)\cdot s} - p(s,h) + p(s,h)e^{-a(t-\tau)\cdot s} \\ &= p(s,h) \cdot \left(e^{-a(t-\tau)s} - e^{-a(t)s}\right) \end{aligned} \tag{6}$$

$$X(t) = \int_0^\infty \int_0^\infty x(s,h,t) ds dh. \tag{7}$$

The number of new infections per unit time is:

$$\begin{aligned}\frac{dX(t)}{dt} &= \int_0^\infty \int_0^\infty \frac{dx(s,h,t)}{dt} dsdh \\ &= \int_0^\infty \int_0^\infty -\left(\alpha s x(s,h,t) \int_0^\infty \int_0^\infty r \cdot y(q,r,t) dqdr\right) dsdh \\ &= -\alpha \left(\int_0^\infty \int_0^\infty sx(s,h,t)dsdh\right) \cdot \left(\int_0^\infty \int_0^\infty h \cdot y(s,h,t)dsdh\right). \end{aligned} \tag{8}$$

Let $S(t)$ denote the mean susceptibility of the uninfected and $I(t)$ the mean infectivity of the infected; then

$$S(t) = \frac{\int_0^\infty \int_0^\infty sx(s,h,t)dsdh}{\int_0^\infty \int_0^\infty x(s,h,t)dsdh} = \frac{\int_0^\infty \int_0^\infty sx(s,h,t)dsdh}{X(t)} \tag{9}$$

and similarly

$$I(t) = \frac{\int_0^\infty \int_0^\infty h \cdot y(s,h,t)dsdh}{Y(t)}; \tag{10}$$

thus, multiplying equation (9) by $X(t)$ and equation (10) by $Y(t)$ and substituting the results into equation (8),

$$\frac{dX(t)}{dt} = -\alpha X(t)S(t)Y(t)I(t). \tag{11}$$

The specific formulae used from here depend on the specific choice assumed for $p(s,h)$. The ratio $\frac{p(s,h)}{P}$ is the bivariate probability density function for s and h in the population. Let $f(s,h) = \frac{p(s,h)}{P}$. Obviously, if s and h are independently distributed, $I(t)$ will be a constant. However, remember that s and h include individual variation in behavior. Epidemiological evidence on the infectivity of different behaviors suggests that, whereas some behaviors may be more likely to transmit the HIV virus in one direction than the reverse (for example, anal intercourse from the insertive to the receptive partner), almost all risky behaviors can transmit in either direction. Further, behavioral data suggest wide variation in the frequency of risky behaviors overall (Turner, Miller, and Moses, 1989). Thus, we can expect substantial variation in s, and h positively correlated with s.

Let us first consider a particularly simple case: let s and h be identical and exponentially distributed, so that (under our normalization) $f(s,h) = f(s) = e^{-s}$ and $h \equiv s$. (Alternatively, we could write $f(s,h) = \delta(h-s)e^{-s}$ where δ is the Dirac delta function.) Thus we have

$$S(t) = \frac{\int_0^\infty s e^{-\left(a(t)+1\right)s} ds}{\int_0^\infty e^{-\left(a(t)+1\right)s} ds} = \frac{\left(\frac{1}{a(t)+1}\right)^2}{\frac{1}{a(t)+1}} \tag{12}$$

$$= \frac{1}{a(t)+1} \equiv \frac{X(t)}{P}, \tag{13}$$

the proportion uninfected.

$$I(t) = \frac{\int_0^\infty h\left(e^{-\left(a(t-\tau)+1\right)h} - e^{-\left(a(t)+1\right)h}\right)dh}{\int_0^\infty \left(e^{-\left(a(t-\tau)+1\right)h} - e^{-\left(a(t)+1\right)h}\right)dh}$$

$$= \frac{\left(\frac{1}{a(t-\tau)+1}\right)^2 - \left(\frac{1}{a(t)+1}\right)^2}{\frac{1}{a(t+\tau)+1} - \frac{1}{a(t)+1}}$$

$$= \frac{1}{a(t-\tau)+1} + \frac{1}{a(t)+1}$$

$$\equiv \frac{Y(t)}{P} + 2\frac{X(t)}{P} = 1 + \frac{X(t)}{P} - \frac{Z(t)}{P}. \tag{14}$$

Note that early in the epidemic (i.e., $\frac{X(t)}{P} \approx 1$) $S(t)$ is approximately the population average ($\bar{s} \equiv 1$), while $I(t)$ is approximately twice the population average ($I(t) \approx 2 \equiv 2\bar{h}$); both $S(t)$ and $I(t)$ decline over the course of the epidemic. Obviously, the exponential distribution is a particularly simple case. One convenient generalization is the Γ distribution. The shape parameter can be chosen to give varying degrees of concentration of the distribution in the "low risk" end while maintaining a significant fraction at very high risk. (Exponential is Γ with shape parameter 1).

Let s be Γ with shape parameter c normalized to a mean of 1, i.e.,

$$f(s) = \frac{c^c s^{c-1} e^{-cs}}{\Gamma(c)}.$$

Then,

$$S(t) = \frac{\int_0^\infty c^c s^c e^{-\left(c+a(t)\right)s} ds}{\int_0^\infty c^c s^{c-1} e^{-\left(c+a(t)\right)s} ds}$$

$$= \frac{\left(\frac{c}{c+a(t)}\right)^{c+1} \cdot \Gamma(c)}{\left(\frac{c}{c+a(t)}\right)^{c} \cdot \Gamma(c)} = \frac{c}{c+a(t)}, \tag{15}$$

while

$$\frac{X(t)}{P} = \left(\frac{c}{c+a(t)}\right)^c, \tag{16}$$

hence

$$S(t) = \left(\frac{X(t)}{P}\right)^{1/c}. \tag{17}$$

If c is taken less than one, the bulk of the population has susceptibility less than the (arithmetic) average. We use $c = \frac{1}{3}$ for the base case in our elaborated model (Cardell et al., 1987). If we kept $h \equiv s$ we would have

$$I(t) = \left(1 + \frac{X(t)}{P} - \frac{Z(t)}{P}\right)\left(\left(1 - \frac{Z(t)}{P}\right)^2 + \left(\frac{X(t)}{P}\right)^2\right). \tag{18}$$

However, $h \equiv s$ is not plausible, particularly when s is assumed to have a wide variation. Let h now denote the common factors that influence both susceptibility and infectivity. We will show that under this altered definition, h plays exactly the same role in our simplified model as under the definition just considered. Susceptibility and infectivity depend primarily on frequencies of risky behaviors. Since transmission can only occur in the presence of risky behaviors, we can conclude that susceptibility and infectivity should vary through some limited range conditional on h. (For instance, the probability per month of an individual becoming infected, or if infected, infecting someone else, can never exceed his probability of engaging in at least one risky behavior). We reflect this conclusion in the structure of equations. Let

$$s = h \cdot u$$
$$i = h \cdot v$$

where

h, u, v are independent random variables,
$h, u, v \geq 0$,
u, v with finite ranges,
i is individual infectivity (temporarily).

Let $f(h)$, $f(u)$ and $f(\nu)$ be the respective marginal distribution functions. Without loss of generality, we normalize h, u, ν so:

$$E(h) = E(u) = E(\nu) = 1.$$

Similarly, as before,

$$S(t) = \frac{\int_0^\infty \int_0^\infty h \cdot u f(h) f(u) e^{-a(t)h \cdot u} dh du}{\frac{X(t)}{P}} \tag{19}$$

$$\left(\frac{Y(t)}{P}\right) \cdot I(t) = \int_0^\infty \int_0^\infty \int_0^\infty h\nu f(h) f(u) f(\nu) \left(e^{-a(t-\tau)hu} - e^{-a(t)hu}\right) dh du d\nu$$

$$= \int_0^\infty \nu f(\nu) d\nu \int_0^\infty \int_0^\infty h f(h) f(u) (e^{-a(t-\tau)hu} - e^{-a(t)hu}) dh du \tag{20}$$

but

$$\int_0^\infty \nu f(\nu) d\nu \equiv E(\nu) \equiv 1.$$

Thus,

$$I(t) = \frac{\int_0^\infty \int_0^\infty hf(h)f(u)(e^{-a(t-\tau)hu} - e^{-a(t)hu})dhdu}{\left(\frac{Y(t)}{P}\right)} \tag{21}$$

$$\frac{X(t)}{P} = \int_0^\infty \int_0^\infty f(u)f(h)e^{-a(t)hu}dhdu \tag{22}$$

$$\frac{Z(t)}{P} = 1 - \int_0^\infty \int_0^\infty f(u)f(h)e^{-a(t-\tau)hu}dhdu \tag{23}$$

$$\frac{Y(t)}{P} = 1 - \frac{X(t)}{P} - \frac{Z(t)}{P}. \tag{24}$$

Note that the ν and functions of ν drop out of all the final computations. That is, random variations in infectivity that are unrelated to susceptibility have no effect on model results. Thus, we can ignore ν, take $i \equiv h$, and consider h to be individual infectivity as before.

Before proceeding, let us consider a simple choice for $f(u)$ and $f(h)$. Let h be gamma with shape parameter 2 and u be uniform $[0, 2]$; then

$$f(h) = 4he^{-2h}$$

$$f(u) = \begin{cases} \frac{1}{2} & 0 \le u \le 2 \\ 0 & u > 2 \end{cases}$$

$$\begin{aligned} \frac{X(t)}{P} &= \int_0^2 \int_0^\infty \left(\frac{1}{2}\right) 4he^{-2h}e^{-a(t)hu}dhdu = \int_0^\infty 2he^{-2h}\frac{1}{a(t)h}\left(1 - e^{-a(t)h2}\right)dh \\ &= \frac{2}{a(t)}\int_0^\infty \left(e^{-2h} - e^{-2h\left(1+a(t)\right)}\right)dh \\ &= \frac{2}{a(t)} \cdot \left(\frac{1}{2} - \frac{1}{2(1+a(t))}\right) = \frac{1}{1+a(t)}, \end{aligned} \tag{25}$$

and

$$\begin{aligned} \frac{X(t)}{P}S(t) &= \int_0^\infty \int_0^\infty hu \cdot 2he^{-2h}e^{-a(t)hu}dudh \\ &= \int_0^\infty 2h^2e^{-2h}\left(\frac{1}{a(t)^2h^2} - \frac{e^{-a(t)h\cdot 2}}{a(t)^2h^2} - \frac{2e^{-a(t)h\cdot 2}}{a(t)h}\right)dh \\ &= \frac{1}{a(t)^2} - \frac{1}{a(t)^2} \cdot \frac{1}{1+a(t)} - \frac{1}{a(t)}\frac{1}{\left(1+a(t)\right)^2} \\ &= \frac{1}{\left(1+a(t)\right)^2}. \end{aligned} \tag{26}$$

Thus[2]

$$\frac{X(t)}{P} = \frac{1}{1+a(t)}$$

$$S(t) = \frac{1}{1+a(t)} = \frac{X(t)}{P}. \tag{27}$$

$$\frac{Y(t)}{P} = \frac{1}{1+a(t-\tau)} - \frac{1}{1+a(t)} \tag{28}$$

$$\begin{aligned}
\frac{Y(t)}{P} I(t) &= \int_0^\infty \int_0^2 h \cdot 2he^{-2h} \left(e^{-a(t-\tau)hu} - e^{-a(t)hu} \right) du dh \\
&= \int_0^\infty 2h^2 e^{-2h} \Big(\frac{1}{a(t-\tau)h} (1 - e^{-a(t-\tau)h \cdot 2}) - \frac{1}{a(t)h} (1 - e^{-a(t)h \cdot 2} \Big) dh \\
&= \int_0^\infty 2h \Big(\frac{1}{a(t-\tau)} e^{-2h} - \frac{1}{a(t-\tau)} e^{-2\left(1+a(t-\tau)\right)h} \\
&\quad - \frac{1}{a(t)} e^{-2h} + \frac{1}{a(t)} e^{-2\left(1+a(t)\right)h} \Big) dh \\
&= \frac{1}{2} \frac{1}{a(t-\tau)} - \frac{1}{2} \frac{1}{a(t-\tau)} \frac{1}{\left(1+a(t-\tau)\right)^2} - \frac{1}{2} \frac{1}{a(t)} + \frac{1}{2} \frac{1}{a(t)} \frac{1}{\left(1+a(t)\right)^2} \\
&= \frac{1 + \frac{a(t-\tau)}{2}}{\left(1+a(t-\tau)\right)^2} - \frac{1 + \frac{a(t)}{2}}{\left(1+a(t)\right)^2} \\
&= \frac{1}{2} \left(\frac{1}{1+a(t-\tau)} - \frac{1}{1+a(t)} + \frac{1}{\left(1+a(t-\tau)\right)^2} - \frac{1}{\left(1+a(t)\right)^2} \right) \qquad (29) \\
\Longrightarrow I(t) &= \frac{1}{2} + \frac{1}{2} \left(\frac{1}{1+a(t-\tau)} + \frac{1}{1+a(t)} \right) \\
&= 1 + \frac{1}{2} \left(\frac{X(t)}{P} - \frac{Z(t)}{P} \right). \qquad (30)
\end{aligned}$$

Note that by comparison to the case where s is exponential (as it is here) and $h \equiv s$, the selection effect on $I(t)$ has been halved: that is, the effect of the fact that the most susceptible tend to become infected first on the average infectivity of the infected is one half of the earlier result.

[2]It is no coincidence that these results are the same as for the case where s is exponentially distributed. $f(h)$ and $f(u)$ are convenient in part because they result in an exponentially distributed s.

We have normalized h and u so that

$$1 \equiv \int_0^\infty \int_0^\infty f(h)f(u)hu\ dhdu$$

$$= \int_0^\infty \int_0^\infty \frac{x(h,u,t)}{P} hu\ dhdu + \int_0^\infty \int_0^\infty \frac{y(h,u,t)}{P} hu\ dhdu$$

$$+ \int_0^\infty \int_0^\infty \frac{z(h,u,t)}{P} hu\ dhdu$$

and

$$1 \equiv \int_0^\infty \int_0^\infty f(h)f(u)h \cdot dhdu$$

$$= \int_0^\infty \int_0^\infty \frac{x(h,u,t)}{P} h \cdot dhdu + \int_0^\infty \int_0^\infty \frac{y(h,u,t)}{P} h \cdot dhdu$$

$$+ \int_0^\infty \int_0^\infty \frac{z(h,u,t)}{P} h \cdot dhdu.$$

For the following discussion it is convenient to think of susceptibility and infectivity as aggregate quantities. Thus, the aggregate susceptibility of the uninfected population is $S(t)X(t)$. Let $Q(t)$ be the proportion of the initial aggregate susceptibility that remains in the uninfected population, then:

$$Q(t) = \frac{1}{P} X(t)S(t) = \int_0^\infty \int_0^\infty h \cdot u \cdot f(h)f(u)e^{-a(t)hu} dhdu. \tag{31}$$

Similarly, recall that h characterizes an individual, so we can consider the aggregate latent infectivity of the uninfected population. Let $R(t)$ be the proportion of this aggregate latent infectivity that remains in the uninfected population, then:

$$R(t) = \int_0^\infty \int_0^\infty hf(h)f(u)e^{-a(t)hu} dhdu. \tag{32}$$

We can now write:

$$S(t) = \frac{Q(t)}{\left(\frac{X(t)}{P}\right)} \tag{33}$$

$$I(t) = \frac{R(t-\tau) - R(t)}{\frac{X(t-\tau)}{P} - \frac{X(t)}{P}}. \tag{34}$$

In order to allow generalizations to a multiple-population model and to allow for convenient computer implementation, it is desirable to limit ourselves to functional form choices that allow Q and R to be solved for as simple functions of $\frac{X}{P}$. For the base case in our elaborated model (Cardell et al., 1987), as in the simplified simulation presented ahead, $Q(t) = \left(\frac{X(t)}{P}\right)^4$ and $R(t) = \left(\frac{X(t)}{P}\right)^2$. Note that $R(t)$ declines more slowly than $Q(t)$ over the course of the epidemic. This is a natural consequence of the fact that the infection process directly selects out the most susceptible, but only indirectly selects out the most infectious (through the relationship between infectivity and susceptibility). We now demonstrate that $R(t)$ must be between $\frac{X(t)}{P}$ and $Q(t)$. That is, $Q(t) \leq R(t) \leq \frac{X(t)}{P}$. For simplicity, assume the moments of the h distribution are all finite.

Let
$$B(u,t) = \int_0^\infty hf(h)e^{-a(t)hu}dh. \tag{35}$$

Then
$$R(t) = \int_0^\infty f(u)B(u,t)du, \tag{36}$$

and
$$Q(t) = \int_0^\infty uf(u)B(u,t)du \tag{37}$$

$$\frac{\partial B(u,t)}{\partial u} = -\int_0^\infty a(t)h^2 f(h)e^{-a(t)hu}dh < 0. \tag{38}$$

For all $u > 0$, all t, all $B(u,t) > 0$, and all $f(u) > 0$ then $u \leq 1$ implies $uf(u) \leq f(u)$, and $u \geq 1$ implies $uf(u) \geq f(u)$. Recall

$$\int_0^\infty f(u)du \equiv 1 \equiv \int_0^\infty uf(u)du$$
$$\Longrightarrow \int_0^1 (1-u)f(u)du = \int_1^\infty (u-1)f(u)du \tag{39}$$

$$R(t) = \int_0^1 (1-u)f(u)B(u,t)du + \int_0^1 uf(u)B(u,t)du + \int_1^\infty f(u)B(u,t)du \tag{40}$$

$$Q(t) = \int_1^\infty (u-1)f(u)B(u,t)du + \int_0^1 uf(u)B(u,t)du + \int_1^\infty f(u)B(u,t)du \tag{41}$$

$$\begin{aligned} R(t) &\geq \left(\int_0^1 (1-u)f(u)du\right) \cdot B(1,t) + \int_0^\infty \min\left(f(u), uf(u)\right)B(u,t)du \\ &= \left(\int_1^\infty (u-1)f(u)du\right) \cdot B(1,t) + \int_0^\infty \min\left(f(u), uf(u)\right)B(u,t)du \qquad (42) \\ &\geq Q(t), \end{aligned}$$

since for $0 \leq u \leq 1$, it follows that $(1-u) \geq 0$ and $B(u,t) \geq B(1,t)$ while for $u \geq 1$, it follows that $(u-1) \geq 0$ and $B(u,t) \leq B(1,t)$. Thus $R(t) \geq Q(t)$ and since $\frac{\partial B(u,t)}{\partial u} < 0$, for any nondegenerate distribution of u (that is, $\int_0^{1-e} f(u)du > 0$, or equivalently, $\int_{1+e}^\infty f(u)du > 0$, some $e > 0$), $R(t) > Q(t)$.

Similar to the above argument, let

$$B(h,t) = \int_0^\infty f(u)e^{-a(t)hu}du. \tag{43}$$

Then

$$\frac{\partial B(h,t)}{\partial h} = -\int_0^\infty a(t)uf(u)e^{-a(t)hu}du < 0, \tag{44}$$

$$\frac{X(t)}{P} = \int_0^\infty f(h)B(h,t)dh, \tag{45}$$

$$R(t) = \int_0^\infty hf(h)B(h,t)dh. \tag{46}$$

Recall $\int_0^\infty f(h)dh \equiv 1 \equiv \int_0^\infty hf(h)dh$. Thus

$$\begin{aligned}\frac{X(t)}{P} &= \int_0^1 (1-h)f(h)B(h,t)dh + \int_0^\infty \min\big(f(h), hf(h)\big)B(h,t)dh \\ &\geq \left(\int_0^1 (1-h)f(h)dh\right)\cdot B(1,t) + \int_0^\infty \min\big(f(h), hf(h)\big)B(h,t)dh \\ &= \left(\int_1^\infty (h-1)f(h)dh\right)\cdot B(1,t) + \int_0^\infty \min\big(f(h), hf(h)\big)B(h,t)dt \\ &\geq R(t),\end{aligned} \tag{47}$$

thus $\frac{X(t)}{P} \geq R(t)$ and for $f(h)$ nondegenerate $\frac{X(t)}{P} > R(t)$.

Note that the above gives us four cases:

1) No susceptibility variation (h and u degenerate) $\frac{X(t)}{P} \equiv R(t) \equiv Q(t)$, $S(t) \equiv I(t) \equiv 1$.
2) Susceptibility varies and is identical to infectivity (h nondegenerate, u degenerate) $\frac{X(t)}{P} > R(t) \equiv Q(t)$.
3) Susceptibility variation only (h degenerate, u nondegenerate) $\frac{X(t)}{P} \equiv R(t) > Q(t)$, $I(t) \equiv 1$.
4) Susceptibility and infectivity vary and are related but not identical (h and u nondegenerate, $\frac{X(t)}{P} > R(t) > Q(t)$.

Obviously, the one-population model above is overly simplified. However, some generalizations are direct. Assume that there are J interacting groups, and that individuals in group j interact with individuals in group k for a proportion of their total activity θ_{jk} $\left(\sum_{k=1}^{J} \theta_{jk} \equiv 1\right)$. Then, equation 11 generalizes directly to:

$$\frac{dX(t)}{dt} = -\alpha_j X_j(t)S_j(t)\cdot\sum_k \theta_{jk}Y_k(t)I_k(t), \tag{48}$$

where S and I can be computed from Q, R and X above. This is basically the form used in the RAND HIV model (Cardell et al., 1987). If HIV-transmitting behavior is treated as symmetric, then it is necessary to impose constraints to ensure that the total amount of intergroup activity is the same for each group in the interacting pair jk (Blythe and Castillo-Chavez, 1989; Hethcote and Yorke, 1984; Nold, 1980).

In the epidemic of HIV infection, it is clear that susceptibility and infectivity vary considerably among individuals within identifiable groups (Padian et al., 1987). These variations certainly have behavioral components, which are positively correlated, resulting in a positive correlation between susceptibility and infectivity. There may also be a biological component (Wiley, Herschkorn, and Padian, 1989). The consequences of heterogeneity are that the most susceptible tend to become infected first; the mean susceptibility of the uninfected declines over time; the mean infectivity of those first infected exceeds the mean infectivity of the population that would occur if all were infected; and the mean infectivity of the infected declines over time. These consequences in turn result in an epidemic curve that initially (i.e., when the proportion infected is small) grows faster than the corresponding logistic curve (i.e., the epidemic curve when there is no variation in susceptibility or infectivity), and that later grows more slowly than the corresponding logistic curve.

We have shown that the simple theory developed above yields a practical and plausible representation of the effects of heterogeneity in epidemic models. This representation is an appropriate choice in a variety of situations. For instance, if the interaction between individuals of different susceptibility/infectivity is not random, the interpretation of $S(t)$ and $I(t)$ is more complex, but the same basic phenomena hold, and one can apply formulae 11, 33 and 34 with Q and R chosen as appropriate functions of $\frac{X(t)}{P}$. To apply the above technique the modeler simply chooses appropriate functions $R(t) = f_1\left(\frac{X(t)}{P}\right)$ and $Q(t) = f_2\left(\frac{X(t)}{P}\right)$ such that $\frac{X(t)}{P} > R(t) > Q(t)$. These choices are then used in formulae 33 and 34, and the results used in formulae 11 or 48. The choice $R(t) = \left(\frac{X(t)}{P}\right)^2$ and $Q(t) = \left(\frac{X(t)}{P}\right)^4$ has worked well in the RAND HIV model. We expect that this or a similar choice would work well in other diseases, including conventional STDs, where the behavior that makes one susceptible varies substantially at the individual level.

4. A One-Population Simulation

These dynamics and their consequences can be readily seen in the results of a simulation that introduces heterogeneity into a simple one-population SI model. In this simulation, the starting condition is a 1% prevalence of infection and a value of α that leads to a 23% growth rate for the no-variation case in the first month. Figure 1 shows the cumulative proportion infected at various points over an eight-year period for populations with differing amounts of variation in susceptibility and infectivity. The first column sketches the epidemic growth curve in a population that is homogeneous in susceptibility and infectivity; in this case, the high growth rate results in nearly universal infection in about three years. The second column shows the consequences of introducing variation in susceptibility. (The parameterization chosen for this case is the one used in the "base case" of our epidemiological model, and is described more fully below). In this case, the epidemic grows much more slowly than in the homogeneous case, so that after eight years nearly a third of the population remains uninfected.

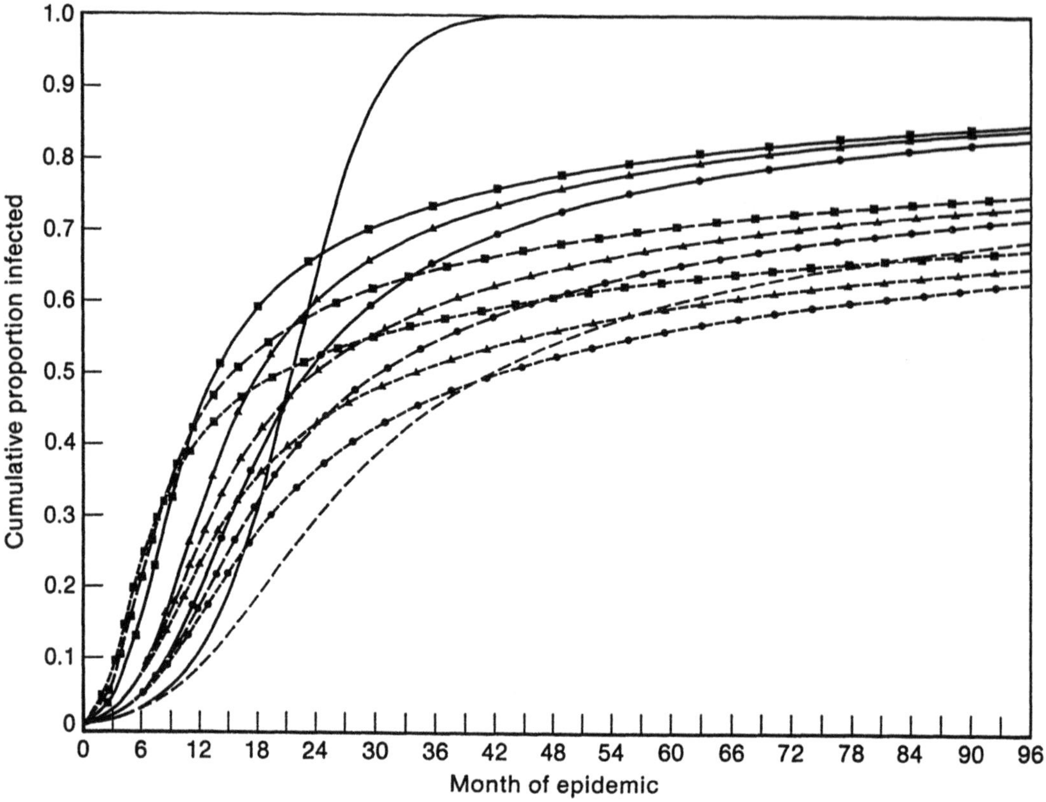

NN = no infectivity or susceptibility variation
NM = no infectivity variation, medium susceptibility variation
LL = low infectivity variation, low susceptibility variation
LM = low infectivity variation, medium susceptibility variation
LH = low infectivity variation, high susceptibility variation
ML = medium infectivity variation, low susceptibility variation
MM = medium infectivity variation, medium susceptibility variation
MH = medium infectivity variation, high susceptibility variation
HL = high infectivity variation, low susceptibility variation
HM = high infectivity variation, medium susceptibility variation
HH = high infectivity variation, high susceptibility variation

NOTE: Low, medium and high susceptibility variation are identified respectively as mean relative susceptibility of the uninfected equals the square, cube or fourth power of the proportion uninfected. Low and medium infectivity variation are defined respectively as mean relative infectivity of the infected equals one plus one half the proportion uninfected or one plus the proportion uninfected. High infectivity variation is defined as infectivity perfectly correlated with susceptibility.

Figure 1
Effects of Variation in Infectivity and Susceptibility
in a Single High Growth Rate Population

The rightmost three columns at the top of Figure 1 show epidemic growth scenarios when both susceptibility and infectivity are allowed to vary (and are positively correlated). The effects of a low level of variation in infectivity are shown for three different levels of variation in susceptibility. Note that the growth rates in the first 12 to 18 months are higher than when there is no variation. These initially higher growth rates soon moderate, however, so that by 24 months, the epidemic is growing more slowly than it would in the absence of variation. Note also that the effect of introducing infectivity variation along with a given level of variation in susceptibility is to increase the epidemic growth rate. The columns at the bottom of the table provide similar results in cases of "medium" or "high" variation in infectivity. The "high" infectivity variation cases are especially interesting, because in these cases infectivity is defined as perfectly correlated with susceptibility. The effect of their variation is first to increase and then to moderate the epidemic growth rate relative to the case of no variation.

One way of gauging how important heterogeneity may be in modeling the spread of HIV infection is to assess how much difference alternative assumptions about heterogeneity make in the range of future projections that are consistent with a particular observed history. As a simple illustration of this, Figure 2 shows the results of a simulation identical to that presented in Figure 1, except that all cases are initialized to have the same growth rate assumed in the "no variation" case in Figure 1 (23% in the first month). Note that infectivity variation now reduces the rate of epidemic growth for all periods after the initial "observed history". The reason is that variation in infectivity results in a decline over time in the mean infectivity of the infected, and we have now adjusted to start at the same level.

The main point of Figure 2, of course, is that variations in infectivity and susceptibility make a substantial difference in the subsequent epidemic growth rate, even after one has taken the initial growth rate into account. A pragmatic implication is that the absence of good information about the extent of population heterogeneity can be an important source of uncertainty in fitting a model to an observed epidemic growth curve. This will be especially true in the early stages of the epidemic, when there is little indication as to whether and how rapidly the growth rate will moderate as the mean levels of infectivity of the infected and susceptibility of the uninfected decline over time.

5. Discussion

Although our focus in this paper has been on parametric representation of heterogeneity within a single population, we noted at the outset that models may also deal with heterogeneity by partitioning the population into risk groups that differ in their behavior. Indeed, for addressing certain types of heterogeneity, partitioning is the preferred approach. Consider four ways in which subgroups of a population may differ: in the *type* of behavior in which they engage, in their *patterns of interaction* with other subgroups, in the *frequency* of their relevant behaviors and interactions, and in the *consequences* attendant on those behaviors. The first two sources of heterogeneity, type of behavior and patterns of interaction, can best be addressed in a model by partitioning the population into discrete groups rather than by paramcterization. For example, group boundaries in the RAND HIV model are defined by participation in

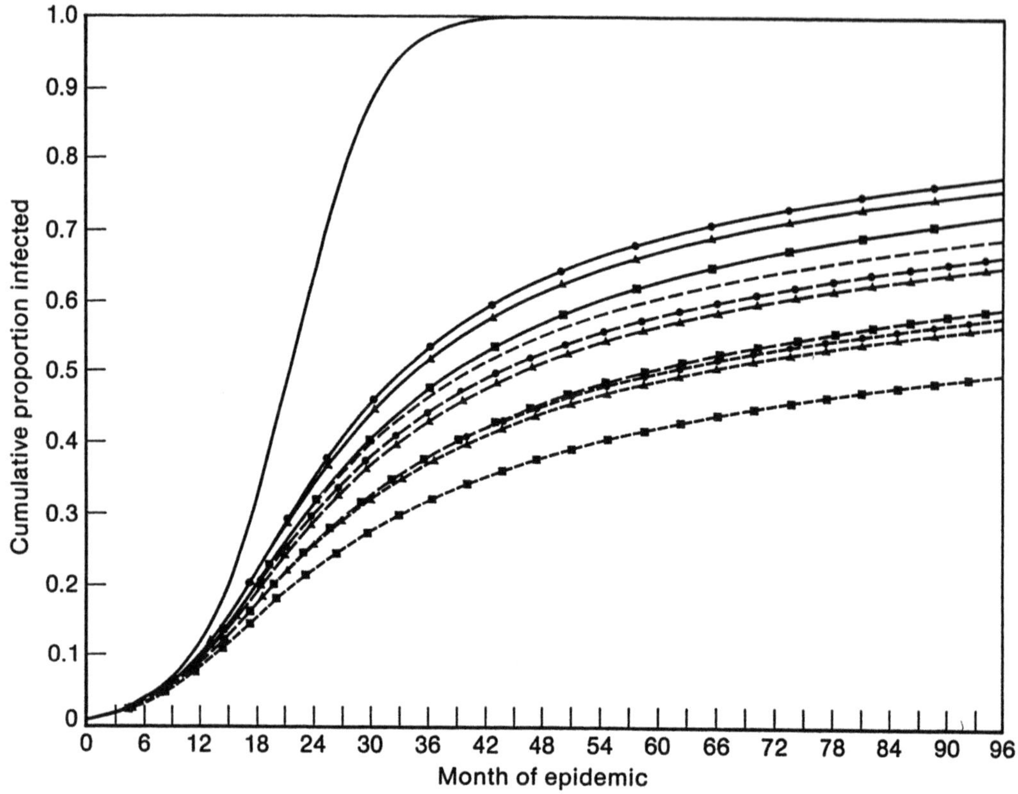

NN = no infectivity or susceptibility variation
NM = no infectivity variation, medium susceptibility variation
LL = low infectivity variation, low susceptibility variation
LM = low infectivity variation, medium susceptibility variation
LH = low infectivity variation, high susceptibility variation
ML = medium infectivity variation, low susceptibility variation
MM = medium infectivity variation, medium susceptibility variation
MH = medium infectivity variation, high susceptibility variation
HL = high infectivity variation, low susceptibility variation
HM = high infectivity variation, medium susceptibility variation
HH = high infectivity variation, high susceptibility variation

NOTE: Susceptibility and infectivity are defined as in Figure 1. Initial prevalence of infection (1%) and initial growth rate in new infections (23% in first month) are defined as the same in all cases. Differences in growth rates thereafter reflect differences in population heterogeneity.

Figure 2
Effects of Variation in Infectivity and Susceptibility
After Initial Growth Rate Has Been Normalized

each of the key risk behaviors (homosexual contact, heterosexual contact, and needle sharing). Heterogeneity in behavioral frequency and epidemiological consequences can be addressed either through categorization or parameterization, but most effectively through both. If we assume proportionate mixing within groups, groups should be defined in such a way that selection of partners for risky behaviors tends to occur within rather than between groups. For that reason, age and geographic location were the other primary determinants of group boundaries in the RAND HIV model.

A full model of HIV spread within the overall population must address many complexities besides heterogeneity. For example, the infected stage is not uniform and the induction time from infection to death is not a constant as assumed above. Most of these complexities, however, need not affect the way that within-group heterogeneity is handled within a model. The technique we have described in this paper allows a simple and plausible representation of the effects of heterogeneity in epidemiological models, including a full model of HIV spread.

Our analysis suggests a number of conclusions. First, the extent of within-group variation in infectivity and susceptibility can have a substantial effect on the dynamics of the growth rate in epidemics of this type. Second, epidemiological projections for HIV are quite sensitive to the amount of variation that is explicitly assumed, and therefore to the amount implicitly assumed where such variation is not explicitly considered. Third, heterogeneity in susceptibility and infectivity naturally slows the epidemic growth rate over time. Such slowing could rather easily be confused with the effects of behavior change, which are similar. The implications of the two processes are quite different, however, and it is important to distinguish them both in modeling work and in monitoring and interpreting actual incidence data. In modeling work, the use of a disaggregated model makes it possible to distinguish the effects of behavior change from the selection effects that result from heterogeneity. Fourth, the importance of heterogeneity in modeling transmission dynamics suggests the importance of gathering data that would permit empirically-based estimation of these parameters. At present, it is difficult to find relevant data for this purpose, but it is possible to describe the types of studies that would be useful. These include studies of the distribution and patterning of risk behaviors in populations and studies that seek to identify and quantify biological markers of infectivity or susceptibility in individuals. Fifth, it is important to consider the potential effects of policy options on the variation in susceptibility and infectivity as well as on their mean levels.

Acknowledgments

This paper is based in part on a presentation at the annual meetings of the Population Association of America, April 1988. This research was supported by RAND corporate funds. We are grateful to Audrey Cardell, James Hammitt, Albert Williams, and two anonymous reviewers for comments on an earlier draft.

REFERENCES

Blythe, S.P. and R.M. Anderson. (1988). Distributed incubation and infectious periods in models of the transmission dynamics of the human immunodeficiency virus (HIV). *IMA J. Math. Biol. Med.*, 5, 1-19.

Blythe, S.P. and C. Castillo-Chavez. (1989). Like-with-like preference and sexual mixing models. Submitted, *Math. Biosci.*

Cardell, N.S., D.E. Kanouse, E.M. Gorman, C. Serrato, P.H. Reuter, and A.P. Williams. (1987). Modeling the spread of human immunodeficiency virus in the United States. Presented to III International Conference on AIDS, Washington, D.C.

Castillo-Chavez, C., K. Cooke, W. Huang, and S.A. Levin. (1989). The role of long periods of infectiousness in the dynamics of acquired immunodeficiency syndrome (AIDS). In *Mathematical Approaches to Resource Management and Epidemiology.* In press, Lecture Notes in Biomathematics, Springer-Verlag.

Curran, J.W., H.W. Jaffe, A.M. Hardy, M. Morgan, R.M. Selik, and T.J. Dondero. (1988). Epidemiology of HIV infection and AIDS in the United States. *Science*, 239, 610-616.

Friedland, G.H, and R. S. Klein. (1987). Transmission of the human immunodeficiency virus. *N. Engl. J. Med.*, 317, 1125-1135.

Hethcote, H.W. (1976). Qualitative analysis of communicable disease models. *Math Biosciences*, 28, 335-356.

Hethcote, H.W. and J.W. Van Ark. (1987). Epidemiological models for heterogeneous populations: proportionate mixing, parameter estimation, and immunization programs. *Math. Biosci.*, 84, 85-118.

Hethcote, H.W. and J.A. Yorke. (1984). *Gonorrhea, transmission dynamics and control.* Lecture Notes in Biomathematics 56, Springer-Verlag, Berlin, Heidelberg, New York, Tokyo.

Hyman, J.M. and E.A. Stanley. (1988). Using mathematical models to understand the AIDS epidemic. *Math. Biosci.*, 90, 415-473.

Jacquez, J.A., C.P. Simon, J. Koopman, L. Sattenspiel, and T. Perry. (1988). Modeling and analyzing HIV transmission: the effect of contact patterns. *Math. Biosci.*, 92, 119-199.

Nold, A. (1980). Heterogeneity in diseases-transmission modeling. *Math. Biosci.*, 52, 227-240.

Padian, N., J. Wiley, and W. Winkelstein. (1987). Male to female transmission of human immunodeficiency virus (HIV): Current results, infectivity estimates, and San Francisco population seroprevalence estimates. Presented to III International Conference on AIDS, Washington, D.C.

Sattenspiel, L. and C.P. Simon. (1988). The spread and persistence of infectious diseases in structured populations. *Math. Biosci.*, 90, 341-366.

Turner, C.F., H.G. Miller, and L.E. Moses (eds.). (1989). *AIDS: Sexual Behavior and Intravenous Drug Use.* National Academy Press, Washington, D.C.

Wiley, J. (1987). Models for estimation of transmission probabilities of HIV in epidemiologic studies. Presented at Conference on Statistical and Mathematical Modeling of the AIDS Epidemic, Johns Hopkins University, Baltimore, MD.

Wiley, J.A., S.J. Herschkorn, and N.S. Padian. (1989). Heterogeneity in the probability of HIV transmission per sexual contact: The case of male-to-female transmission in penile-vaginal intercourse, *Stat. Med.*, 8, 93-102.

ON THE ROLE OF VARIABLE INFECTIVITY IN THE DYNAMICS OF THE HUMAN IMMUNODEFICIENCY VIRUS EPIDEMIC

Horst R. Thieme
Department of Mathematics
Arizona State University
Tempe, AZ 85287

Carlos Castillo-Chavez
Biometrics Unit & Center for Applied Math.
341 Warren Hall, Cornell University
Ithaca NY 14853-7801

Abstract

In this paper, we study the effects of variable infectivity in combination with a variable incubation period on the dynamics of HIV (the human immunodeficiency virus, the etiological agent for AIDS, the acquired immunodeficiency syndrome) in a homogeneously mixing population. In the model discussed here, the functional relationship between mean sexual activity and size of the population is assumed to be nonlinear and to saturate at high population sizes. We identify a basic reproductive number R_0 and show that the disease dies out if $R_0 < 1$. If $R_0 > 1$ the incidence rate converges to or oscillates around a uniquely determined nonzero equilibrium, the stability of which is studied. Our findings provide the analytical basis for exploring the parameter range in which the equilibrium is locally asymptotically stable. Oscillations cannot be excluded in general, and may occur in particular, if the variable infectivity is concentrated at an earlier part of the incubation period. Whether they can also occur for the reported two peaks of infectivity observed in HIV-infected individuals has to be the subject of future numerical investigations.

1. Introduction

Most epidemiological models for the transmission of infectious diseases have assumed that all infectious individuals are equally so. This assumption has proved to be reasonable in the study of the dynamics of communicable diseases such as influenza (see Castillo-Chavez *et al.* 1988, 1989 and references therein) or in the study of sexually transmitted diseases such as gonorrhea (see Hethcote and Yorke 1984 and references therein).

The AIDS epidemic, however, has forced researchers to look more closely at the role played by variable infectivity in the transmission of HIV. The experimental work reported in Francis *et al.* (1984), Salahuddin *et al.* (1984), and Lange *et al.* (1986) has begun to clarify the possible shape of the infectivity curve, supporting the hypothesis that there are two infectivity peaks. Once an individual has been infected, s/he experiences a short latency period of about two months, followed by a rise of virus titer (first peak). This period of infectivity is believed to last about six months, after which the individual's virus titer decreases and stays at a reduced level for a long period of time (presumably for an average of about seven to eight years). Finally, about a year before the onset of "full-blown" AIDS, a substantial increase in virus titer is observed (second peak). Though it may be premature to identify virus titer levels with infectivity levels, there is reason enough to study the possible effects of variable infectivity at this stage of affairs in order to clarify how important a good knowledge of the infectivity curve is for the understanding of the dynamics of the epidemic.

Numerical simulations of models that incorporate variable infectivity (see Anderson and May (1989); Hyman and Stanley 1988, 1989; Blythe and Anderson 1988b) demonstrate that the initial (transient) dynamics are very sensitive to the shape and timing of the first infectivity peak. Furthermore, all the published numerical simulations show the same qualitative dynamics, namely a steady approach to a unique endemic equilibrium. Hyman and Stanley's simulations (1988, 1989) indicate the same qualitative dynamics even in the presence of a high degree of heterogeneity in sexual behavior. The mathematical analysis of Castillo-Chavez *et al.* (1989a, b, c, and this volume) proves that the interactions between a distributed incubation period and a nonlinear mean sexual activity (as a function of population size) are not enough to excite undamped oscillations (at least not by a Hopf Bifurcation). In this paper, we will discuss whether and how these results change if we add variable infectivity results for the special case of a homogeneously mixing homosexual population.

The main body of the paper is organized as follows: Section 2 introduces a model for the sexual transmission of HIV that incorporates age of infection and variable infectivity and shows that this model is well-posed (i.e, its solutions exist and make epidemiological sense). Section 3 discusses the existence of stationary states and disease persistence in connection with the basic reproductive number, while Section 4 presents our stability results as well as the discussion of the possibility of sustained oscillatory behavior. The technical details will be published elsewhere. In the concluding discussion, we briefly review conditions upon which epidemiological models have been found to exhibit sustained oscillations, compare them to our results, and project future work.

2. Model description and well-posedness

In order to mimic HIV dynamics in a homogeneously mixing male homosexual population, we incorporate the following particular ingredients in our mathematical model:

- A nonlinear functional relationship between mean sexual per capita activity and the size of the sexually active population.
- A stratification of the infected part of the sexually active population according to infection age, i.e., time since the moment of infection.
- An infection-age-dependent rate of leaving the sexually active population due to disease progression.
- An infection-age-dependent infectivity .

The model considered here shares the first three features with the models considered by Castillo-Chavez *et al.* (1989 a, b, c and this volume) though the stratification according to infection age is not explicit there. The fourth feature has been added in order to study the kind of effects infection-age-dependent infectivity produces in combination with the other mechanisms. The model does not include heterogeneities other than infection-age-dependent infectivity and, by restricting itself to the homosexual part of a population which is replenished by constant recruitment, does not reflect the mutual effects of HIV dynamics and the dynamics of the total population (see Anderson and May 1989; Busenberg *et al.* 1989).

More specifically, we divide the population into three groups: S (uninfected, but susceptible), I (HIV infected), and A (fully developed AIDS symptoms). A-individuals are assumed to be sexually inactive and sexually active individuals (S and I) are supposed to choose their partners at random.

In our model, t denotes time, whereas τ denotes time since the moment of being infected, i.e., infection-age. As time unit we choose the average length of the period of sexual activity for healthy individuals. Individuals are recruited into the sexually active population at a constant rate Λ. We assume that the length of the sexually active period is exponentially distributed such that healthy individuals become sexually inactive at a constant rate μ. As we have chosen the average length $1/\mu$ of the activity period to be 1, $\mu = 1$. Infected individuals with infection-age τ stop being sexually active by force of the disease at a rate $\alpha(\tau)$. So the chance of an individual still being sexually active if he has been infected τ time units ago is given by

$$\exp\left(-\tau - \int_0^\tau \alpha(\rho)\mathrm{d}\rho\right).$$

We stratify the infected part of the population according to age of infection such that

$$\mathrm{I}(t) = \int_0^\infty \mathrm{i}(t,\tau)\mathrm{d}\tau ,$$

with $i(t,\tau)$ denoting the infection-age density. The chance that a randomly chosen partner is infected and has infection-age τ is

$$\frac{i(t,\tau)}{T(t)},$$

with T + S + I being the size of the sexually active population. We assume that an average susceptible contracts the disease from an infected partner with age of infection τ at a mean risk $\lambda(\tau)$. So the chance of an average susceptible individual being infected at time t (under the condition that he has had a sexual contact at that time) is given by

$$\frac{W(t)}{T(t)},$$

where

$$T = S + I,$$

$$W(t) = \int_0^\infty \lambda(\tau)i(t,\tau)d\tau .$$

The mean per capita sexual activity is measured in terms of the mean number of sexual contacts C(T) that an average individual has per unit of time. We assume that this number is a function of the size of the sexually active population: T = S + I.

We arrive at the following expression for the incidence rate (number of new cases of infection per unit time):

$$B(t) = C(T(t))S(t)\,\frac{W(t)}{T(t)} .$$

The dynamical model can now be formulated as follows:

$$\frac{dS(t)}{dt} = \Lambda - B(t) - S(t) ; \qquad (1)$$

$$\left(\frac{\partial}{\partial t} + \frac{\partial}{\partial \tau}\right) i(t,\tau) = -\Big(1 + \alpha(\tau)\Big)i(t,\tau) ; \qquad (2)$$

$$i(t,0) = B(t) = S(t)C(T(t))\,\frac{W(t)}{T} ; \qquad (3)$$

$$T = I + S ; \qquad (4)$$

$$I(t) = \int_0^\infty i(t,\tau)d\tau ; \qquad (5)$$

$$W(t) = \int_0^\infty \lambda(\tau)i(t,\tau)d\tau ; \qquad (6)$$

$$\frac{d}{dt}A(t) = \int_0^\infty \alpha(\tau)i(t,\tau)d\tau - (1+\nu)A(t) .$$

Though A, the number of individuals with fully developed AIDS symptoms (that are supposed to be too ill to be sexually active), is not assumed to play any further role in the dynamics of the epidemic, we give the formula here because it is one of the epidemiological entities which can be compared to data. ν denotes the rate at which an individual with fully developed AIDS symptoms dies from the disease.

Note that, in contrast to Anderson and May (1987), Blythe and Anderson (1988a), and Castillo-Chavez *et al.* (1989a, b), this model does not assume that at the moment of infection, an individual follows a severe or a mild course of the disease. By assuming that

$$\int_0^\infty \alpha(\tau)d\tau < \infty ,$$

this model, albeit with a different mechanism, takes into account the possibility that some individuals may not develop "full-blown" AIDS. Also, note that this model extends that of Blythe and Anderson (1988b). Furthermore, when this approach is combined with that of Castillo-Chavez *et al.* (this volume), the resulting model generalizes that of Hyman and Stanley (1988, 1989). We do not write a model of this generality because this paper is concerned with the mathematical analysis of the least complex model. Once we fully understand the dynamics of this model, we will proceed to the analysis of more detailed models.

Throughout this paper, we assume that $\alpha(\tau)$ is a nonnegative measurable function; $\lambda(\tau)$ is a nonnegative integrable function of infection age. C(T) is assumed to be a nondecreasing function of T, where $C(T) > 0$ whenever $T > 0$. Later we will assume that

$$M(T) = \frac{C(T)}{T}$$

is a nonincreasing function of T, i.e., C increases in a sublinear way reflecting some kind of saturation effect.

There are different ways of handling problem (1),$\cdots$,(6), each of which has its definite advantages. The first approach reformulates (1),$\cdots$,(6) as an abstract ordinary differential equation. See Thieme (1989a, b), in particular Section 7. This approach provides a dynamical system in terms of S and I useful in proving instability and persistence. A second approach consists of integrating (1),$\cdots$,(6) along characteristic lines (see Webb 1985) generating the same dynamical system but in a different way. Thirdly, one can use integration along characteristic lines to reduce the system (1),$\cdots$,(6) to the following set of integral equations:

$$S = \Lambda - B * P_1 + f_1 , \qquad (7)$$

$$V = B * P_{\alpha+1} + f_2 , \qquad (8)$$

$$W = B * Q + f_3 , \qquad (9)$$

$$B = SM(S + V)W . \qquad (10)$$

Here we have used the following notation:

$$P_\alpha(\tau) = \exp\left(-\int_0^\tau \alpha(s)ds \right) , \qquad (11)$$

$$Q(\tau) = \lambda(\tau)P_{\alpha+1}(\tau) , \tag{12}$$

$$(B * P)(t) = \int_0^t B(t-s)P(s)ds , \tag{13}$$

$$f_1(t) = \left(S(0) - \Lambda\right)e^{-t} , \tag{14}$$

$$f_2(t) = \int_t^\infty i(0,\tau-t)\frac{P_{\alpha+1}(\tau)}{P_{\alpha+1}(\tau-t)}d\tau , \tag{15}$$

$$f_3(t) = \int_t^\infty i(0,\tau-t)\lambda(\tau)\frac{P_{\alpha+1}(\tau)}{P_{\alpha+1}(\tau-t)}d\tau , \tag{16}$$

$$M(T) = \frac{C(T)}{T} . \tag{17}$$

Note that

$$f_j \to 0, \quad t \to \infty . \tag{18}$$

P_1 and $P_{\alpha+1}$ are defined in analogy to P_α.

Some of the entities defined above have an intuitive meaning. We mention that $P_1(s) = e^{-s}$ gives the chance a healthy individual has of still being sexually active s time units after having entered the active population. $P_{\alpha+1}(\tau)$ gives the chance an infected individual of infection age τ has of still being sexually active. Fitting Equation (10) into Equations (7), (8), and (9) yields a system of Volterra integral equations of convolution form for which a well-developed theory is available. See Miller (1971), or Londen (1981). Substituting Equations (7), (8), and (9) into equation (10) yields an integral equation which is not of common Volterra type, but has the advantage of being scalar.

From (1) we realize that S(t) remains positive (nonnegative) if S(0) has the corresponding property. We can then easily check, from the various equations, that nonnegativity is preserved under the solution flow. Integrating (2) over τ and combining it with (1) yields the differential inequality:

$$\frac{d}{dt}T \leq \Lambda - T , \tag{19}$$

and, as a result, the *a priori* estimate

$$S(t),I(t) \leq T(t) = S(t) + I(t) \leq \Lambda + \left(T(0) - \Lambda\right)e^{-t} . \tag{20}$$

By using the theory found in Webb (1985) or Thieme (1989a, b) 1985) or by applying standard fixed point arguments to (7),$\cdots$,(10), it is shown that the model is well posed (i.e., there is a unique nonnegative solution for given nonnegative initial conditions). Furthermore, the solution depends continuously on the initial conditions, and the functions S, I, W, B are continuous and satisfy the estimate given by (20).

3. Stationary states, the basic reproductive number, and disease persistence

This section begins with a discussion of possible stationary states: the infection-free state and the endemic state. These solutions are important because their feasibility (i.e., existence) is usually intimately connected to the basic reproductive number R_0, (which can be determined in terms of model parameters and is a starting point for the development and evaluation of control measures) and because they are candidates for the asymptotic behavior of the model. We show that, for $R_0 < 1$, the disease dies out while, for $R_0 > 1$, the disease persists in the population. In the latter case, there is a unique endemic equilibrium which is locally asymptotically stable for R_0 being slightly larger than 1, but which might lose stability if R_0 increases (see Section 4). Even if possibly unstable, the endemic equilibrium may be an indicator of the severity of the disease because (as we show) the incidence rate fluctuates around the endemic equilibrium value.

We start our analysis by noting that the system (1),$\cdots$,(6) always has the infection-free state

$$S_0 = \Lambda, \quad I_0 = 0, \quad W_0 = 0, \quad B_0 = 0, i_0 = 0 . \tag{21}$$

In order to determine the existence of the endemic equilibria of (1),$\cdots$,(6) we have to look for solutions of the following algebraic system of equations:

$$S^* = \Lambda - B^* , \tag{22}$$

$$I^* = B^*\hat{P}_{\alpha+1}(0) , \tag{23}$$

$$W^* = B^*\hat{Q}(0) , \tag{24}$$

$$B^* = \frac{S^*}{T^*}C(T^*)W^*, \quad T^* = S^* + I^* . \tag{25}$$

Here we have used the *Laplace* transform notation, i.e.,

$$\hat{Q}(z) = \int_0^\infty e^{-z\tau}Q(\tau)d\tau , \tag{26}$$

$$\hat{P}_{\alpha+1}(z) = \int_0^\infty e^{-z\tau}\hat{P}_{\alpha+1}(\tau)d\tau . \tag{27}$$

Substituting Equation (24) into (25) and dividing by B^* (which is assumed to be positive), we obtain the following:

$$1 = \frac{S^*}{T^*}C(T^*)\hat{Q}(0), \quad T^* = S^* + I^* . \tag{28}$$

We introduce a dimensionless quantity, namely the fraction of infected individuals,

$$\xi = \frac{I^*}{T^*} , \tag{29}$$

and note from (22), (23), and the second equation in (27) that

$$\frac{S^*}{T^*} = 1 - \xi, \quad T^* = \frac{\Lambda}{1 + \left(\frac{1}{\hat{P}_{\alpha+1}(0)} - 1\right)\xi} . \tag{30}$$

Fitting these into (28) we arrive at

$$1 = (1-\xi)C\left(\frac{\Lambda}{1 + \left(\frac{1}{\hat{P}_{\alpha+1}(0)} - 1\right)\xi}\right)\hat{Q}(0) . \tag{31}$$

Recalling that C(T) is a monotone nondecreasing function and that $1 > \hat{P}_{\alpha+1}(0)$, we realize that the right-hand side of (31) is a strictly decreasing function of ξ. For $\xi = 0$, the right-hand side of (31) gives the basic reproductive number R_0 of the disease-free population (in its equilibrium):

$$R_0 = C(\Lambda)\hat{Q}(0) . \tag{32}$$

R_0 gives the average number of secondary infections that a typical infectious individual can produce if it is introduced into the disease-free population. From the intermediate value theorem we arrive at the following result:

Theorem 1. If $R_0 \le 1$, there exists only the disease-free equilibrium. If $R_0 > 1$, there is a unique endemic equilibrium.

Theorem 1 does not provide us with a relation between the basic reproductive number and the actual disease dynamics. It only provides information regarding the existence of a state in which the disease persists. The next theorem, however, partially connects the basic reproductive number.

Theorem 2. Let $R_0 < 1$. Then the disease-free equilibrium is globally attractive. In particular we have

$$B(t), I(t), W(t) \to 0, \quad S(t) \to \Lambda \quad \textit{for } t \to \infty .$$

Proof. Applying Fatou's lemma to (9) and (10) and using the estimate (20) and the fact that C is nondecreasing, we obtain

$$\limsup_{t\to\infty} B(t) \le R_0 \limsup_{t\to\infty} B(t) .$$

This implies the assertion.

In general, it is not possible to obtain a global convergence result if $R_0 > 1$. One can show, however, that if a trajectory is not attracted to the endemic equilibrium, it has to oscillate around it.

Theorem 3. *Let $R_0 > 1$. The following holds:*

a)
$$\limsup_{t\to\infty} B(t) \le B^* .$$

b) Let $\lambda(\tau) \not\equiv 0$ and $\tau_\dagger$ be the smallest $\bar{\tau}$ such that $\lambda(\tau) = 0$ for a.a. $\tau \ge \bar{\tau}$. *Let*
$$\int_0^{\tau_\dagger} i(0,\tau)d\tau > 0 .$$
Then
$$\limsup_{t\to\infty} B(t) \ge B^* .$$
The proof of this result can be found in Thieme and Castillo-Chavez (1989).

Analogous statements can now be derived for S, I, and W. Note, however, that Theorem 3 does not yet answer the question of whether I, the total number of infected individuals, is bounded away from zero whenever $R_0 > 1$, as well as whether or not this bound depends on the initial conditions. To address this question, it is better to look at the initial formulation (1),⋯,(6) given in a framework suitable for dynamical systems theory. See Hale and Waltman's (1989) theory of persistence and note that part b of our Theorem 3 implies the satisfaction of condition (4.2) of their Theorem 4.1. Combining these observations with Equation (20), we see that the solution flow has a bounded attractor. Using the approach found in Webb (1985, proposition 3.16) we can show also that the solution flow is asymptotically smooth. Furthermore, the boundary flow, i.e., i = 0, is attracted to the infection-free state. Hale and Waltman's result (1989, Theorem 4.2) leads us to the following result:

Theorem 4. *Let $R_0 > 1$ and $\lambda(\tau) \not\equiv 0$, and let $\tau_\dagger$ be the smallest $\bar{\tau}$ such that $\lambda(\tau) = 0$ for* a.a. $\tau \ge \bar{\tau}$. *If*
$$\int_0^{\tau_\dagger} i(0,\tau)d\tau > 0 .$$
Then
$$\liminf_{t\to\infty} I(t) > \epsilon > 0 ,$$
with ϵ not depending on the initial conditions.

Unfortunately, the dynamical systems persistence theory does not give us information as to whether or not B and W are bounded away from zero.

4. Stability of the endemic equilibrium

The stability of the endemic equilibrium is of epidemiological interest for two reasons:

First, in the case of local asymptotic stability, there is some reason to believe that it really is the ultimate state of the epidemic because the disease-free equilibrium is a repellor and there is no third equilibrium. But only global stability could answer this question (e.g., there could be a "blue sky" bifurcation of periodic orbits). Secondly, if the endemic equilibrium is unstable, this strongly suggests undamped oscillations of the disease dynamics around the equilibrium. Recall Theorem 3.2. Intuitively, local asymptotic stability means that, once the course of the disease comes close to the endemic equilibrium, it remains close and finally approaches it. The model formulation (1),⋯,(6) is the most appropriate framework for a precise definition.

Definition. a) The endemic equilibrium S^*, I^*, W^*, B^*, i^* of (1),⋯,(6) with

$$i^*(\tau) = B^* P_{\alpha+1}(\tau)$$

is *locally asymptotically stable* if and only if the following two properties hold:

(i) For any $\epsilon > 0$ there is some $\delta > 0$ such that if

$$|S(0) - S^*| + \int_0^\infty |i(0,\tau) - i^*(\tau)| d\tau \leq \delta ,$$

then

$$|S(t) - S^*| + \int_0^\infty |i(t,\tau) - i^*(\tau)| d\tau \leq \epsilon, \quad \text{for all } t \geq 0 .$$

(ii) There exists $\delta_0 > 0$ with the property that if

$$|S(0) - S^*| + \int_0^\infty |i(0,\tau) - i^*(\tau)| d\tau \leq \delta_0 ,$$

then

$$|S(t) - S^*| + \int_0^\infty |i(t,\tau) - i^*(\tau)| d\tau \quad \to 0 \quad \text{for} \quad t \to \infty .$$

b) The endemic equilibrium is called *unstable* if there exists a sequence of solutions S_n, I_n to (1),⋯,(6), a sequence of times $t_n \to \infty$, and a positive number $\epsilon_0 > 0$ such that

$$|S_n(0) - S^*| + \int_0^\infty |i_n(0,\tau) - i^*(\tau)| d\tau \quad \to 0 \quad \text{for} \quad n \to \infty ,$$

but

$$|S_n(t_n) - S^*| + \int_0^\infty |i_n(t_n,\tau) - i^*(\tau)| d\tau \geq \epsilon_0, \quad \text{for all } n \in N .$$

To facilitate the discussion of the stability and instability of the endemic equilibria, we switch from the original parameters of the model to the following nondimensional ones:

$$\xi = \frac{I^*}{T^*} = \frac{I^*}{S^* + I^*} , \tag{33}$$

$$\gamma := - \frac{T^* M'(T^*)}{M(T^*)} , \tag{34}$$

and

$$\sigma := \frac{1}{\hat{P}_{\alpha+1}(0)} . \tag{35}$$

ξ, the fraction of infected individuals in the sexually active population, is a very convenient dimensionless parameter satisfying

$$0 < \xi < 1 .$$

Note that all ξ in the interval $0 < \xi < 1$ are feasible (as one can see from (31), (32) by choosing $R_0 > 1$ accordingly) albeit not all are realistic. In addition, we observe that $\frac{1}{\sigma} = P_{\alpha+1}(0)$ denotes the average length of the sexually active period of infected individuals (relative to the average length of the sexually active period of healthy individuals, our time unit). Hence it is intuitively clear (and this follows from the definition of $P_{\alpha+1}$ - see (11)) that $\sigma > 1$. The average infection has been estimated to be about 10 years (see May and Anderson 1989 and references therein). If we assume that the mean of the sexually active period lies in the interval [15 years, 30 years], then we obtain values of σ in the interval [1.5, 3]. γ is a dimensionless parameter also, and since $M(T) = \frac{C(T)}{T}$ is nonincreasing and C is nondecreasing, we see that

$$0 \leq \gamma \leq 1 .$$

The following choices for C(T) may give us a feeling for a reasonable range for γ.

a) Mass action type contact law

The classical epidemiological contact law is $C(T) = \beta T$, i.e., M = constant and $\gamma = 0$. This contact law is more appropriate for casual contact diseases like influenza (see Castillo-Chavez *et al.* 1988, 1989).

b) C = constant

If the number of available partners is large enough and everybody can make more contacts than is practically feasible, this may be a good approximation in some situations. In this case $\gamma = 1$.

c) Michaelis Menton type contact law

The Michaelis Menton type contact law (or Holling functional response type 1) combines the two previous approaches by assuming that, if the number of available partners is low, the number of actual per capita partners C(T) is proportional to T, whereas, if the number of available partners is large, there is a saturation effect which makes the number of actual partners constant. We may take

$$C(T) = \frac{\beta T}{1 + \kappa T} .$$

In this case,

$$\gamma = \frac{kT^*}{1 + \kappa T^*} ,$$

and γ covers the range from 0 to 1 when T^* covers the range from 0 to ∞. Therefore any value of γ is feasible (as one can see from (30), although not necessarily realistic).

In view of this discussion, we call γ the saturation index of the number of partners at the endemic equilibrium. If $\gamma = 0$, there is no saturation at all because the number of actual partners is proportional to the number of available partners. If $\gamma = 1$, there is a complete saturation because the number of actual partners hardly changes if the number of available partners does. Thieme and Castillo-Chavez (1989) prove the following result.

Theorem 5. *The endemic equilibrium is locally asymptotically stable if one of the following holds:*

a) ξ *is sufficiently close to* 0 *or to* 1.

b) σ *is sufficiently large.*

c) γ *is sufficiently close to* 0.

d) $\lambda = const.$

e) $P_{\alpha+1}$ *is convex.*

Thus the endemic equilibrium is locally asymptotically stable if the fraction of infected individuals is either low or high, or if the length of the sexually active period of infected individuals is short compared with the length of the sexually active period of the healthy individuals, or if the saturation index is low. Further, we have local stability if the infectivity is evenly distributed over the period of sexual activity. $P_{\alpha+1}$ may be convex (e.g., if the length of the sexually active period of infected individuals is exponentially distributed). This of course, may not be the case.

Conversely, the following holds (see Thieme and Castillo-Chavez 1989):

Theorem 6. *Let* $\gamma > 0$ *and*

$$\int_0^\infty cos(sy)P_{\alpha+1}(s)ds < 0 \quad \text{for some } y \,. \tag{36}$$

If Q is concentrated sufficiently close to 0, *one can find* ξ *and* σ $(0 < \xi < 1, \sigma > 1)$ *such that the corresponding endemic equilibrium is unstable.*

Actually, the saturation index has a destabilizing effect. The closer it is to 1, the more likely the endemic equilibrium will be unstable. The requirement that Q is concentrated at 0, i.e., that the infectivity is concentrated in the early part of the incubation period, emphasizes the importance of an infection-age-dependent infectivity. Future numerical studies have to show whether more realistic infectivity distributions (one early and one late peak) induce instability. An example for which (36) holds is given in Thieme and Castillo-Chavez (1989).

Theorems 5 and 6 follow from studying the roots of the characteristic equation

$$1 = -\frac{\sigma\xi}{1+z}\left(\frac{1}{1-\xi} - \gamma\right) - \xi\gamma\hat{p}(z) + \hat{q}(z) \tag{37}$$

with

$$p(s) = \frac{P_{\alpha+1}}{\hat{P}_{\alpha+1}(0)}, \tag{38}$$

and

$$q(s) = \frac{Q(s)}{\hat{Q}(0)}. \tag{39}$$

Actually they represent special cases of the following more technical result which follows from linearizing (1),···,(6) around the endemic equilibrium and applying Theorem 4.13 in Webb (1985) or Corollary 4.3 and Section 7 in Thieme (1989 a, b) (see Thieme and Castillo-Chavez 1989):

Theorem 7. *a) The endemic equilibrium is locally asymptotically stable if all the roots of the characteristic equation* (37) *have strictly negative real parts.*

b) The endemic equilibrium is unstable if the characteristic equation has at least one root with strictly positive real part.

The characteristic equation can be used to trace the parameters ξ, σ for which the endemic equilibrium changes (if at all) its stability. In this case, the root of the characteristic equation with largest real part crosses the imaginary axis. Setting $z = jy$ with $j = \sqrt{-1}$ being the imaginary unit and separating real and imaginary part of the characteristic equation, we obtain

$$1 - \int_0^\infty \cos(sy)q(s)ds = -\frac{1}{1+y^2}\,\sigma\xi\left(\frac{1}{1-\xi} - \gamma\right) - \xi\gamma\int_0^\infty \cos(sy)p(s)ds \tag{40}$$

$$\int_0^\infty \sin(sy)q(s)ds = \frac{y}{1+y^2}\,\sigma\xi\left(\frac{1}{1-\xi} - \gamma\right) + \xi\gamma\int_0^\infty \sin(sy)p(s)ds\,. \tag{41}$$

We can solve for ξ by multiplying (40) by y and adding the two equations together:

$$\xi = \frac{y\left(1 - \int_0^\infty \cos(sy)q(s)ds\right) + \int_0^\infty \sin(sy)q(s)ds}{\gamma\left(\int_0^\infty \sin(sy)p(s)ds - y\int_0^\infty \cos(sy)p(s)ds\right)}\,. \tag{42}$$

Fitting (42) into (41) makes it possible to solve for σ:

$$\sigma = \frac{\int_0^\infty \sin(sy)q(s)ds - \xi\gamma \int_0^\infty \sin(sy)p(s)ds}{\frac{y}{1+y^2}\left(\frac{\xi}{1-\xi} - \xi\gamma\right)} . \tag{43}$$

Note that only ξ, γ and σ satisfying $0 < \xi < 1$, $0 \leq \gamma \leq 1$ and $\sigma > 1$ make epidemiological sense in the framework of our model. Hence equations (40),$\cdots$,(43) provide the following technical stability result which implies Theorem 5 d, e.

Theorem 8. *The endemic equilibrium is locally asymptotically stable if there is no $y > 0$ satisfying the following simultaneously:*

$$\int_0^\infty \cos(sy)q(s)ds > 0 ,$$

$$\int_0^\infty \sin(sy)q(s)ds > 0 ,$$

$$\int_0^\infty \cos(sy)p(s)ds < 0 ,$$

$$0 < y\left(1 - \int_0^\infty \cos(sy)q(s)ds\right) + \int_0^\infty \sin(sy)q(s)ds$$

$$< \gamma\left(\int_0^\infty \sin(sy)p(s)ds - y \int_0^\infty \cos(sy)p(s)ds\right).$$

The equations (42), (43) provide a curve $\xi = \xi(y)$, $\sigma = \sigma(y)$, $y > 0$ which traces the parameters ξ, σ for which the characteristic equation has roots on the imaginary axis. From the shape of this curve, it should be possible to decide in which ξ, σ range, for given γ, p and q, the characteristic equation has roots z in the right-half plane implying that the endemic equilibrium is unstable. Again one has to keep in mind that only ξ, σ satsifying $0 < \xi < 1$, $\sigma > 1$ are meaningful, and the realistic parameter range is much narrower than this. It is not too difficult to see from (42), (43) that the endemic equilibrium is unstable for realistic values of ξ, σ if the assumptions of Theorem 5 are satisfied.

5. Discussion and projected future work

The mathematical analysis of epidemic models has identified both mechanisms capable and incapable of generating sustained oscillations (see Hethcote *et al.* 1981, and Hethcote and Levin 1989 for a survey). One of the most common mechanisms known to be capable of exciting oscillations derives from the return of infectives into a susceptible class (with or without having experienced a period of temporary immunity). Anderson *et al.* (1981) found, for a fox rabies model, that sustained oscillations can be generated by the combined effects of a rapid turnover of the fox population and the relatively long latency and the high fatality of fox rabies. Liu *et al.* (1986, 1987), in their work on influenza, have shown that generalized nonlinear incidence rates can also generate sustained oscillations. Castillo-Chavez *et al.* (1988, 1989) and Andreasen's (1988, 1989) work on influenza strongly suggests that the interaction between multiple viral related strains of influenza type A, the host immune system (cross-immunity), and age-dependent host's mortality are needed to generate sustained oscillations. Epidemic models which incorporate time since infection - age of infection - do or do not exhibit sustained oscillations: this depends on the form of the infection-age dependent infectivity curve and the distribution of the length of the infection period (see Diekmann *et al.* 1982, 1984; Gripenberg 1980, 1981; Hethcote and Thieme 1985).

The mechanisms found to generate sustained oscillations for the models described above do not operate in the case of HIV dynamics. But these models (rabies exempted) are different from any realistic HIV model in one respect: they assume that the disease is essentially nonfatal and the population size is constant. Though our model assumes a constant recruitment rate into the sexually active population, the population size will vary with time due to the disease fatalities. So how the per capita number of sexual contacts C = C(T) depends on the number of sexually active individuals T becomes crucial for the dynamics of the disease. For sexually transmitted diseases, it seems reasonable to assume a saturation effect for partner acquisition, namely that C(T) becomes largely independent of T if the population size T is large.

In our model, the saturation of mean per capita sexual activity interacts with an infection-age-dependent rate (at which infected individuals are sexually inactivated by the disease) and an infection-age-dependent infectivity of infected individuals. We find that the endemic equilibrium can lose its stability (thus generating sustained oscillations) by a rather unique combination of conditions:

(i) The probability that an infected individual is still sexually active is sufficiently far away from being a convex function of infection age.

(ii) There is sufficient saturation in partner acquisition, i.e., the number C(T) of actual partners per capita is largely independent of slight changes in the number of available partners T.

(iii) The period of sexual activity is not too short for infected individuals in relation to uninfected ones.

(iv) The fraction of infected individuals in the sexually active population is neither too low nor too high.

(v) The infection-age-distributed infectivity is concentrated at any early part of the incubation period.

Sustained oscillations can be ruled out if any of the conditions (i), (ii), (iii), or (iv) are not satisfed. But actually, they do not seem unreasonable for a model of HIV transmission. Condition (v) represents our first step towards an analysis of the effects of variable infectivity on HIV dynamics. As sustained oscillations can be ruled out if the infectivity is rather evenly distributed over the activity period (as suggested by the analysis in Castillo-Chavez *et al.* 1989 a, b, c, and this volume, where it is assumed to be constant), condition (v) emphasizes the possible relevance of variable infectivity for the dynamics of the epidemic. Relying on analytical techniques, so far we have found sustained oscillations only if the infectivity distribution has one (early) peak instead of one early and one late peak. But this is warning enough not to take stability of the endemic equilibrium for granted. Actually, stability will depend on the choice of the model parameters. Future numerical work will attempt to see whether or not undamped oscillations also occur for models with an early and a late infectivity peak. The above mentioned stability criterion will be the analytical basis for numerically exploring the parameter range in which oscillations occur. The ξ, σ curves generated by equations (42) and (43) will help to find the boundary of the ξ, σ region within which (if at all) the endemic equilibrium is unstable. This procedure has to be repeated for different choices of γ, p and q producing different curves, of course. A saturation index $\gamma = 1$ will be a reasonable first choice (see our discussion in the previous section). Whether the endemic equilibrium is unstable in a realistic ξ, σ range will crucially depend on the shape of p, q as we recognize from (i) and (v). The shape of p, q for which the endemic equilibrium is unstable may or may not be realistic. Our analytic results so far suggest instability if the age-infected infectivity is concentrated at an early part of the incubation period. The numerical simulations of models that incorporate variable infectivity by Anderson and May (1989), Hyman and Stanley (1988, 1989), Blythe and Anderson (1988b) rather suggest that the endemic equilibrium is stable for realistic infectivity functions.

Here further investigations are needed. These can be done much easier and more effectively by first exploring the parameter range of possible sustained oscillations using the ξ, σ curves just described. Although simulations of the full model are indispensable for showing whether the amplitudes of the oscillations are large enough to be epidemiologically significant, they need to be guided by the previous exploration of the critical parameter range.

The uncertainty of whether or not the endemic equilibrium is stable raises the question of whether it has to be totally discarded as some kind of measure of the severity of the disease when unstable. We have shown, however, that the incidence rate either converges to its (uniquely determined) endemic equilibrium or fluctuates around it (provided that an endemic equilibrium exists). This at least gives some information. It would be more useful to know whether the time averages converge (as time tends to infinity) towards the endemic equilibrium. This stronger statement may or may not be true.

ACKNOWLEDGMENTS

This research has been partially supported by NSF grant DMS-8906580, NIAID grant R01 A129178-01, and Hatch project grant NYC 151-409, USDA awarded to Carlos Castillo-Chavez. We are extremely grateful to K. L. Cooke for his stimulating conversations and his comments in this manuscript.

REFERENCES

Anderson, R.M., H.C. Jackson, R.M. May, and A.D.M. Smith. (1981). Population dynamics of fox rabies in Europe. *Nature* 289, 765-771.

Anderson, R.M. and R.M. May. (1987). Transmission dynamics of HIV infection. *Nature* 326, 137-142.

Anderson, R.M., R.M. May, and G.F. Medley. (1986). A preliminary study of the transmission dynamics of the human immunodeficiency virus (HIV), the causative agent of AIDS. *IMA J. Math. Med. Biol.* 3, 229-263.

Andreasen, V. (1988). Dynamical models of epidemics in age-structured populations: Analysis and simplifications. Ph.D. Thesis, Cornell University.

Andreasen, V. (1989). Multiple time scales in the dynamics of infectious diseases. In *Mathematical Approaches to Problems in Resource Management and Epidemiology*, C. Castillo-Chavez, S.A. Levin, and C. Shoemaker (eds.). Lecture Notes in Biomathematics 81. Springer-Verlag, Berlin, Heidelberg, New York, Tokyo.

Blythe, S.P. and R.M. Anderson. (1988a). Distributed incubation and infectious periods in models of the transmission dynamics of the human immunodeficiency virus (HIV). *IMA J. Math. Med. Bio.* 5, 1-19.

Blythe, S.P. and R.M. Anderson. (1988b). Variable infectiousness in HIV transmission models. *IMA J. of Mathematics Applied in Med. and Biol.* 5, 181-200.

Busenberg, S., K.L. Cooke, and H.R. Thieme. (1989). Interaction of population growth and disease dynamics for HIV/AIDS in a heterogeneous population. (Preprint.)

Castillo-Chavez, C., K.L. Cooke, W. Huang, and S.A. Levin. (1989a). On the role of long periods of infectiousness in the dynamics of acquired immunodeficiency syndrome (AIDS). In *Mathematical Approaches to Problems in Resource Management and Epidemiology*, C. Castillo-Chavez, S.A. Levin, and C. Shoemaker (eds.). Lecture Notes in Biomathematics 81, Springer-Verlag,.

Castillo-Chavez, C., K.L. Cooke, W. Huang, and S.A. Levin. (1989b). One the role of long incubation periods in the dynamics of acquired immunodeficiency syndrome (AIDS), Part 1. Single population models. *J. Math. Biol.* 27, 373-398.

Castillo-Chavez, K.L. Cooke, W. Huang, and S.A. Levin. (1989c). Results on the dynamics for models for the sexual transmission of the human immunodeficiency virus. *Applied Mathematics Letters.* (In press.)

Castillo-Chavez, C., K.L. Cooke, W. Huang, and S.A. Levin. (1989d). On the role of long incubation periods in the dynamics of acquired immunodeficiency syndrome (AIDS), Part 2. Multiple group models. In *Mathematical and Statistical Approaches to AIDS Epidemiology,* C. Castillo-Chavez (ed.). Lecture Notes in Biomathemtics, Springer-Verlag. (This volume.)

Castillo-Chavez, C., H.W. Hethcote, V. Andreasen, S.A. Levin, and W.M. Liu. (1989). Epidemiological models with age structure, proportionate mixing, and cross-immunity. *J. Math. Biol.* 27, 233-258.

Castillo-Chavez, C., H.W. Hethcote, V. Andreasen, S.A. Levin, and W.M. Liu. (1988). Cross-immunity in the dynamics of homogeneous and heterogeneous populations. In *Mathematical Ecology,* L. Gross, T.G. Hallam, and S.A. Levin (eds.). Proceedings of the Autumn Course Research Seminars, Trieste 1986 and World Scientific Publ. Co., Singapore.

Diekmann, O. and S.A. van Gils. (1984). Invariant manifolds for Volterra integral equations of convolution type. *J. Diff. Equa.* 54, 189-190.

Diekmann, O. and R. Montijn. (1982). Prelude to Hopf bifurcation in an epidemic model: analysis of a characteristic equation associated with a nonlinear Volterra integral equation. *J. Math. Biol.* 14, 117-127.

Francis, D.F., P.M. Feorino, J.R. Broderson, H.M. McClure, J.P. Getchell, C.R. McGrath, B. Swenson, J.S. McDougal, E.L. Palmer, A.K. Harrison, F. Barré-Sinoussi, J.C. Chermann, L. Montagnier, J.W. Curran, C.D. Cabradilla, and V.S. Kalyanaraman. (1984). Infection of chimpanzees with lymphadenopathy-associated virus. *Lancet* 2, 1276-1277.

Gripenberg, G. (1980). Periodic solutions to an epidemic model. *J. Math. Biol.* 10, 271-280.

Gripenberg, G. (1981). On some epidemic model. *Appl. Math.* 39, 317-327.

Hale, J.K. and P. Waltman. (1989). Persistence in infinite-dimensional systems. *SIAM J. Math. Anal.* 20, 388-395.

Hethcote, H.W. and S.A. Levin. (1989). Periodicity in epidemiological models. In *Applied Mathematical Ecology,* S.A. Levin, T.G. Hallam, and L.J. Gross (eds.). Biomathematics 18, Springer-Verlag, Heidelberg.

Hethcote, H.W., H.W. Stech, and P. van den Driessche. (1981). Periodicity and stability in epidemic models: a survey. In *Differential Equations and Applications in Ecology, Epidemics and Population problems,* S. Busenberg and K.L. Cooke (eds.). Academic Press, New York.

Hethcote, H.W. and H.R. Thieme. (1985). Stability of the endemic equilibrium in epidemic models with subpopulations. *Math. Biosci.* 75, 205-227.

Hethcote, H.W. and J.A. Yorke. (1984). Gonorrhea, transmission dynamics, and control. Lecture Notes in Biomathematics 56. Springer-Verlag, Berlin, Heidelberg, New York, Tokyo.

Holling, C.S. (1966). The functional response of invertebrate predators to prey density. *Mem. Ent. Soc. Canada* 48.

Hyman, J.M. and E.A. Stanley. (1988). A risk base model for the spread of the AIDS virus. *Math. Biosci.* 90, 415-473.

Hyman, J.M. and E.A. Stanley. (1989). The effects of social mixing patterns on the spread of AIDS. In *Mathematical Approaches to Problems in Resource Management and Epidemiology*, C. Castillo-Chavez, S.A. Levin, and C. Shoemaker (eds.). Lecture Notes in Biomathematics 81, Springer-Verlag, Berlin, Heidelberg, New York and Tokyo.

Lange, J.M.A., D.A. Paul, H.G. Huisman, F. De Wolf, H. Van den Berg, C.A. Roel, S.A. Danner, J. Van der Noordaa, and J. Goudsmit. (1986). Persistent HIV antigenaemia and decline of HIV core antibodies associated with transition to AIDS. *Brit. Med. J.* 293, 1459-1462.

Liu, W-m., H.W. Hethcote, and S.A. Levin. (1987). Dynamical behavior of epidemiological models with nonlinear incidence rates. *J. Math. Biol.* 25(4), 359-380.

Liu, W-m., S.A. Levin, and Y. Iwasa. (1986). Influence of nonlinear incidence rates upon the behavior of SIRS epidemiological models. *J. Math. Biol.* 23, 187-204.

Londen, S.O. (1981). Integral equations of Volterra type. *Mathematics of Biology.* Liguori Editore, Napoli, Italia.

May, R.M. and R.M. Anderson. (1989). The transmission dynamics of human immunodeficiency virus (HIV). *Phil. Trans. R. Soc. London B* 321, 565-607.

May, R.M., R.M. Anderson, and A.R. McLean. (1988). Possible demographic consequences of HIV/AIDS epidemics: I. Assuming HIV infection always leads to AIDS. *Math. Biosci.* 90, 475-506.

May, R.M., R.M. Anderson, and A.R. McLean. (1989). Possible demographic consequences of HIV/AIDS epidemics: II. Assuming HIV infection does not necessarily lead to AIDS. In *Mathematical Approaches to Problems in Resource Management and Epidemiology.* C. Castillo-Chavez, S.A. Levin, and C. Shoemaker (eds). Lecture Notes in Biomathematics 81, Springer-Verlag, Berlin, Heidelberg, New York and Tokyo.

Miller, R.K. (1971). *Nonlinear Volterra Integral Equations.* Benjamin, Menlo Park.

Salahuddin, S.Z., J.E. Groopman, P.D. Markham, M.G. Sarngaharan, R.R. Redfield, M.F. McLane, M. Essex, A. Sliski, and R.C. Gallo. (1984). HTLV-III in symptom-free seronegative persons. *Lancet* 2, 1418-1420.

Thieme, H.R. (1989a). Semiflows generated by Lipschitz perturbations of non-densely defined operators. I. The theory. (Preprint.)

Thieme, H.R. (1989b). Semiflows generated by Lipschitz perturbations of non-densely defined operators. II. Examples. (Preprint.)

Thieme, H.R. and C. Castillo-Chavez. (1989). On the possible effects of infection-age-dependent infectivity in the dynamics of HIV/AIDS. (Manuscript.)

Webb, G.F. (1985). *Theory of Nonlinear Age-Dependent Population Dynamics.* Marcel Dekker, New York.

III. Heterogeneity and HIV Transmission Dynamics

ASSESSMENT OF THE RISK OF HIV SPREAD VIA NON-STEADY HETEROSEXUAL PARTNERS IN THE U.S. POPULATION

Joan L. Aron and P. Sankara Sarma
Dept. of Population Dynamics
School of Hygiene and Public Health
The Johns Hopkins University
615 N. Wolfe St.
Baltimore, MD 21205

Abstract

We evaluate the conditions for the initial spread of HIV infection via non-steady heterosexual partners in the U.S. population. The main source of data is a 1988 U.S. survey on sexual partners in the 12 months prior to the survey. The behavioral data are coupled with a multi-state life table constructed from 1985 U.S. rates of marriage, divorce and mortality. The life table allows for projections that take age, sex and marital status into account.

We consider the basic reproductive rate of HIV infection from the most sexually active group of adults, 18-year-old unmarried males. Using a period of infectivity of 10 years, an HIV-infected 18-year-old unmarried male might contact, on average, around 100 males via his non-steady female sexual partners and their non-steady male sexual partners. This estimate does depend on the age and marital status of the chosen partners. However, the most important parameter is the product of per-partner probabilities of male-to-female and female-to-male transmission. This quantity would have to exceed roughly 1/100 in order for the epidemic to spread via non-steady heterosexual partners. Although current estimates suggest this is unlikely, major uncertainties remain concerning HIV transmission to both steady and non-steady heterosexual partners.

1. Introduction

The possibility of substantial spread of human immunodeficiency virus (HIV) into the general heterosexual population in the U.S. is a persistent concern. Seeding of the heterosexual population has already occurred through exposures such as blood transfusions and intravenous injections of drugs. Moreover, many instances of HIV transmission to heterosexual partners are well documented. This paper will analyze demographically a

1988 U.S. survey on sexual behavior in order to better assess the conditions for growth of heterosexual transmission of HIV.

2. General Social Survey

Every year, the General Social Survey (GSS) seeks to interview a probability sample of people who are at least 18 years old and living in U.S. households (Davis and Smith 1988). In 1988, the interview was supplemented by a short self-administered questionnaire on sexual behavior. The four questions in the supplement are listed in Table 1.

Table 1

Questions on Sexual Behavior

Q.1 How many sex partners have you had in the last 12 months?
Responses are 0, 1, 2, 3, 4, 5-10, 11-20, 21-100 or 100+.

Q.2 Was one of the partners your husband or wife or regular sex partner?
Responses are yes or no.

Q.3 If you had other partners, please indicate all categories that apply to them - close personal friend; neighbor, co-worker, or long-term acquaintance; casual date or pick-up; person you paid or paid you for sex; other.
Responses are yes or no for each of the five categories.

Q.4 Have your sex partners in the last 12 months been exclusively male, both male and female, or exclusively female?
Responses are exclusively male, both male and female or exclusively female.

In 1988, the overall response rate was 77.3% and resulted in 1481 interviews; 93.9% of those interviewed also responded to the sexual behavior questionnaire. The remaining 6.1% that did not respond appeared to be similar in sex, age, race and marital status but were slightly less well educated (Michael et al. 1988).

Of the 1390 individuals who filled out the sexual behavior questionnaire, 17 were excluded from subsequent analysis on the basis of their answers to the last question: 14 men who reported their partners were exclusively male, 1 woman who reported her partners were exclusively female and 2 men who reported their partners were male and female. The remaining respondents are presumed to be exclusively heterosexual. This group includes not only people who explicitly reported that their partners were of the opposite sex, but also people who reported no partners at all (93 men and 225 women) or left the last question blank (28 men and 25 women). In this group are 581 men of whom 350 are currently married with spouse present and 792 women of whom 384 are currently married with spouse present.

The purpose of this analysis is to project the number of heterosexual partners that might be contacted by an infected person taking into account age, sex and marital status. Ideally, these calculations should utilize the number of new sexual partners each year. Data on all sexual partners in the past year considerably overestimate the number of new partners. We choose to discard apparently steady sexual partners and focus on non-steady sexual partners. Operationally, we define the annual number of non-steady partners to be one less than the total number of partners (see Q.1 in Table 1) if there is a regular partner (see Q.2 in Table 1). The annual numbers of non-steady partners as a function of age for married men, unmarried men, married women and unmarried women form the basis for projecting the risk of spreading HIV. Ultimately, a full analysis of heterosexual contacts must address long-term relationships, but the limited nature of the GSS dataset does not permit this.

Before constructing an annual number of non-steady partners, it is necessary to impute values to fill in some gaps in responses to particular questions. However, the common practice of imputing a single value does not capture the sensitivity of conclusions to the use of imputation; a modest number of multiple imputations is recommended for this purpose (Rubin 1987). Selection of the number of multiple imputations must weigh the information to be gained against the time and effort taken to analyze an additional imputed dataset. As a compromise, this analysis will use three imputations.

The first type of gap is a missing answer to Q.1 or Q.2. For each missing answer, a matching pool of questionnaires form a sample of possible answers which can be imputed to the missing answer. The matching process utilizes responses to Q.1, Q.2 and Q.3, where the responses to Q.3 are abbreviated to a single "yes" if there is a "yes" response in any of the five categories (details in Appendix). Table 2 shows the results of imputations for missing data for males. Since imputation is performed three times, all imputed items have three values. The ID is the public use tape identification number of the respondent in the 1988 GSS. The "*" for Q.1 means that imputation for an interval response was performed (see Table 4). Table 3 shows the results of imputations for missing data for females. Females are treated similarly except that two unknown ages must also be filled in (details in Appendix).

The second type of imputation is used to handle interval responses to Q.1. These include 5-10, 11-20, 21-100 and 100+. Clearly, in order to take averages, some number must be assigned to the interval data for more than

Table 2

Imputed Missing Data for Males

ID	Q.1	Q.2	Q.3
213	1,1,1	Yes	No Answer
444	1,1,1	Yes	No Answer
631	1,1,1	Yes	No Answer
1264	2,2,2	Yes	Yes
1327	3,3,2	Yes	Yes
234	1	Yes,Yes,Yes	No Answer
335	1	Yes,Yes,Yes	No Answer
714	1	Yes,Yes,Yes	No Answer
1006	5-10*	Yes,No,No	Yes
1062	1	Yes,Yes,Yes	No Answer

Table 3

Imputed Missing Data for Females

ID	Age	Q.1	Q.2	Q.3
39	55	1,1,1	Yes	No Answer
53	26	1,1,1	Yes	No Answer
931	55	1,1,1	Yes	No Answer
1170	28	1,1,1	Yes	No Answer
29	73,65,43	0	No Answer	No Answer
192	20,44,27	1	Yes	No Answer
365	54	2	Yes,Yes,Yes	No Answer
429	48	1	Yes,Yes,Yes	No Answer
763	61	1	Yes,Yes,Yes	No Answer
976	31	1	Yes,Yes,Yes	No Answer
1091	29	1	Yes,Yes,Yes	No Answer
1148	20	2	No,Yes,Yes	Yes

four partners. To make this assignment, we assume that the underlying distribution for large numbers of partners, n, decays as n^{-3}. There is some justification for this exponent based on Kinsey data (Colgate et al. 1988), but this choice is best considered as a reasonable attempt to characterize the underlying variation in the absence of good models. The distribution was truncated at 500 partners and a constant term was added to fit the GSS data on numbers of partners. Without the constant term, the theoretical distribution would have placed too little probability on having very large numbers of partners (details in Appendix). The resulting distribution for males is proportional to $(5.1 + n)^{-3}$ and the resulting distribution for females is proportional to $(3.2 + n)^{-3}$. For each of the intervals 5-10, 11-20, 21-100 and 101-500, the conditional distribution for that interval was used for sampling (details in Appendix). Table 4 shows the results of three imputations for males. The "*" for Q.2 means that imputation for a missing response was performed (see Table 2). Females are treated similarly in Table 5. The algorithm for missing data for Q.1 also drew from the full partner distribution from 5 to 500 in the event that the initial selection of an imputed partner number was not 1,2,3 or 4; however, that event never occurred.

Table 4

Imputed Interval Data for Males

ID	Q.1	Q.1 Imputed	Q.2	Q.3
10	11-20	19,11,17	No	Yes
56	5-10	6,9,7	Yes	Yes
87	5-10	5,6,6	Yes	Yes
117	5-10	5,5,6	Yes	Yes
149	11-20	11,12,15	No	No Answer
152	100+	130,173,109	Yes	Yes
153	11-20	16,11,12	No	Yes
172	5-10	8,6,9	Yes	Yes
318	5-10	9,5,7	No	No Answer
466	21-100	29,44,26	No	Yes
516	5-10	7,6,5	No	Yes
565	5-10	5,5,5	Yes	Yes
578	5-10	9,5,8	Yes	Yes
580	5-10	5,7,9	No	Yes
607	5-10	7,6,7	Yes	Yes
667	5-10	10,9,5	Yes	Yes
727	5-10	7,8,6	No	Yes
832	21-100	39,31,21	Yes	No Answer
834	21-100	24,22,58	Yes	Yes
1006	5-10	7,6,8	*	Yes
1188	5-10	5,5,5	Yes	Yes
1426	5-10	7,5,9	No	No Answer
1444	5-10	5,7,5	Yes	Yes
1452	5-10	7,8,6	Yes	Yes

Table 5

Imputed Interval Data for Females

ID	Q.1	Q.1 Imputed	Q.2	Q.3
113	21-100	31,27,25	Yes	No Answer
312	5-10	5,7,5	Yes	No Answer
945	5-10	8,5,5	No	Yes
1142	5-10	8,5,5	Yes	Yes
1160	5-10	6,5,6	Yes	Yes
1420	11-20	13,13,20	Yes	No Answer

The annual number of non-steady partners by age, sex and marital status is calculated by treating each imputation as a different version of the dataset. That is, all of the first, second and third imputations for a response are taken as the first, second and third versions of the dataset, respectively. Consequently, every empirical relationship has three different versions. It is clear from inspection of all of the datasets that the dependence of the annual number of non-steady partners on age is not the same for married and unmarried people. As an illustration, Table 6 shows the results of the first imputation for younger married and unmarried males. The form (β_0 exp (- β_1 * age)) is chosen to express the rela-

Table 6

Distribution of Annual Number of Non-Steady Partners
First Imputed Dataset

Age	Unmarried Males Non-Steady Partners					Married Males Non-Steady Partners				
	0	1-2	3-4	5+	All	0	1-2	3-4	5+	All
<22	19	11	7	10	47	4	0	1	0	5
23-27	16	14	9	2	41	22	3	0	0	25
28-32	25	5	2	1	33	38	0	0	0	38
33-37	8	5	2	1	16	47	1	0	1	49
38-42	15	9	3	1	28	49	2	0	0	51
43-47	8	5	1	0	14	35	1	1	0	37
48-52	2	1	1	1	5	17	2	0	0	19
53-57	2	2	0	0	4	21	1	0	1	23
Total	95	52	25	16	188	233	10	2	2	247

Table 7

Regression Estimates for Annual Number of Non-Steady Partners

	β_0	$SE(\beta_0)$	β_1	$SE(\beta_1)$
Unmarried Males	6.3324	3.1855	.04130	.01903
	6.8321	3.7186	.04541	.02103
	4.0002	1.9757	.02476	.01657
Unmarried Females	2.2415	.7214	.04199	.01071
	2.0760	.6383	.04115	.01013
	2.0483	.7531	.03930	.01195
Married Males	.0504	1.1386	.00882	.02273
	.0523	1.5175	.01156	.03029
	.07165	.9549	.00717	.01906
Married Females	.03877	.2330	.00186	.00487
	.02058	.2062	.00215	.00431
	.03967	.1887	.00149	.00395

tionship for the unmarried males and females, while the form (β_0 + β_1* age) is chosen for married males and females. Nonlinear and linear regression procedures in SAS (SAS 1985) were used to estimate the parameters β_0 and β_1 and their corresponding standard errors (Table 7). Figure 1 graphs the results for males which clearly show the difference between the unmarried and the married. Figure 2 likewise graphs the results for females. Although females, on average, report fewer partners, the dependence on age is similar in shape to that of males. In particular, note that there appears to be a strong decline with age for unmarried people but relatively little dependence on age (if anything, a slight rise) for married people.

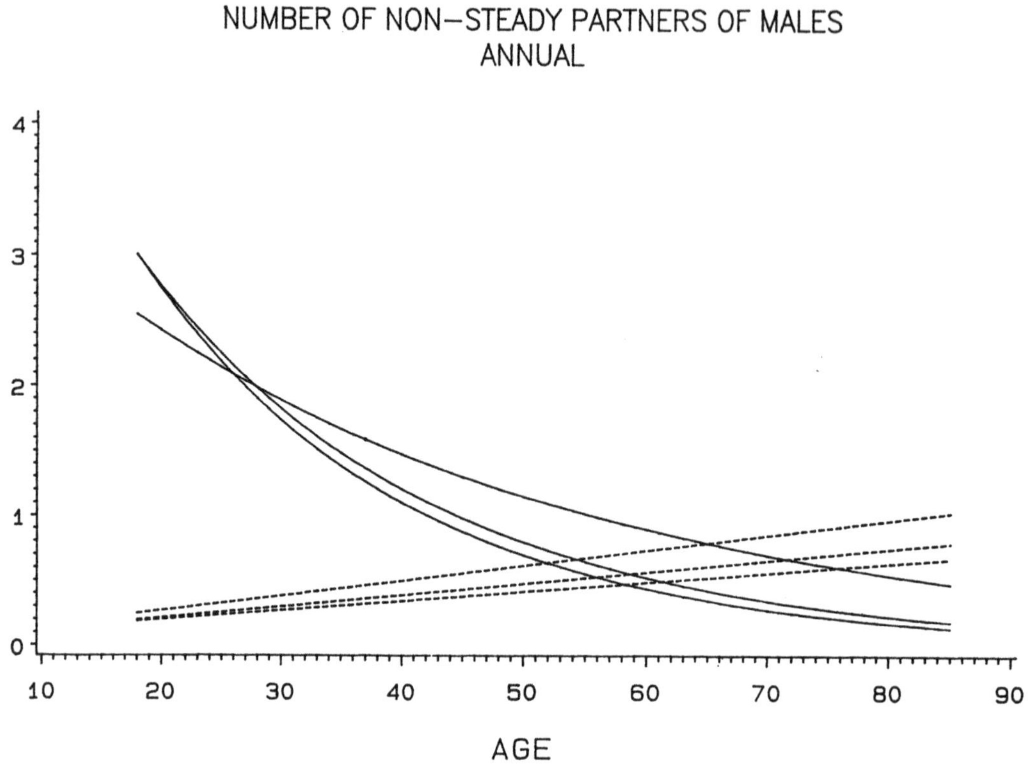

Figure 1. Curves showing the number of annual non-steady partners of males by age, estimated by fitting curves to number of non-steady partners as a function of age. For unmarried (——) and married (----), the curves are given for 3 imputed data sets.

3. Multi-State Life Table

Projections of the risk of spread of HIV cumulate possible exposures over time. However, since sexual behavior in both men and women varies by age and marital status, a dynamic model of these factors is required. The multi-state life table provides a framework for characterizing transitions in marital status and age for the U.S. population.

The approach is to combine age-specific transitions between married and unmarried states with a mortality schedule (Schoen 1975; Schoen and Land 1979). For each sex separately, it is possible to calculate the probability of being alive and married, alive and unmarried or dead at a certain age conditional on a starting age and marital status. The sources of data are national rates of mortality, marriage and divorce for 1985,

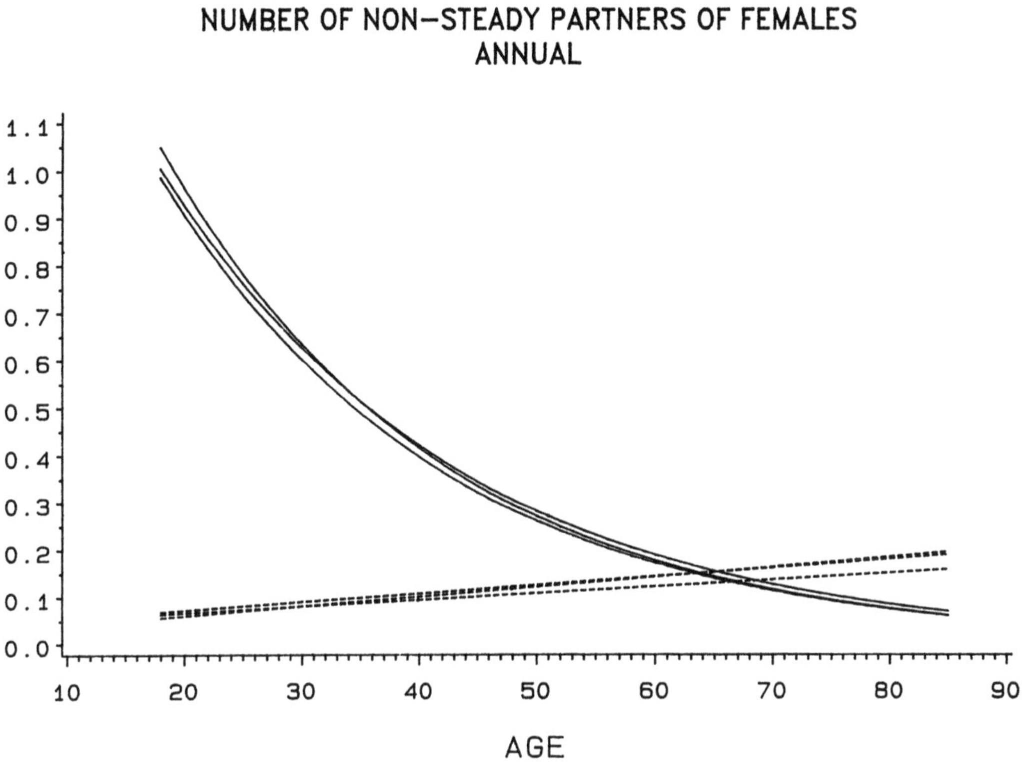

Figure 2. Curves showing the number of annual non-steady partners of females by age, estimated by fitting curves to number of non-steady partners as a function of age. For unmarried (——) and married (----), the curves are given for 3 imputed data sets.

the most recent year for which data are available. The mortality rates are provided in single-year age groups and are used regardless of marital status (National Center for Health Statistics 1988a). The marriage (National Center for Health Statistics 1988b) and divorce (National Center for Health Statistics 1989) rates are provided in five-year age groups; in this analysis, the five-year average is applied to each year in the age interval. Widowhood rates are constructed using mortality rates. For married men, the widowhood rate is the rate of mortality for women two years younger. For married women, the widowhood rate is the rate of mortality for men two years older. More details can be found in the Appendix.

The focus is on 18-year-olds because, among adults, they offer the greatest potential for heterosexual spread of HIV. For males at age 18, the probability of being alive and married at subsequent ages can depend on whether they are initially married or unmarried (Figure 3). The depen-

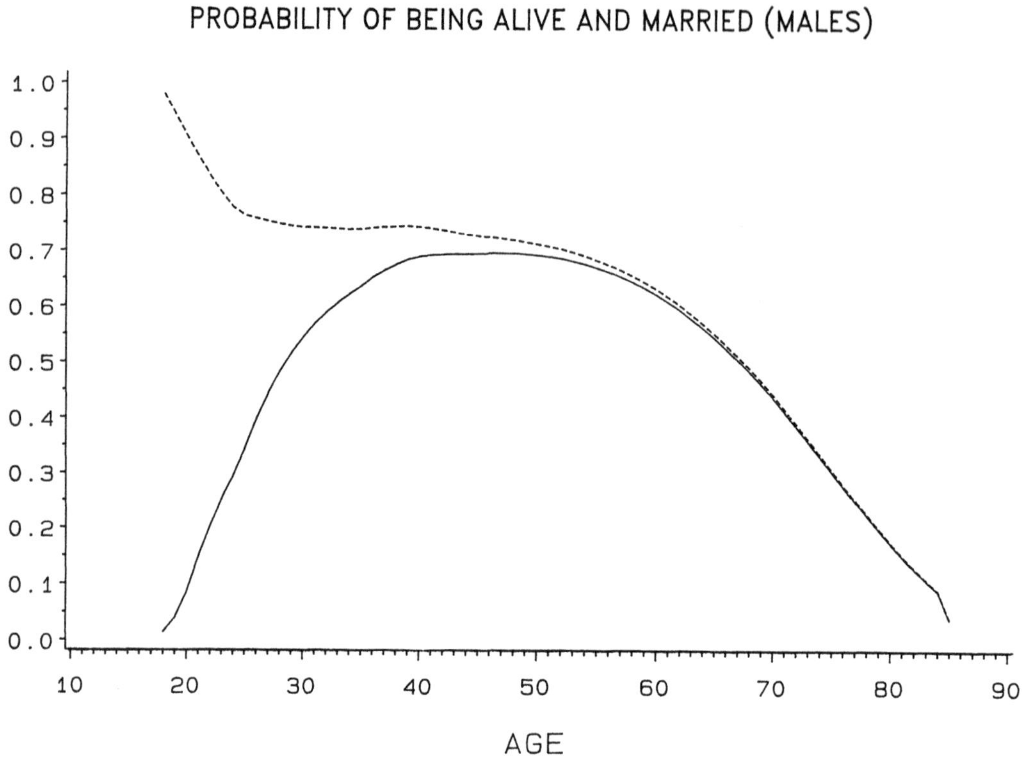

Figure 3. Curves showing the probability that an unmarried male aged 18 (———) and a married male aged 18 (----) will be alive and in the married state at subsequent ages. The probabilities are calculated from a multi-state life table constructed with 3 states: unmarried, married and dead.

dence on the initial state lasts for decades. The probability of being alive and unmarried at subsequent ages complements the previous picture (Figure 4). Note that the probabilities of being alive and married or alive and unmarried both decline at older ages because of the growing probability of death. For females at age 18, the probability of being married or unmarried at subsequent ages can depend on whether they are initially married or unmarried (Figures 5,6). As with males, the dependence on the initial state lasts for decades.

4. Heterosexual Partners at Risk

All heterosexual partners of an HIV-infected individual are presumed to be at risk of HIV infection. The cumulative number of heterosexual

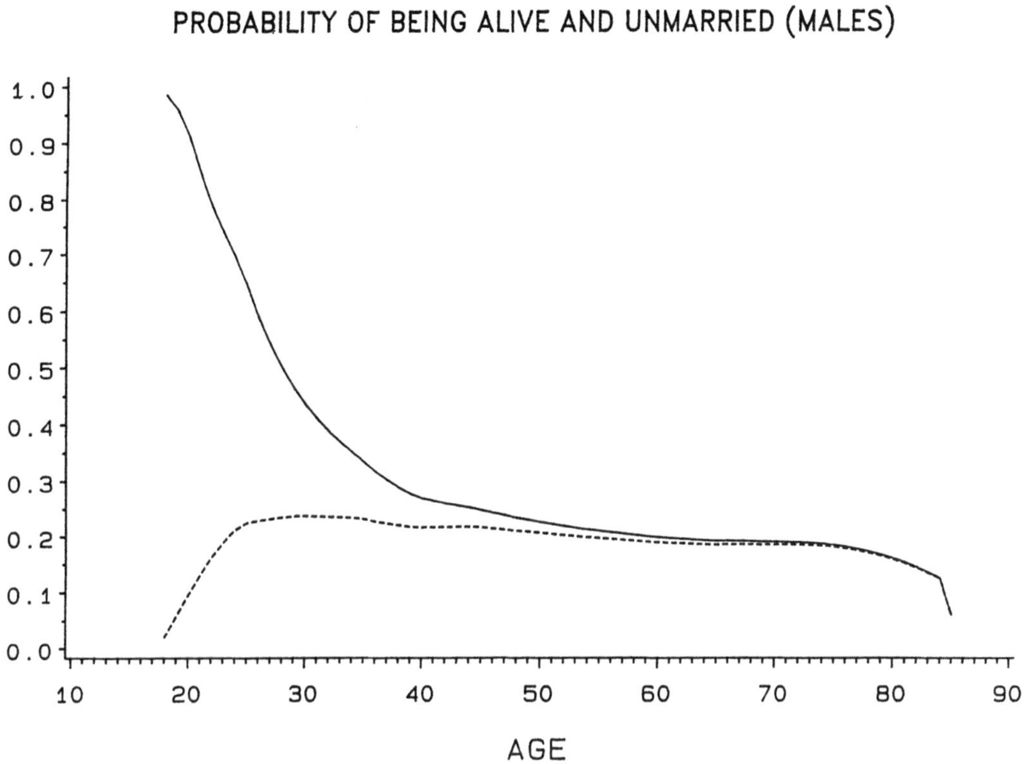

Figure 4. Curves showing the probability that an unmarried male aged 18 (———) and a married male aged 18 (----) will be alive and in the unmarried state at subsequent ages. The probabilities are calculated from a multi-state life table constructed with 3 states: unmarried, married and dead.

partners at risk is estimated from projections of marital status, the annual number of non-steady partners and the duration of infectivity. The projection includes non-steady partners acquired while married and non-steady partners acquired while unmarried. More details can be found in the Appendix.

Although these calculations can be performed for any age group, we restrict our attention to the 18-year-olds because they provide the greatest potential for HIV spread. Figures 7 and 8 show, for males and females, respectively, the cumulative number of non-steady partners up to a given age for a person infected at age 18. The calculations are performed both with and without marital transitions. It is clear that the cumulative number of non-steady partners by any age depends on whether or not a person is married at age 18. However, the difference between married

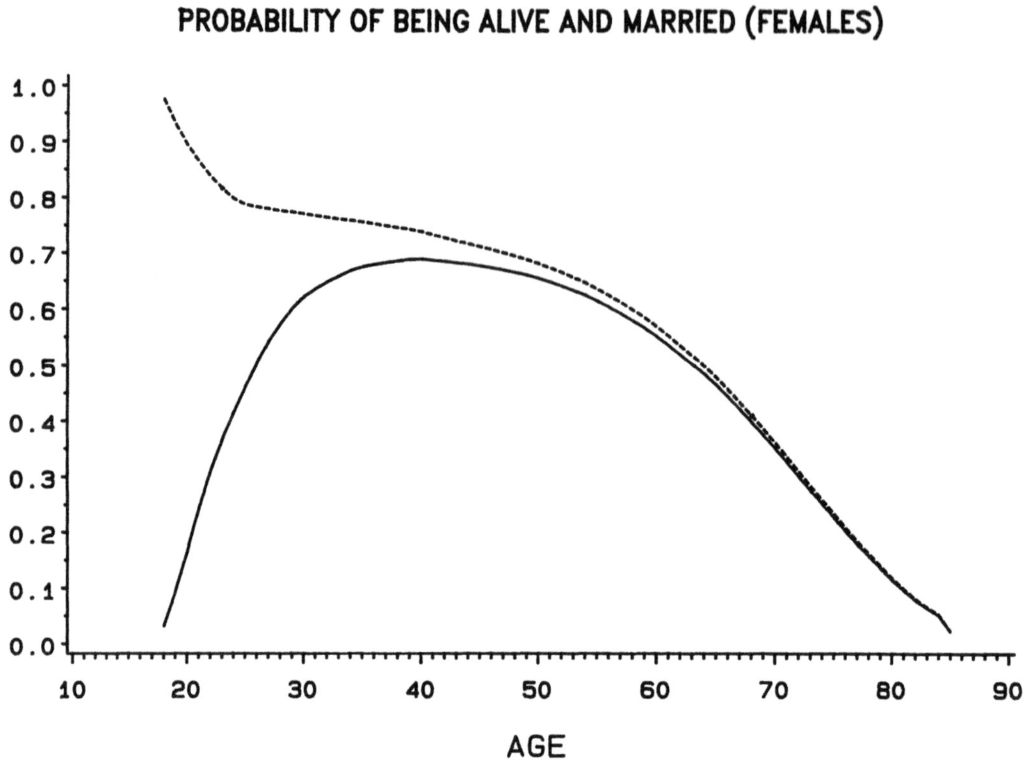

Figure 5. Curves showing the probability that an unmarried female aged 18 (——) and a married female aged 18 (----) will be alive and in the married state at subsequent ages. The probabilities are calculated from a multi-state life table constructed with 3 states: unmarried, married and dead.

and unmarried individuals is greater in the absence of marital transitions. Overall, the patterns for males and females are similar except that the total number of partners is considerably lower for females than for males.

5. Basic Reproductive Rate

The basic reproductive rate of infection measures the average number of infections produced by an infected individual when virtually everyone is susceptible. This number must be greater than unity for an epidemic to spread. This concept can profitably be used to understand the epidemic potential of HIV (Anderson and May 1988). In its simplest form, the basic

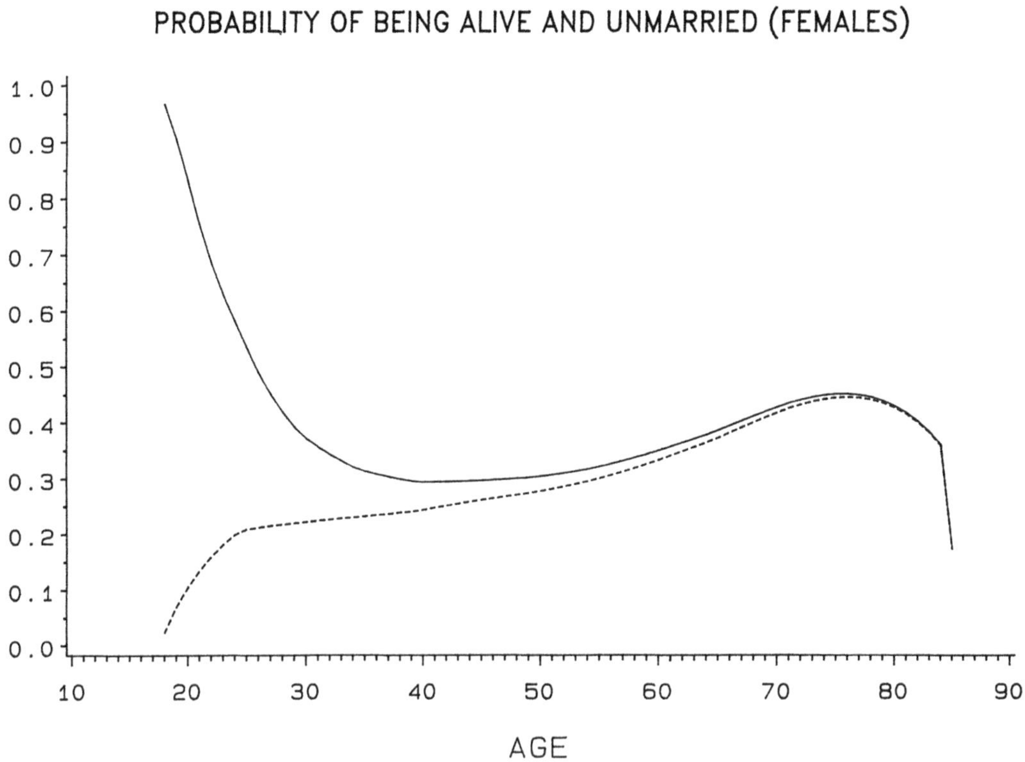

Figure 6. Curves showing the probability that an unmarried female aged 18 (———) and a married female aged 18 (----) will be alive and in the unmarried state at subsequent ages. The probabilities are calculated from a multi-state life table constructed with 3 states: unmarried, married and dead.

reproductive rate is the product of three components: 1) the average number of new sexual partners per unit time, 2) the average probability that an infected person will infect his/her partner over the course of their relationship, and 3) the average duration of infectiousness. In applying this concept to heterosexual spread, the direct contacts must be extended to include partners of partners. That is, the basic reproductive rate is the number of new male infectives generated by a male infective or the number of new female infectives generated by a female infective (Hethcote and Yorke 1984). The basic reproductive rate must be further qualified to take into account heterogeneity in the population.

We examine the potential for HIV spread specifically for the most sexually active group of adults, 18-year-old unmarried males. A critical parameter is the duration of infectivity. This analysis uses 10 years,

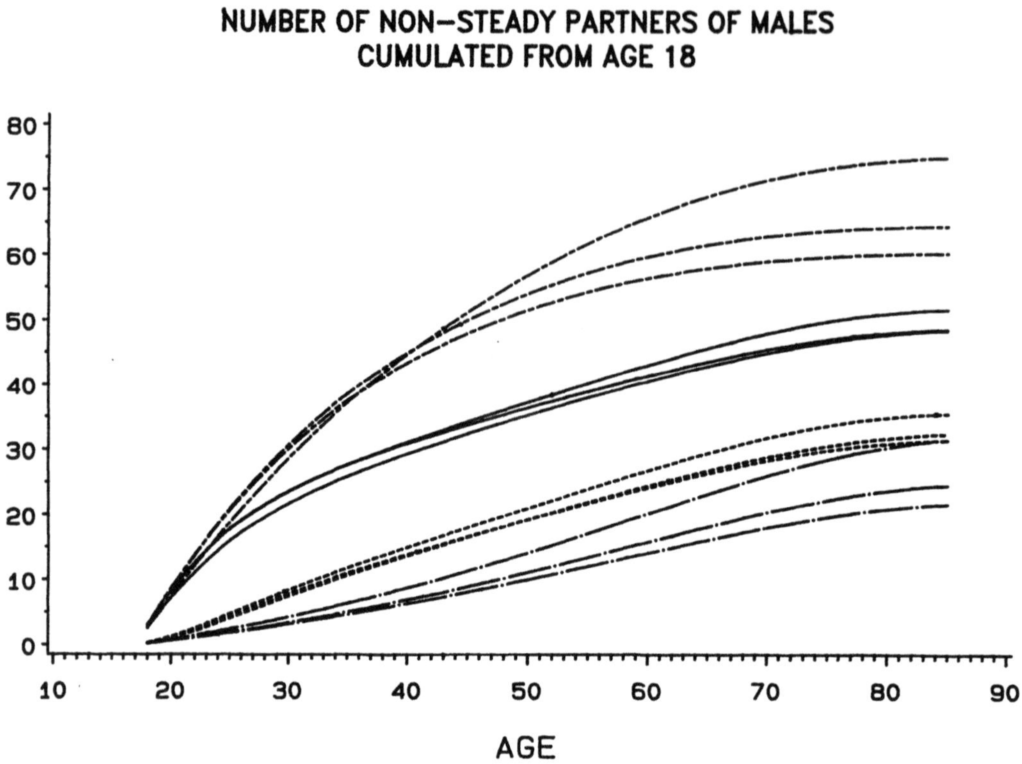

Figure 7. Curves showing the number of non-steady sexual partners of males, cumulated from age 18 to subsequent ages. The second (——) and third (----) set of curves from the top are for those unmarried and married at age 18, respectively, and take marital transitions into account. The curves at the top (– — –) and the bottom (·——·) are also for those unmarried and married at age 18, respectively, but marital transitions are not incorporated.

which allows for some lengthening beyond current estimates of a 7 to 8 year incubation period (Anderson and May 1988). We thus use behavioral data and the multi-state life table to calculate the number of non-steady partners of non-steady partners over 10 years. (More details on the computation may be found in the Appendix). An unmarried male of age 18 is expected to have around 20 non-steady female partners by the time he is age 27 (20.4293, 20.3252 and 18.4908 in the 3 imputations). Assuming those partners are unmarried females of age 18, then each female partner will have around 6 non-steady male partners over a period of 10 years (i.e., through age 27) from the time of contact with the index male (6.4484, 6.0607 and 6.2259 in the 3 imputations). Taken all together, the number

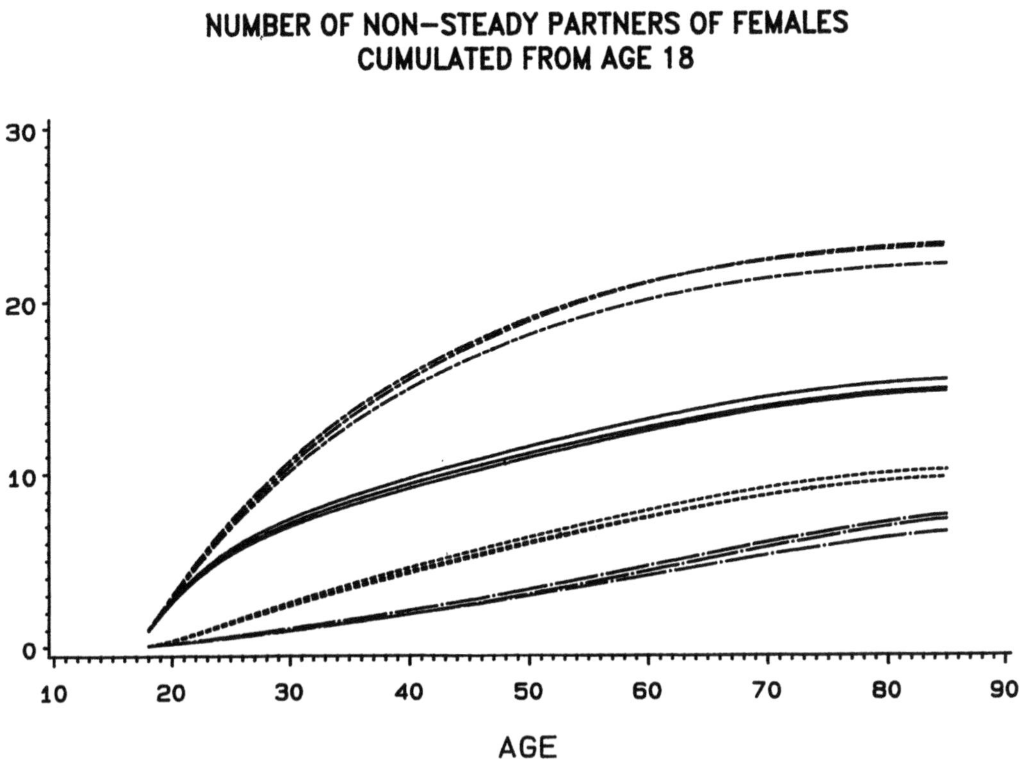

Figure 8. Curves showing the number of non-steady sexual partners of females, cumulated from age 18 to subsequent ages. The second (——) and third (----) set of curves from the top are for those unmarried and married at age 18, respectively, and take marital transitions into account. The curves at the top (– — –) and the bottom (·——·) are also for those unmarried and married at age 18, respectively, but marital transitions are not incorporated.

of males indirectly contacted by an 18-year-old unmarried HIV-infected male is around 120 (131.74, 123.18 and 115.12 in the 3 imputations). However, an approximate 30% reduction is obtained by assuming that, as the 18-year-old male ages, his female partners are the same age (but still unmarried). The number of males indirectly contacted is then around 85 (93.54, 87.54 and 81.07 in the 3 imputations). A further reduction could be obtained by including married female partners. Thus, choices of sexual contacts substantially affect the potential for HIV spread.

In the absence of detailed information on the patterns of sexual contacts, a rough idea of epidemic potential emerges from the observation that the average number of heterosexual males at risk of HIV infection from an 18-year-old unmarried male is at most on the order of 100 males.

The remaining parameter of the basic reproductive rate is the product of per-partner probabilities of male-to-female and female-to-male transmission. This quantity would have to exceed .01 in order for the epidemic to spread via non-steady heterosexual partners.

Current estimates of the probability of heterosexual transmission suggest this is unlikely. The average transmission probability for long-term heterosexual relationships is around 0.1 to 0.2 (Anderson and May 1988). It is not unreasonable to expect the probability of transmission for short-term relationships to be smaller by an order of magnitude. By this reasoning, the product of male-to-female and female-to-male transmission probabilities is .0001 to .0004. An alternative line of argument adopts a probability of .002 per unprotected sexual act for a heterosexual couple (Dietz 1988). This too would suggest a probability of transmission on the order of .01 for short-term relationships, which corresponds to .0001 for the product of probabilities. Thus, if a random sample of 18-year-old unmarried U.S. males were infected with HIV, current estimates suggest that a heterosexual HIV epidemic would be unlikely.

6. Future Studies

The analysis in this paper was designed to take advantage of available data on recent U.S. sexual behavior and marriage formation. Their limitations should provide the spur for improvements in future studies. A major assumption is that the respondents to the questionnaires are a good sample of the U.S. population. Bias in the non-respondents could be a serious problem. There could also be bias in the pattern of missing data for those who did respond. For example, although the prevalence of male homosexuality in the 1988 GSS survey is consistent with a 1970 survey, overall levels are probably under-reported (Fay et al. 1989). Even where responses are provided, problems remain. Interval responses had to be converted into a number under an assumption of a particular distribution of the number of annual partners. The responses themselves could also be inaccurate due to deliberate or inadvertent misreporting. For example, it is curious that the highest partner counts for a male and female are provided by middle-aged married people although, as a group, young unmarried people have the most partners. And, of course, the survey totally excludes adolescents. Further, the form of the marriage model ignores effects of marital history and the multiple groups within the unmarried population. It is especially poor for widowhood, which does not generate a public record. The generic problem of using period data to project the experience of cohorts is also well known (Keyfitz 1988).

The very nature and duration of sexual partnerships is another major area of concern. Although marital status has a strong association with behavior in the survey, the link between formal marriage and cohabitation has been growing weaker (U.S. Bureau of the Census 1988; Bumpass and Sweet 1988). Uncertainty about the type and frequency of sexual practices could be partially resolved through a proposed national survey on health and sexual behavior although political opposition may block the survey (Specter 1989). It has also been shown here and elsewhere (Hyman and Stanley 1988; Jacquez et al. 1988; Blythe and Castillo-Chavez 1989) that the selection of sexual partners influences the dynamics of spread. Such effects could be very important since it appears that the potential for heterosexual spread in the U.S. is at or below the critical threshold. Near the threshold, small changes in the conditions can have a large effect (Dietz 1988). Patterns of self-selection also create subpopulations for which the dynamics may be quite different from the larger population. For example, marriage rates in the U.S. black population have been diverging from rates in the U.S. white population (Schoen and Kluegel 1988). Formal modeling of these processes must take into account the "two-sex" problem in which "per-male" and "per-female" rates of male-female pairing events may produce inconsistent results (Yellin and Samuelson 1977; Schoen 1983).

Finally, the problem of uncertainty and variability in the likelihood of transmission remains. For example, there is growing evidence that infectivity may increase late in the course of HIV infection (Curran et al. 1988). Several have pointed out the corresponding potential for a delay in the appearance of a heterosexual epidemic and for the estimates of heterosexual infectivity to be misleadingly low (Hyman and Stanley 1988; May and Anderson 1987; DeGruttola and Mayer 1988). Further, the variable pattern of infectivity interacts with age-dependent patterns of partner selection. For instance, an 18-year-old infected male might be most likely to infect someone when he is 27 years old. The role of potentiating co-factors, such as other sexually transmitted diseases, is also cause for concern (Pepin et al. 1989). Recent increases in syphilis in the U.S. are particularly disturbing (Centers for Disease Control 1988). Thus, while preliminary evidence suggests that a heterosexual epidemic of HIV is unlikely in the U.S., more attention needs to be paid to elucidating the behavioral and biological factors that determine the dynamics of HIV transmission.

APPENDIX

A. Imputation for Missing Data

Individuals who did not answer any of the questions on sexual behavior described in Table 1 were excluded from further analysis. The 17 individuals who directly reported homosexuality or bisexuality were also excluded. For the remaining 1373 individuals (581 men and 792 women), imputations were performed for non-responses to two of the questions on sexual behavior and for unknown ages. It should be noted that a person who reported zero sexual partners in the last 12 months did not have to answer any of the other questions on sexual behavior. That is, blanks were not considered to be non-responses.

Of the 1373 respondents analyzed, 5 men and 4 women did not answer Q.1. These 9 individuals were matched to other respondents based on gender and the responses to Q.2 and Q.3. There were 3 separate matching groups. The first group is men who answered yes to Q.2 but did not answer yes to any of the 5 parts of Q.3 (370 men who responded to Q.1 and 3 men who did not). The second group is men who answered yes to Q.2 and to at least 1 of the 5 parts of Q.3 (60 men who responded to Q.1 and 2 men who did not). The third group is women who answered yes to Q.2 but did not answer yes to any of the 5 parts of Q.3 (482 women who responded to Q.1 and 4 women who did not). For each matching group, the number of respondents reporting 1, 2, 3, 4 and 4+ partners were counted. The resulting empirical distributions were sampled using random numbers in the interval [0,1] generated by the "S" package (Becker and Chambers 1984). For each missing response, three values from the corresponding empirical distribution were drawn. The category 4+ was so rare that it was never selected; if it had been selected, imputation for the interval 5 to 500 would have been performed as described in the next section of the Appendix. The results of the imputation process are shown in the first 5 lines of Table 2 and the first 4 lines of Table 3.

Of the 1373 respondents analyzed, 5 men and 6 women did not answer Q.2. These 11 individuals were matched to other respondents based on gender and the responses to Q.1 and Q.3. There were 5 separate matching groups. The first group is men who reported exactly 1 partner and did not answer yes to any of the 5 parts of Q.3 (363 men who responded to Q.2 and 4 men who did not). The second group is men who reported 5-10 partners and answered yes to at least 1 of the 5 parts of Q.3 (14 men who responded to Q.2 and 1 man who did not). The third group is women who reported exactly 1 partner and did not answer yes to any of the 5 parts of Q.3 (474 women who responded to Q.2 and 4 women who did not). The fourth group is women who reported exactly 2 partners and did not answer yes to any of the 5 parts of Q.3 (15 women who responded to Q.2 and 1 woman who did not). The fifth group is women who reported exactly 2 partners and answered yes to at least 1 of the 5 parts of Q.3 (27 women who responded to Q.2 and 1 woman who did not). For each matching group, the number of respondents answering yes or no to Q.2 was counted. The resulting empirical distributions were sampled using random numbers in the interval [0,1] generated by the "S" package (Becker and Chambers 1984). For each missing response, three values from the corresponding empirical distribution were drawn. The results of the imputation process are shown in the last 5 lines of Table 2 and the last 6 lines of Table 3.

Age was missing for 2 of the 792 female respondents. Each woman with a missing age was matched to a group of other female respondents based on marital status and responses to Q.1 and Q.2. The first group is married women who reported no sexual partners (35 women of known age and 1 woman of unknown age). The second group is never married women who reported exactly 1 sexual partner and answered yes to Q.2 (52 women of known age and 1 woman of unknown age). For each matching group, the number of respondents in single-year ages was counted. The resulting empirical distributions were sampled using random numbers in the interval [0,1] generated by the "S" package (Becker and Chambers 1984). For each missing age, three values from the corresponding empirical distribution were drawn. The results of the imputation process are shown in lines 5 and 6 of Table 3.

B. Imputation for Interval Data

Imputations were performed for interval responses to Q.1. The intervals 5-10, 11-20, and 21-100 were replaced by numbers from 5 to 10, 11 to 20, and 21 to 100, respectively. The interval 100+ was truncated to 101-500 and handled accordingly. For males and females separately, the underlying distribution of partners was assumed to be proportional to the form $(a+n)^{-3}$, $n=5,6,\ldots,500$, where n is the annual number of sexual partners. The parameter a is chosen to minimize the Chi-square statistic for the four interval categories. The parameter a is 5.1 and 3.2 for males and females, respectively. For each interval response, the conditional discrete distribution from the lower bound to the upper bound of the interval was sampled 3 times using random numbers in the interval [0,1] generated by the "S" package (Becker and Chambers 1984). The results of the imputation process are shown in Table 4 and Table 5.

C. Multi-State Life Table

The multi-state life table combines age-specific transitions between the unmarried state (state 1) and the married state (state 2) with an age-specific mortality schedule. A separate life table is constructed for each sex using 1985 U.S. data on marriage rates, divorce rates and mortality rates. As described in the text, widowhood rates are constructed from mortality rates. The results of the life table are expressed in terms of ${}_{a}^{i}\Pi_{x}^{j}$, the probability that a person in state i at age x will be in state j at age x+a. The calculations are for single years of age with a maximum age of 86 years. The formulae are provided in Equations 5.6, 5.12, 5.13 and 6.1 of Schoen and Land (1979). Figures 3 and 5 show ${}_{a}^{1}\Pi_{18}^{2}$ and ${}_{a}^{2}\Pi_{18}^{2}$ for males and females, respectively. Figures 4 and 6 show ${}_{a}^{1}\Pi_{18}^{1}$ and ${}_{a}^{2}\Pi_{18}^{1}$ for males and females, respectively.

D. Cumulative Number of Non-Steady Partners

The annual number of non-steady partners is calculated for each age, sex and marital status according to the fitted relationships whose coefficients are listed in Table 7. For the sake of simplicity, the following discussion will be in terms of males. If we let n^{i}_{x+a} be the number of non-steady partners for a male of age x+a in state i, then the cumulative number of non-steady partners up to age x+a for a male who is initially in state i at age x is

$$\sum_{y=0}^{a} {}_{y}^{i}N_{x}, \qquad i=1,2,$$

where

$${}_{a}^{1}N_{x} = {}_{a}^{1}\Pi_{x}^{1}\; n^{1}_{x+a} + {}_{a}^{1}\Pi_{x}^{2}\; n^{2}_{x+a}$$

and

$${}_{a}^{2}N_{x} = {}_{a}^{2}\Pi_{x}^{1}\; n^{1}_{x+a} + {}_{a}^{2}\Pi_{x}^{2}\; n^{2}_{x+a}.$$

The results for the initial age of 18 years are shown for males in Figure 7. Another set of values, neglecting the marital status transitions, are also shown in Figure 7. Without the marital transitions, the probabilities of survival from age 18 are used to generate the probability of being in the same state at subsequent ages; there is no chance of switching states. The results repeated for females are shown in Figure 8.

E. Non-Steady Partners of Non-Steady Partners

The calculation of the spread of HIV by unmarried 18-year-old males depends on

$$\sum_{y=0}^{9} {}_{y}^{1}N_{18}^{m} ,$$

the number of female partners cumulated over 10 years. The spread of HIV also depends on the male partners of the female partners. If all the female partners chosen are 18-year-old unmarried females, then the cumulative number of males indirectly contacted by an 18-year-old unmarried HIV-infected male is

$$\left(\sum_{y=0}^{9} {}_{y}^{1}N_{18}^{m}\right)\left(\sum_{y=0}^{9} {}_{y}^{1}N_{18}^{f}\right).$$

If, instead, the female partners chosen are unmarried females of the same age as the male, then the cumulative number of males indirectly contacted by an 18-year-old unmarried male is

$$\sum_{y=0}^{9} \left({}_{y}^{1}N_{18}^{m} \left(\sum_{z=0}^{9} {}_{z}^{1}N_{18+y}^{f} \right)\right).$$

ACKNOWLEDGMENTS

We thank Terri Singer and Judy Gehret of the Hopkins Population Center for providing bibliographic assistance and computer advice and Bettie Martin for carefully preparing the camera-ready copy. We also thank anonymous reviewers for helpful criticism. P. Sankara Sarma was supported by the Hewlett Foundation.

REFERENCES

Anderson, R.M. and R.M. May. (1988). Epidemiological parameters of HIV transmission. Nature 333, 514-519.

Becker, R.A. and J.M. Chambers. (1984). S: An Interactive Environment for Data Analysis and Graphics, Wadsworth, Belmont, California.

Blythe, S.P. and C. Castillo-Chavez. (1989). Like-with-like preference and sexual mixing models. Math. Biosci. In press.

Bumpass, L.L. and J.A. Sweet. (1988). Preliminary evidence on cohabitation. National Survey of Families and Households Working Paper No. 2. Center for Demography and Ecology, University of Wisconsin-Madison.

Centers for Disease Control. (1988). Syphilis and congenital syphilis-United States, 1985-1988. MMWR 37, 486-489.

Colgate, S.A., E.A. Stanley, J.M. Hyman, S.P. Layne and C. Qualls. (1988). A behavior based model of the initial growth of AIDS in the United States. Los Alamos National Laboratory Report LA-UR-88-2396.

Curran, J.W., H.W. Jaffe, A.M. Hardy, W.M. Morgan, R.M. Selik and T.J. Dondero. (1988). Epidemiology of HIV infection and AIDS in the United States. Science 239, 610-616.

Davis, J.A. and T.W. Smith. (1988). General Social Surveys, 1972-1988: Cumulative Codebook, NORC, Chicago.

DeGruttola, V. and K.H. Mayer. (1988). Assessing and modeling heterosexual spread of the human immunodeficiency virus in the United States. Rev. Infect. Dis. 10, 138-150.

Dietz, K. (1988). On the transmission dynamics of HIV. Math. Biosci. 90, 397-414.

Fay, R.E., C.F. Turner, A.D. Klassen and J.H. Gagnon. (1989). Prevalence and patterns of same-gender sexual contact among men. Science 243, 338-348.

Hethcote, H.W. and J.A. Yorke. (1984). Gonorrhea Transmission Dynamics and Control. Lect. Notes in Biomathematics, Vol. 56, Springer-Verlag, Berlin.

Hyman, J.M. and E.A. Stanley. (1988). Using mathematical models to understand the AIDS epidemic. Math. Biosci. 90, 415-473.

Jacquez, J.A., C.P. Simon, J. Koopman, L. Sattenspiel and T. Perry. (1988). Modeling and analyzing HIV transmission: the effect of contact patterns. Math. Biosci. 92, 119-199.

Keyfitz, N. (1988). A Markov chain for calculating the durability of marriage. Math. Pop. Stud. 1, 101-121.

May, R.M. and R.M. Anderson. (1987). Transmission dynamics of HIV infection. Nature 326, 137-142.

Michael, R.T., E.O. Laumann, J.H. Gagnon and T.W. Smith. (1988). Number of sex partners and potential risk of sexual exposure to human immunodeficiency virus. MMWR 37, 565-568.

National Center for Health Statistics. (1988a). Vital Statistics of the United States, 1985 Life Tables, Vol. 2, Section 6, U.S. Department of

Health and Human Services, Hyattsville, Maryland.

National Center for Health Statistics. (1988b). Advance report of final marriage statistics, 1985. Monthly Vital Statistics Report, 37(1), Supplement, U.S. Department of Health and Human Services, Hyattsville, Maryland.

National Center for Health Statistics. (1989). Vital Statistics of the United States, Vol. 3, Marriage and Divorce, 1985. U.S. Department of Health and Human Services, Hyattsville, Maryland. In press.

Pepin, J., F.A. Plummer, R.C. Brunham, P. Piot, D.W. Cameron and A.R. Ronald. (1989). The interaction of HIV and other sexually transmitted diseases: an opportunity for intervention. AIDS 3, 3-9.

Rubin, D.B. (1987). Multiple Imputation for Nonresponse in Surveys. Wiley and Sons, New York.

SAS. (1985). SAS User's Guide: Statistics, Version 5 Edition. SAS, Institute, Cary, North Carolina.

Schoen, R. (1975). Constructing increment-decrement life tables. Demography 12, 313-324.

Schoen, R. (1983). Measuring the tightness of a marriage squeeze. Demography 20, 61-78.

Schoen, R. and J.R. Kluegel. (1988). The widening gap in black and white marriage rates: the impact of population composition and differential marriage propensities. Amer. Soc. Rev. 53, 895-907.

Schoen, R. and K.C. Land. (1979). A general algorithm for estimating a Markov-generated increment-decrement life table with applications to marital-status patterns. J. Amer. Stat. Assn. 74, 761-776.

Specter, M. (1989). Funds for sex survey blocked by house panel. Washington Post July 26, 1989, A3.

U.S. Bureau of the Census. (1988). Marital Status and Living Arrangements: March 1987, Current Population Reports, Series P-20, No.423, U.S. Government Printing Office, Washington, D.C.

Yellin, J. and P.A. Samuelson. (1977). Comparison of linear and nonlinear models for human population dynamics. Theor. Pop. Biol. 11, 105-126.

ON THE ROLE OF LONG INCUBATION PERIODS IN THE DYNAMICS OF ACQUIRED IMMUNODEFICIENCY SYNDROME (AIDS). PART 2: MULTIPLE GROUP MODELS.

Carlos Castillo-Chavez
Biometrics Unit
Cornell University
Ithaca, NY 14853

Kenneth L. Cooke
Department of Math.
Pomona College
Claremont, CA 91711

Wenzhang Huang
Claremont Grad. Sch.
Claremont, CA 91711

Simon A. Levin
Center for Env. Res.
Cornell University
Ithaca, NY 14853

Abstract

In this paper, we restate previously obtained results on homogeneously-mixed single-group models for HIV (human immunodeficiency virus) with distributed waiting times in the infectious class. We also present some simulations that illustrate the effects of a changing mean sexual activity in the dynamics of HIV, and formulate a single group model for a heterogeneously mixed population with continuously-distributed sexual activity. This model forms the basis for our formulation of an N-group model with arbitrary social/sexual mixing. The local stability analysis of this N-group model is discussed. A two-group example under preferred mixing that has multiple endemic equilibria is presented, as well as an example for an N-group model, under proportionate mixing, possessing multiple endemic equilibria.

1. Introduction

The social/sexual mixing structure of a population or a group of interacting populations plays a crucial role in the dynamics of disease transmission (see Kaplan *et al.* 1989; Jacquez *et al.* 1988, 1989; Sattenspiel 1987; Sattenspiel and Simon 1988; May and Anderson 1989; Hyman and Stanley 1988, 1989; Blythe and Castillo-Chavez 1989; and Castillo-Chavez and Blythe 1989). These heterogeneities, combined with the effects of the initial conditions and varying epidemiological and behavioral parameters, can significantly affect the rates of disease spread within populations and among interacting populations.

An increased qualitative understanding of the role that social dynamics, variable infectivity (and other epidemiological parameters), asymptomatic carriers, age structure, socio-economic structure, race, sexual preference, sexual behaviors (such as frequency of anal sex), sharing of needles, and intervention programs (such as the generalized use of AZT) play in the dynamics of HIV is necessary for the development, testing, and evaluation of control programs to slow down the AIDS epidemic at local and global scales.

The increased quantitative evaluation of the effects of these factors in the dynamics of HIV within and between specific populations is of importance in the generation, through transmission models, of mid- and long-term predictions of the number of AIDS cases and the number of HIV infectives among these populations. In this paper, we introduce some fairly general models that incorporate some of the important features just discussed in a systematic way. The achievement of a qualitative understanding of the dynamics of this type of model through a combination of numerical simulations and mathematical analysis would represent a very important step toward their future validation.

This paper is organized into four sections. Section 2 introduces our basic single group model for a homogeneously mixed population. Our recent analytical results are stated, and the results of a few numerical simulations are presented to illustrate the effect of a varying mean sexual activity (a function of the effective sexually-active population size) in the dynamics of HIV. Section 3 introduces heterogeneous mixing through a continuous distribution of sexual activity: i.e., we divide our population by their degree (partners per unit time) of sexual activity. This approach is sometimes equated with the construction of a multiple group model. Although this is a valid interpretation, it may not be the most useful, since epidemiological data (such as AIDS incidence) are usually collected or aggregated by other criteria such as race, geographic location, socioeconomic background, drug use, sexual preference, etc. Of course, what is needed is a mixed approach where modelers, behaviorists, and epidemiologists work together to construct "strategic" models that attempt to define the aggregation scheme (during the initial stages of research) and therefore have a direct input into experimental design (such as questionnaire development, or simply the gathering of data).

An aggregation scheme provides us with a collection of groups, each with its own distribution of sexual activity. A standard approach consists of assigning the mean sexual activity of its corresponding distribution to all members of such socially-defined groups. It is then assumed that group members mix at random within their own group, and a rule for intergroup mixing is then postulated (for a discussion on the limitations of this approach, see Sattenspiel 1987; Sattenspiel and Simon 1988). Of course, nobody prevents the modeler from constructing a more detailed multigroup model incorporating the distribution of sexual activity for each group. This last approach increases the level of detail and is important for theoretical reasons, as it allows us to determine the effects of some neglected features. However, it also has the disadvantage of increasing the number of parameters that will have to be estimated, and hence its value is diminished when we attempt to use it for predictive purposes. Since models can be used for very different purposes (see Hethcote and Yorke 1984), it is obvious that a balance has to be reached between the level of detail that one wishes to incorporate, the number of parameters that may be possible to estimate, and the effect of the level of aggregation that is considered appropriate for the question under consideration.

Section 4 states our recent analytical results for multiple group models. A key result states that multiple group models can have multiple endemic equilibria even under the assumption of proportionate mixing. These results contradict the "generalized" thinking that epidemiological models of the SIR (susceptible, infected and removed) type have at most two equilibria, an infection-free and an endemic state. Two examples, for which two endemic equilibria are possible, are included in Section 5. A detailed technical exposition of these results will be published elsewhere (see Huang *et al.* 1989).

2. Single Population Models

A sexually active homosexual population is subdivided into three groups: S (susceptible), I (HIV infectious), and A (AIDS infectious). We assume that A-individuals are sexually inactive and hence do not contribute to disease dynamics. Furthermore, we assume that sexually active individuals choose their partners at random. The demographic parameters are given by Λ, the recruitment rate into S; μ, the sexual activity removal rate; and d, the AIDS-induced mortality rate. In addition, λ, which denotes the transmission rate per infectious partner, is assumed to be given by the product of two constant parameters: i, the average proportion of contacts with an infectious individual necessary for transmission, and ϕ, the average number of contacts per sexual partner. C(T) denotes the mean number of sexual partners that an average individual has per unit time, given that the sexually active population is $T = S+I$. It is reasonable to expect that in general C(T) increases linearly for small T and saturates for large T. We further assume that the incidence rate B(t)—the number of new cases per unit time—is proportional to C(T), to S, and to the sexually active infected fraction:

$$B(t) = \lambda C(T)S(t)\frac{I(t)}{T(t)}. \tag{1}$$

The proportionality constant is given by λ (the transmission coefficient). Finally, we let P(s) denote the proportion of individuals that are infected at time t and that, if alive, are still infectious at time t+s. P(s) is nonnegative, and nonincreasing, and $P(0) = 1$. We assume that

$$\int_0^\infty P(s)ds<\infty,$$

and observe that $-P'(s)$ denotes the removal rate from group I into group A, s time units after infection. The distributed-delay model for the sexual spread of HIV/AIDS is therefore given by the following system of integro-differential equations:

$$\frac{dS(t)}{dt} = \Lambda - B(t) - \mu S(t) , \tag{2}$$

$$I(t) = I_0(t) + \int_0^t B(x)\, e^{-\mu(t-x)} P(t-x)dx , \tag{3}$$

$$A(t) = A_0(t) + A_1 e^{-dt} + \int_0^t \left\{ \int_0^\tau B(x) e^{-\mu(\tau-x)} \left[-P'(\tau-x) e^{-d(t-r)} \right] dx \right\} d\tau, \tag{4}$$

where the functions (with compact support) $I_0(t)$, $A_0(t)$, and the constant A_1, are introduced to take initial conditions into account.

This model generalizes the models developed by Anderson *et al.* (1986), Anderson and May (1987), and Blythe and Anderson (1988a). In Blythe and Anderson (1988a), a submodel was studied numerically for various survivorship functions and the local asymptotic stability analysis was completed for a specific family of survivorship functions. We (Castillo-Chavez *et al.* 1989a, b, c) have shown that this model has at most two equilibria, which correspond to the infection-free state and the endemic state. In addition, we have completed a global stability analysis of the infection-free attractor for arbitrary survivorship functions. We have only been able to study the asymptotic local stability of the endemic attractor. We present here an outline of our results.

When $P(s) = e^{-\alpha s}$, the disease-free state $\left(\frac{\Lambda}{\mu},0\right)$ is a globally asymptotically stable equilibrium if and only if the reproductive number

$$R \equiv \lambda C\left(\frac{\Lambda}{\mu}\right) \frac{1}{\mu+\alpha} \leq 1. \tag{5}$$

If $R > 1$, there is a unique endemic state, which is a global attractor for all positive solutions.

When $P(s)$ is arbitrary, the infection-free state is a global attractor whenever the reproductive number

$$R = \lambda C\left(\frac{\Lambda}{\mu}\right) \int_0^\infty e^{-\mu s} P(s) ds \leq 1; \tag{6}$$

if $R > 1$, then the limiting system

$$\frac{dS(t)}{dt} = \Lambda - B(t) - \mu S(t) , \tag{7}$$

$$I(t) = \int_{-\infty}^t B(x)\, e^{-\mu(t-x)} P(t-x)dx , \tag{8}$$

has a unique endemic state. This endemic state is locally asymptotically stable, provided that

$$\frac{dM(T)}{dT} \leq 0, \text{ where } M(T) = \frac{C(T)}{T}.$$

The meaning of local asymptotic stability for this type of model can be found in Thieme and Castillo-Chavez (1989a).

In order to see the effects of C(T) on the dynamics of model (2)-(4), we simulate a special case, letting P(s) denote a generalized gamma distribution. With this selection, our model reduces to the following system of ordinary differential equations:

$$\frac{dS(t)}{dt} = \Lambda - B(t) - \mu S(t) , \tag{9}$$

$$\frac{dI_1(t)}{dt} = B(t) - (a_1 + \mu)I_1(t) , \tag{10}$$

$$\frac{dI_2(t)}{dt} = a_1 I_1(t) - (a_2 + \mu)I_2(t) , \tag{11}$$

$$\frac{dI_3(t)}{dt} = a_2 I_2(t) - (a_3 + \mu)I_3(t) , \tag{12}$$

$$\frac{dI_4(t)}{dt} = a_3 I_3(t) - a_4 I_4(t) , \tag{13}$$

$$I_4(t) = A(t) , \tag{14}$$

$$\frac{dA_T(t)}{dt} = a_3 I(t), \tag{15}$$

where $a_3 I_3(t)$ is the rate at which new AIDS cases occur, $I_4(t)$ denotes the number of living persons with AIDS, and $A_T(t)$ denotes the total cumulative number of AIDS cases up to time t. The incidence in this case is given by the following expression:

$$B(t) = C(T)S(t)\frac{\lambda_1 I_1(t) + \lambda_2 I_2(t) + \lambda_3 I_3(t)}{T(t)}. \tag{16}$$

Since we intend to use approximately the same infectivity coefficients as those reported by Longini *et al.* (1989), we have taken only four compartments. Our simulations will use some of the current information available on the AIDS epidemic for the homosexual population living in San Francisco. These simulations do not attempt to reproduce the situation in San Francisco and are only used as an exploratory tool to increase our understanding of the mechanisms behind the AIDS epidemic. We note, for example, that the results presented by Hethcote at the 1989 summer meeting of the Society for Industrial and Applied Mathematics (henceforth referred as Hethcote 1989) seemed to show that in order to get a good fit to the San Francisco data (not available to the authors of this article), one needs at least seven compartments are needed and a two-group population with biased mixing. In addition, Hethcote (1989) indicated that changes in behavior also need to be introduced through time-dependent parameters to explain the San Francisco data.

The simulations that follow are based *roughly* on the data presented by Hethcote (1989), the parameters estimated by Longini *et al.* (1989), and the data reported in the Los Angeles Times (December 6, 1988). The main objective is to determine whether or not the simplest model (of the type that we have developed) is capable of fitting the reported data.

The simulation parameters are: $\phi_1 = \phi_2 = \phi_3 = \phi = 3$; $i_1 = 0.004$, $i_2 = 0.000$, $i_3 = 0.007$ $i_4 = 0.0057$; hence $\lambda_1 = 0.012$, $\lambda_2 = 0.000$, $\lambda_3 = 0.021$ $\lambda_4 = 0.0171$. The removal rates (following Longini *et al.* 1989) are $a_1 = 5.0$, $a_2 = 0.23$, $a_3 = 0.19$, and $a_4 = 0.5$, and $\mu = 0.05$. We tried several two-parameter functional forms for C(T) such as those described in Thieme and Castillo-Chavez (1989a, b) but a good fit to the number of AIDS cases seems to require an increase in the number of degrees of freedom. In order to do this, an "ad hoc" procedure that maintained the required properties of C(T) was developed. We now let $C(T) \equiv$ denote the number of unsafe contacts per unit time (one year), i.e., we incorporate ϕ into the old definition of C(T). We set $T(0) = 60{,}000$ (the approximate number of sexually active homosexuals in San Francisco, see Hethcote 1989) and assumed that $T(t) \leq T(0)$. C(T), a nondecreasing function of T, is a step function with 15 levels $r_1 \leq r_2 \leq \ldots \leq r_{15}$, with $C(T) = r_1$ whenever $T \leq 50{,}000$ and $C(60{,}000) = r_{15}$. The objective was to choose these 15 (possibly distinct) constants in such a way as to minimize the least square error fit to the number of AIDS cases. Initial simulations (which took up to 8 hours each in a VAX 750) reduced the viable range of T to the T-interval [59,000-60,000]. We then repeated the same procedure in this T-interval but now using 40 "steps" ($r_1 \leq r_2 \leq \ldots \leq r_{40}$). The initial data were chosen as $S(0) = 59{,}600$, $I_1(0) = 29$, $I_2(0) = 180$, $I_3(0) = 161$. $I_4(0) = 30$ gives the reported number of AIDS cases up to 1982 in San Francisco (see Table 1).

The best fit (continuous line) is illustrated in Figure 1. The mean square error is 2024.62, and the standard deviation is 44.996. The fit is excellent at the beginning but not as good over the last two years. In Figure 2 a plot of the best C(T) (actually $\phi C(T)$) is provided. We observe that large change in the mean number of unsafe contacts is needed around 1984 in order to obtain a good fit. The initial point given by $C(T) = 900$ (not in Figure 2) is not indicative of the real situation but, is a consequence of the fitting procedure. C(T) drops immediately to 550 and ends at about 30 unsafe contacts per year. This model predicts approximately 9,000 HIV infecteds by the end of 1987 (Figure 3), which is in substantial disagreement with those reported by Hethcote (1989) of 16,000 to 24,000 HIV infected individuals. We observe that despite the tremendous flexibility of the model (which has a great number of parameters), the method (i.e., differential equations) is very constraining. We need to fit not only AIDS incidence, but also AIDS prevalence, and HIV incidence and prevalence, by means of curves *generated* by these systems of coupled differential equations with appropriately matching parameters. This apparent drawback is actually the biggest strength of the differential equation method in the process of validation of a model.

From these simulations we conclude that using Longini *et al.*'s (1989) data (and hence four compartments) it is not possible to get a reasonable fit to AIDS incidence data using our simple model with homogeneous mixing and a saturating formula for C(T) such as those described in Thieme and Castillo-Chavez (1989a, b). Rather, we have to use a computer intensive "ad hoc" method that properly constrains C(T). Substantial behavioral changes are needed (average number of unsafe contacts per unit time) in order to fit these data. We further noticed that model predictions were somewhat sensitive to initial conditions. The difficulties encountered while trying to fit the AIDS incidence and prevalence, as well as the HIV prevalence data, with this simple model provided us with several important points: more detailed infectivity studies are needed; the assumption of homogeneous mixing is too restrictive. A simple form of mixing, like preferred mixing with two or three groups, may be sufficient to produce a better fit. Unfortunately, data on mixing is lacking. Changes in behavior (i.e., time-dependent parameters) may be critical to explain the data. These results seem to agree generally with those reported by Hethcote (1989). We also note that data sets like the San Francisco data set on homosexual incidence and prevalence of HIV is critical to our fine tuning of AIDS models. This is of particular importance because of the observed sensitivity of these models to initial conditions. Finally, we observe that two-sex "flexible" mixing functions must be developed for the consideration of HIV transmission among heterosexual individuals.

3. Formulation of a model with arbitrary mixing

We consider a sexually active population that is stratified according to a continuous variable s that measures the degree of sexual activity (number of sexual partners per unit time). Hence

$$\int_s^{s+\Delta s} S(n,t)dn, \quad \int_s^{s+\Delta s} I(n,t)dn, \quad \text{and} \quad \int_s^{s+\Delta s} A(n,t)dn$$

denote the number of individuals in each of the epidemiological classifications – susceptible, infected, and "full-blown" AIDS – respectively, with sexual activity in the activity interval $(s, s+\Delta s)$. We again assume that A-individuals are sexually inactive; therefore, if $T(s,t) = S(s,t) + I(s,t)$, then

$$\int_0^\infty T(s,t)ds = \hat{T}(t)$$

denotes the totally sexually active population at time t. Here, the function C(T) of Section 2 is replaced by the function $C(s,W(T(\cdot,t)))$, which denotes the mean number of sexual partners per unit time that an individual with activity level s has, given that the sexually active population is distributed as $T(s,t)$. $W(T(\cdot,t))$ is a measure of total sexual availability at time t, and here is chosen to be a functional of the size of the sexually active population at time t. An example for which W depends only on total sexual availability, and hence is independent of s is given by

$$W(t)=\int_0^\infty h(u)T(u,t)du,$$

where h(u) is an appropriate weighting function. The mixing function $\rho(s, r)$ (Blythe and Castillo-Chavez 1989, Castillo-Chavez and Blythe 1989) is such that

$$\int_r^{r+\Delta r} \rho(s,u)du$$

denotes the fraction of contacts of a person with activity level s with persons with activity levels in $(r,r+\Delta r)$, and therefore satisfies the following constraints for all s, r, and t:

$$\rho(s,r,t) \geq 0\ , \tag{17}$$

$$\int_0^\infty \rho(s, r,t)dr = 1\ , \text{ and} \tag{18}$$

$$\rho(s, r,t)C(s,W(.,t))T(s,t) = \rho(r, s,t)C(r,W(.,t))T(r,t)\ . \tag{19}$$

Conditions (17) and (18) arise because $\rho(s,r,t)$ can be interpreted as a probability density function, while condition (19) expresses a conservation principle; i.e., that the total number of partnerships of s-people with r-people must equal the total number of partnerships of r-people with s-people.

To describe a dynamic model that incorporates a general mixing function, we have to introduce additional notation. We let $\Lambda(s)$ denote the recruitment rate into S(s,t); μ, the sexual removal rate; d, the disease-induced mortality rate; and $\lambda(s,r)$, the transmission coefficient between susceptible individuals with activity s and infective individuals with activity r. Using this notation, we can now derive an expression for the number of new cases per unit time—the incidence B(s,t). First, we observe that $I(r,t)\Delta r$ and $T(r,t)\Delta r$ give the total number of infective and sexually active individuals, respectively, with activity in the activity interval $(r,r+\Delta r)$. Hence,

$$\frac{I(r,t)}{T(r,t)}$$

denotes the infective fraction that has activity level in $(r,r+\Delta r)$. Since $\rho(s,r,t)\Delta r$ denotes the proportion of partnerships that a typical individual with activity level s has with persons with activity levels in $(r,r+\Delta r)$ at time t, $C(s,W(T(.,t))\rho(s,r,t)\Delta r$ denotes the average number of partnerships per person of activity s with persons of activities in $(r,r+\Delta r)$. Furthermore,

$$C(s,W(T(.,t)))\rho(s,r,t)\Delta r\, \frac{I(r,t)}{T(r,t)}$$

denotes the fraction of the average number of partnerships per type s individual that are with infectious individuals with activities in $(r,r+\Delta r)$. The expression for the incidence is therefore given by

$$B(s,t) = S(s,t)C(s,W(T(.,t)))\int_0^\infty \lambda(s,r)\ \rho(s,r,t)\ \frac{I(r,t)}{T(r,t)}dr\ , \tag{20}$$

where $\lambda(s,r)$ is the transmission coefficient from a r-infected individuals to s-susceptible individuals.

To model a population that mixes in proportion to their numbers and their sexual activity (i.e., proportionate mixing), we use the mixing function

$$\rho(s,r,t) = \frac{C(r,W(T(.,t)))T(r,t)}{\int_0^\infty C(u,W(T(.,t)))T(u,t)du}, \tag{21}$$

with its associated incidence rate

$$B(s,t) = \frac{\lambda(s,t)C(s,W(T(.,t)))\int_0^\infty \beta(s,r)C(r,W(T(r,t))I(r,t)dr}{\int_0^\infty C(u,W(T(\cdot,t))T(u,t)du} \tag{22}$$

More general mixing functions can be found in Blythe and Castillo-Chavez (1989) and Castillo-Chavez and Blythe (1989).

The simplest epidemiological model that incorporates these features is given by the following set of equations:

$$\frac{dS(s,t)}{dt} = \Lambda(s) - B(s,t) - \mu S(s,t)\ , \tag{23}$$

$$\frac{dI(s,t)}{dt} = B(s,t) - (\alpha(s) + \mu)I(s,t)\ , \text{ and} \tag{24}$$

$$\frac{dA(s,t)}{dt} = \alpha(s)I(s,t) - d(s)A(s,t)\ . \tag{25}$$

This model, as presented, is not an adequate model for the study of HIV dynamics since it assumes a removal rate from the infective class $\alpha(s)$ independent of time since infection. However, this is not a crucial limitation, as the model can be modified easily to take into account not only time since infection but also different degrees of infectivity in the various infectious categories. The simplest way of doing so is by further subdividing the infectious class into several compartments with different removal rates (Section 2). Also, variable infectivity is easily incorporated into the B(s,t) term. A full model using partial differential equations also can be easily developed via the approach of Blythe and Anderson (1988b),

Hyman and Stanley (1988, 1989), and Thieme and Castillo-Chavez (1989a,b). For extensions of these approaches to age-structured populations, see Busenberg and Castillo-Chavez (1989a,b).

4. Multiple group models

In this section, we describe an N-group model that is contained conceptually in models (23)-(25). A general type of mixing is discussed—biased or preferred mixing—that includes the familiar proportionate mixing. Analytical results for this general model are presented. To describe our N-group model, we proceed by introducing some new notation. Our N sexually active subpopulations are divided into three epidemiological classes: S_i, I_i, and A_i for $i=1,\cdots,N$. Λ_i denotes the constant recruitment rate of susceptibles into class S_i, μ denotes the sexual activity removal rate, d_i denotes the disease-induced mortality in class A_i, and α_i denotes the ith-removal rate of its corresponding infective class. Furthermore, λ_{ij} denotes the transmission coefficient between group i and group j individuals.

To describe the mixing, we let $p_{ij}(t)$ denote the fraction of new partnerships per unit time of individuals in group j with individuals in group i. Then, the p_{ij}'s satisfy the following properties at all times:

$$p_{ij} \geq 0, \qquad i, j = 1,\cdots,N \, , \tag{26}$$

$$\sum_{j=1}^{N} p_{ij} = 1, \qquad i = 1,\cdots,N \, , \tag{27}$$

$$C_i\big(W(T_1,\ldots T_N)\big)T_i p_{ij} = C_j\big(W(T_1,\ldots T_N)\big)T_j p_{ji}, \quad i, j = 1,\cdots,N \, . \tag{28}$$

Proportionate mixing is defined by

$$p_{ij} = \frac{C_j\big(W(T_1,\ldots T_N)\big)T_j}{\sum_{k=1}^{N} C_k\big(W(T_1,\ldots T_N)\big)T_k}, \qquad i,j = 1,\cdots,N \, , \tag{29}$$

whereas preferred or biased mixing is given by

$$p_{ij} = \begin{cases} f_i + (1-f_i) \dfrac{C_i\big(W(T_1,\ldots T_N)\big)(1-f_i)T_i}{\hat{L}}, & i=j \\[2ex] (1-f_i) \dfrac{C_j\big(W(T_1,\ldots T_N)\big)(1-f_j)T_j}{\hat{L}}, & i\neq j \, , \end{cases} \tag{30}$$

where $i,j = 1,\cdots,N$ and $\hat{L} = \sum_{k=1}^{N} (1-f_k)C_k\big(W(T_1,\ldots T_N)\big)T_k$.

In the last definition, f_i denotes the fraction of group i's new partnerships per unit time that are "reserved" within the ith subpopulation; the remaining fraction, $1-f_i$, of group i's new partnerships per unit time is assumed to be distributed according to proportional mixing including some within the ith subpopulation. Note that equation (30) includes proportional mixing (set $f_i = 0$ for $i = 1,\dots,N$).

Following our discussion leading to equation (20), we conclude that the ith-incidence rate is given by

$$B_i(t) = S_i(t)C_i\Big(W(T_1,\dots T_N)\Big)\sum_{j=1}^{N}\lambda_{ij}p_{ij}(t)\,\frac{I_j(t)}{T_j(t)}, \tag{31}$$

where $T_k(t) = S_k(t) + I_k(t)$, $k = 1,\dots,N$.

We set $\sigma_i = \frac{1/\mu}{1/\alpha_i}$ to rescale the dynamics of transmission and arrive at model (32)-(34):

$$\frac{dS_i(t)}{dt} = \Lambda_i - B_i(t) - \mu S_i(t)\ , \tag{32}$$

$$\frac{dI_i(t)}{dt} = B_i(t) - \mu(\sigma_i+1)I_i(t)\ , \tag{33}$$

$$\frac{dA_i(t)}{dt} = \alpha_i I_i(t) - d_i A_i(t), \qquad i=1,2,\cdots,N\ . \tag{34}$$

This model assumes constant removal rates from the infective classes into the AIDS classes. As noted before, this assumption can be relaxed easily by further subdivision of the infective classes, as illustrated in Section 2.

Models (32)-(34) have been analyzed in the case of preferred mixing when

$$W(T_1,\dots T_N) = \hat{T} = \sum_{k=1}^{N} T_k.$$

To describe our results for this model, we define

$$\theta_i(\hat{T}) = f_i\lambda_{ii}C_i(\hat{T}), \qquad r_i(\hat{T}) = (1-f_i)C_i(T)\ ,$$

$$\ell_{ij}(\hat{T}) = C_i(\hat{T})(1-f_i)C_j(\hat{T})(1-f_i)\lambda_{ij} = r_i(\hat{T})r_j(\hat{T})\lambda_{ij},\ i,j = 1,2,\cdots,N\ ,$$

and introduce the matrices $Q(\mu)$ and $H(\mu)$ given by

$$Q(\mu) = \mathrm{diag}\left(\frac{\theta_i(T^*)}{\sigma_i+1}\right) + \mathrm{diag}\left(\frac{\Lambda_i}{K(T^*)(\sigma_i+1)}\right)\Big[\ell_{ij}(T^*)\Big]_{N\times N} \quad \text{and}$$

$$H(\mu) = Q(\mu) - \mu E\ ,$$

where $T^* = \frac{1}{\mu}\sum_{k=1}^{N}\Lambda_k$, $K(T^*) = \sum_{k=1}^{N} r_k(T^*)\Lambda_k$ and E is the $N\times N$ identity matrix.

The following local stability result for the general N-group model was first reported in Castillo-Chavez *et al.* (1989c) for the case of proportionate mixing ($f_i \equiv 0$, $i=1,\cdots,N$). It has since been extended to the case of preferred mixing (see Huang *et al.* 1989). To describe it, we let $M\Big(H(\mu)\Big) = \sup\Big\{\text{Re } \rho : \det\Big(\rho E - H(\mu)\Big) = 0\Big\}$, and assume that $\frac{dC_i(T)}{dT} \geq 0$, $\frac{d}{dT}\left(\frac{C_i(T)}{T}\right) \leq 0$, $T \geq 0$, $i=1,2,\cdots,N$.

There is a unique μ_0 such that

$$M\Big(H(\mu)\Big) = \begin{cases} <0 & \text{if } \mu > \mu_0 \\ 0 & \text{if } \mu = \mu_0 \\ >0 & \text{if } \mu < \mu_0 \end{cases}.$$

Furthermore, the infection-free state $\overline{S} = \left(\frac{\Lambda_1}{\mu},\cdots,\frac{\Lambda_n}{\mu},0,\cdots,0\right)$ is locally asymptotically stable, provided that $M\Big(H(\mu)\Big) < 0$, and unstable if $M\Big(H(\mu)\Big) > 0$.

Bifurcation results for the N-group model were also reported in Castillo-Chavez *et al.* (1989c) for the random mixing case. We have shown that the same results hold for the preferred mixing case under the assumptions in Castillo-Chavez *et al.* (1989c); i.e., $C_i(T) = c_i$ (a constant) for $i=1,2,\cdots,N$, Q is irreducible, and μ_0 is such that $M\Big(H(\mu_0)\Big) = 0$. To state our results, we introduce the expression

$$h(\mu_0) = \sum_{i=1}^{N} \overline{I}_i I_i \left[\frac{K I_i\Big(\mu_0(\sigma_i+1)^2 - \theta_i\sigma_i\Big)}{\Lambda_i^2} - \left(\sum_{j=1}^{N} r_j \sigma_j I_j\right) \frac{\mu_0(\sigma_i+1) - \theta_i}{\Lambda_i} \right],$$

where $K = \sum_{j=1}^{N} r_j \Lambda_j$, $I = (I_1,\cdots,I_n)$ and $\overline{I} = (\overline{I_1},\cdots,\overline{I_n})$ are positive eigenvectors of $H(\mu_0)$ and $H^T(\mu_0)$ corresponding to the zero eigenvalue (T denotes the transpose in this case). The existence of these positive eigenvectors (i.e., all entries are positive) is guaranteed by M-matrix theory. We (Huang *et al.* 1989) have established the following bifurcation results:

If $h(\mu_0) \neq 0$, then μ_0 is a bifurcation point. More specifically, if $h(\mu_0) > 0$ $\Big(h(\mu_0) < 0\Big)$ then there is an $\epsilon > 0$ and unique continuously differentiable functions S and I mapping $(\mu_0\text{-}\epsilon,\mu_0] \rightarrow R_+^n\Big([\mu_0,\mu_0+\epsilon) \rightarrow R_+^n\Big)$ such that $\Big(S(\mu_0),I(\mu_0)\Big) = \left(\frac{\Lambda_1}{\mu},\cdots,\frac{\Lambda_n}{\mu},0,\cdots,0\right)$, and $\Big(S(\mu),I(\mu)\Big)$ is a positive endemic equilibrium of (32–33). This endemic equilibrium is locally asymptotically stable for each μ in $(\mu_0\text{-}\epsilon,\mu_0)$ $\Big($unstable for each μ in $(\mu_0,\mu_0+\epsilon)\Big)$.

For each μ in $(0,\mu_0)$, the system (32–33) has a positive endemic equilibrium; and if $h(\mu_0) < 0$, there is an $\epsilon > 0$, such that the system (32–33) has at least two positive equilibria for each μ in $(\mu_0,\mu_0+\epsilon)$.

Our analytical results for models of the sexual spread of HIV/AIDS show that our single group models are robust, in the sense that only "simple" dynamics are possible. In addition (see Castillo-Chavez *et al.*, 1989a,b), we have shown that the reproductive number is not significantly affected by the shape of the survivorship function, assuming that the survivorship function is biologically reasonable (but see Thieme and Castillo-Chavez 1989a,b). We have also illustrated the effects of a changing mean sexual activity, where the changes are due exclusively to a shrinking sexually active population. These changes allow us to obtain any kind of polynomial growth in the number of AIDS cases after the initial exponential growth phase exhibited by all models of this type. Furthermore, we see that the generalized thinking that S-I-R epidemic models do not have multiple equilibria is inaccurate, and hence the possibility for complex dynamics is certainly real. Our analytical results have been obtained under the assumption of preferred mixing; however, the model formulation is quite arbitrary, as the $p_{ij}(t)$'s can be defined in a variety of ways as long as they satisfy the mixing constraints (25)-(27). Finally, we note that the above models have assumed that all infectious individuals are equally infectious. We have modified our single group model to include variable infectivity, which appears to play a significant role in the qualitative dynamics of our single group model (see Thieme and Castillo-Chavez 1989a, b). In addition, it can affect quantitative values such as the initial rate of spread and the saturation level of cases. The numerical simulations found in Hyman and Stanley (1988, 1989) show that the transient dynamics for a similar model can be very sensitive to changes in the infectivity.

5. N-group model with endemic equilibria: two examples

The examples in this section illustrate the existence of multiple endemic equilibria for the N-group epidemic model (equations 32–34) of Section 3. These examples point to the mechanism responsible for the generation of at least two endemic equilibria: asymmetry. Asymmetry arises through the nature of social/sexual interactions; that is, the mixing or asymmetric epidemiological parameters (here built in the transmission coefficient).

For a two-group example (N=2), let $\mu_0=1$, $\sigma_i=1$, $\Lambda_i=4$, $\theta_i=1$, $\gamma_i=1$, i=1,2 and

$$L = \begin{bmatrix} 1-\epsilon & 0.1\epsilon \\ 1 & 0.9 \end{bmatrix}$$

where $\epsilon > 0$. Lengthy computations then show that $h(\mu_0) < 0$ (see Section 3) if ϵ is sufficiently small.

For our second example, we let $\Lambda_i = r_i = 1$, $\sigma_i = \sigma \;\; 0$, $\theta_i = 0$, $i=1,2,\cdots,N$, and $\ell_{11} > 0$, $\ell_{21} = \ell_{31} = \cdots = \ell_{N1} = \ell > 0$ be fixed such that

$$\frac{\sigma}{N(\sigma+1)} + \frac{(N-1)\ell}{N(\sigma+1)\ell_{11}} > 1 .$$

We let $\ell_{ij} = \epsilon > 0$, $i=1,\cdots,N$, $j=2,\cdots,N$. Using the unique $\mu_0(\epsilon) > 0$ such that $M\Big(H(\mu_0(\epsilon))\Big) = 0$ (see Section 3 for the definition of $M\Big(H(\mu_0)\Big)$) and the above definitions, one can check that

$$\mu_0(\epsilon) = \frac{\ell_{11}}{N(\sigma+1)} + o(\epsilon) ,$$

and that

$$h(\mu_0(\epsilon)) = \ell_{11}\left[1 - \left(\frac{\sigma}{N(\sigma+1)} + \frac{N-1)\ell}{N(\sigma+1)\ell_{11}}\right)\right] + o(\epsilon) .$$

Hence, if ϵ is small enough ($\epsilon>0$), we have that $h(\mu_0(\epsilon)) > 0$. For complete details see Huang *et al.* (1989).

6. Conclusion

In this article, we have restated some of our analytical results on single- and multiple-group models. Of theoretical importance is the fact that multiple group models can possess multiple endemic equilibria. Two examples that illustrate this situation are presented in Section 5. We note, from these two examples, that what appears to be the critical factor in generating multiple endemic equilibria is asymmetry, either in mixing or in infectivity. There are, of course, several situations in which asymmetries of these types exist in the study of sexually transmitted diseases. Examples include the different infectivities for males and females found in gonorrhea research (see Hethcote and Yorke 1984), the (probable) asymmetric mixing between prostitutes and customers, etc.

The theoretical results generated by our models show that these asymmetries have an effect on the qualitative dynamics, and hence the importance of these asymmetries depends on the parameters. Our results strongly suggest that experiments should be conducted to answer important questions such as: How asymmetric is the mixing when one member of a pair is monogamous and the other is not? Is the probability of transmission from males that mostly practice receptive anal sex significantly different to that of males that mostly practice insertive sex? How asymmetric is the use of prophylactics such as condoms among non-monogamous sexual partners that practice receptive anal and insertive intercourse? etc.

We further note that without more detailed data on infectivity and mixing, and without further detailed epidemiological and behavioral studies (accessible to a variety of researchers) such as the San Francisco cohort studies, there is no hope that we can identify the relative effects of these key parameters and therefore increase our understanding of the AIDS epidemic. Predictions that go beyond those currently generated by statistical techniques will be difficult in the absence of these data.

ACKNOWLEDGMENTS

This research has been partially supported by NSF grant DMS-8807478 awarded to Kenneth Cooke and NSF grant DMS-8906580, NIAID grant R01 A129178-01, and Hatch project grant NYC 151-409, USDA awarded to Carlos Castillo-Chavez.

REFERENCES

Anderson, R.M., G.F. Medley, R.M. May and A.M. Johnson. (1986). A preliminary study of the transmission dynamics of the human immunodeficiency virus (HIV), the causative agent of AIDS. *IMA J. of Mathematics Applied in Med. and Biol.* 3, 229-263.

Anderson, R.M. and R.M. May. (1987). Transmission dynamics of HIV infection. *Nature* 326, 137-142.

Blythe, S.P. and R.M. Anderson. (1988a). Distributed incubation and infectious periods in models of transmission dynamics of human immunodeficiency virus (HIV). *IMA. J. of Mathmematics Applied in Med. and Biol.* 5, 1-19.

Blythe, S.P. and R.M. Anderson. (1988b). Variable infectiousness in HIV transmission models. *IMA J. of Mathematics Applied in Med. and Biol.* 5, 181-200.

Blythe, S.P. and C. Castillo-Chavez. (1989). Like-with-like preference and sexual mixing models. *Math. Biosci.* 96, 221-238.

Busenberg, S. and C. Castillo-Chavez. (1989a). Interaction, pair formation and force of infection terms in sexually transmitted diseases. (This volume.)

Busenberg, S. and C. Castillo-Chavez. (1989b). Risk and age-dependent mixing functions and force of infection terms in sexually transmitted diseases. (Submitted.)

Castillo-Chavez, C. and S.P. Blythe. (1989). Mixing framework for social/sexual behavior. (This volume.)

Castillo-Chavez, C., K. Cooke, W. Huang and S.A. Levin. (1989a). On the role of long periods of infectiousness in the dynamics of acquired immunodeficiency syndrome (AIDS). In *Mathematical Approaches to Problems in Resource Management and Epidemiology.* C. Castillo-Chavez, S.A. Levin and C. Shoemaker (eds.). Lecture Notes in Biomathematics 81, Springer-Verlag, Berlin, Heidelberg, New York, Tokyo. (In press.)

Castillo-Chavez, C., K. Cooke, W. Huang and S.A. Levin. (1989b). On the role of long incubation periods in the dynamics of acquired immunodeficiency syndrome (AIDS), Part 1. Single population models. *J. Math. Biol.* 27, 373-398.

Castillo-Chavez, C., K. Cooke, W. Huang and S.A. Levin. (1989c). Results on the dynamics for models for the sexual transmission of the human immunodeficiency virus. *Applied*

Mathematics Letters. (In press.)

Hethcote, H.W. (1989). A dynamic model of HIV transmission and AIDS in San Francisco. Lecture presented at the minisymposium on modeling the epidemiology of AIDS. 1989 SIAM Annual Meeting. July 17–21. San Diego, California.

Hethcote, H.W. and J.A. Yorke. (1984). *Gonorrhea Transmission Dynamics and Control.* Lecture Notes in Biomathematics 56. Spinger-Verlag, Berlin, Heidelberg, New York, Tokyo.

Huang, W., K. Cooke and C. Castillo-Chavez. (1989). Stability and bifurcation for a multiple group model for the dynamics of HIV/AIDS. (Manuscript).

Hyman, J.M. and E.A. Stanley. (1988). Using mathematical models to understand the AIDS epidemic. *Math.Biosci.* 90, 415-473.

Hyman, J.M. and E.A. Stanley (1989). The effect of social mixing patterns on the spread of AIDS. In *Mathematical Approaches to Problems in Resource Management and Epidemiology.* C. Castillo-Chavez, S.A. Levin and C. Shoemaker (eds.). Lecture Notes in Biomathematics 81, Springer-Verlag, Berlin, Heidelberg, New York, Tokyo. (In press.)

Jacquez, J.A., C.P. Simon and J. Koopman. (1989). Structured mixing: heterogeneous mixing by the definition of mixing groups. (This volume.)

Jacquez, J.A., C.P. Simon, J. Koopman, L. Sattenspiel and T. Perry. (1988). Modeling and analyzing HIV transmission: the effects of contact patterns. *Math. Biosci.* 92, 119-199.

Kaplan, E.H., P.C. Cramton and A.D. Paltiel. (1989). Nonrandom mixing models of HIV transmission. (This volume.)

Longini, I.M., Jr., W.S. Clark, M. Haber and C.R. Horsburgh, Jr. (1989). The stages of HIV infection: waiting times and infectious contact rates. (This volume.)

May, R.M. and R.M. Anderson. (1989). The transmission dynamics of human immunodeficiency virus (HIV). *Phil. Trans. R. Soc. London B* 321, 565-607.

Sattenspiel, L. (1987). Population structure and the spread of disease. *Human Biol.* 59, 411-438.

Sattenspiel, L. and C.P. Simon (1988). The spread and persistence of infectious diseases in structured populations. *Math. Biosci.* 90, 341-366.

Thieme, H.R. and C. Castillo-Chavez. (1989a). On the role of variable infectivity in the dynamics of the human immunodeficiency virus. (This volume.)

Thieme, H.R. and C. Castillo-Chavez. (1989b). On the possible effects of infection-age-dependent infectivity in the dynamics of HIV/AIDS. (Manuscript).

Table I.

Observation	Time (6 months)	fitted	observed
1	0	30.590	30.628
2	1	33.095	33.592
3	2	49.861	56.316
4	3	102.916	128.440
5	4	190.765	157.092
6	5	285.253	229.216
7	6	371.723	329.004
8	7	446.573	397.176
9	8	508.933	434.720
10	9	560.226	545.376
11	10	602.764	685.672
12	11	638.707	686.660
13	12	668.015	680.732

Fitted and observed data from the simulation that generated the best fit (standard deviation 44.996).

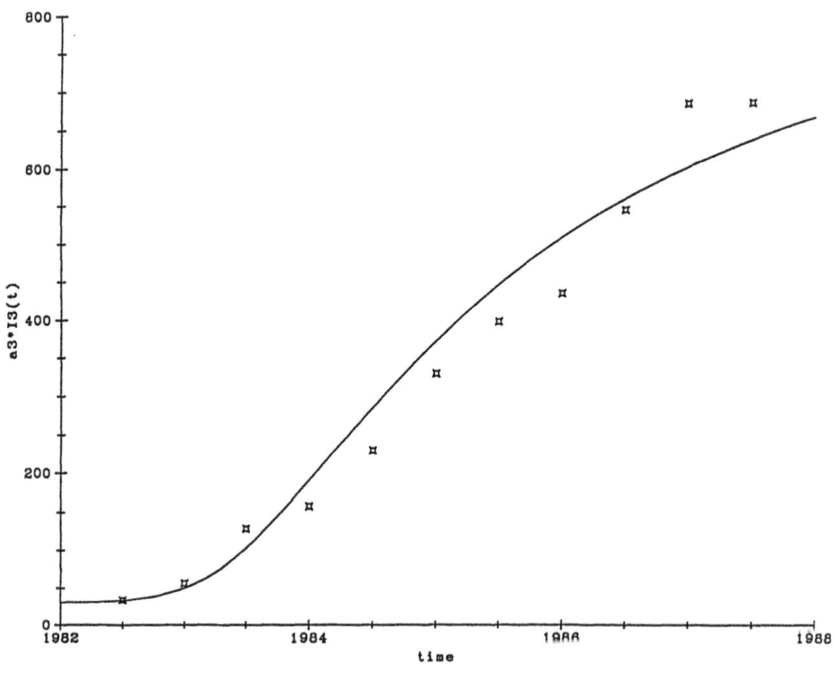

Fig. 1 AIDS incidence as a function of time. The fit is excellent at the beginning but not as good over the last two years. For further details see the text.

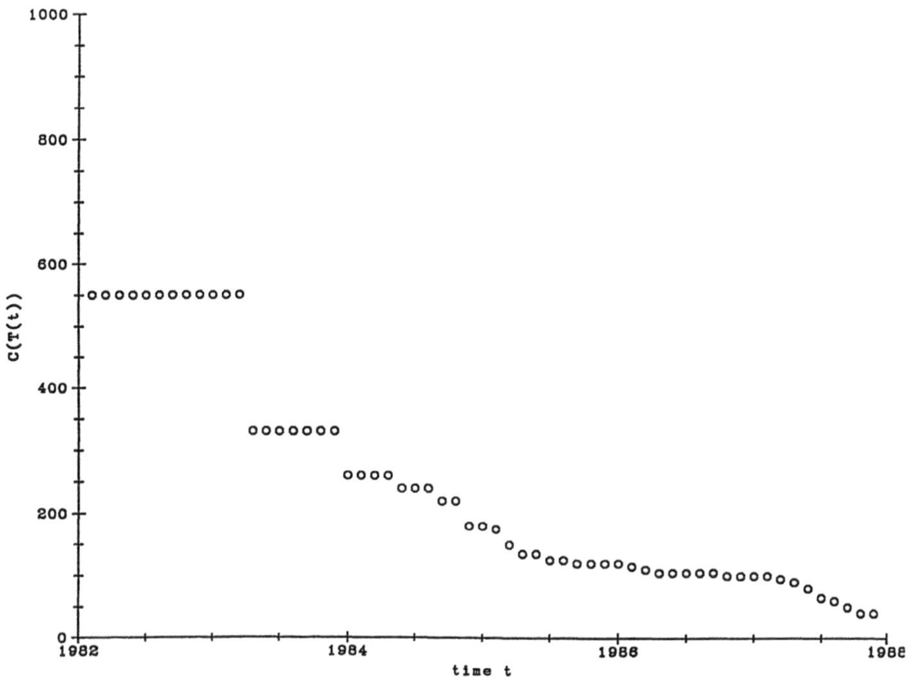

Fig. 2 The optimal $\phi C(T)$ is plotted. A great change in the mean number of unsafe contacts is needed to fit the AIDS incidence.

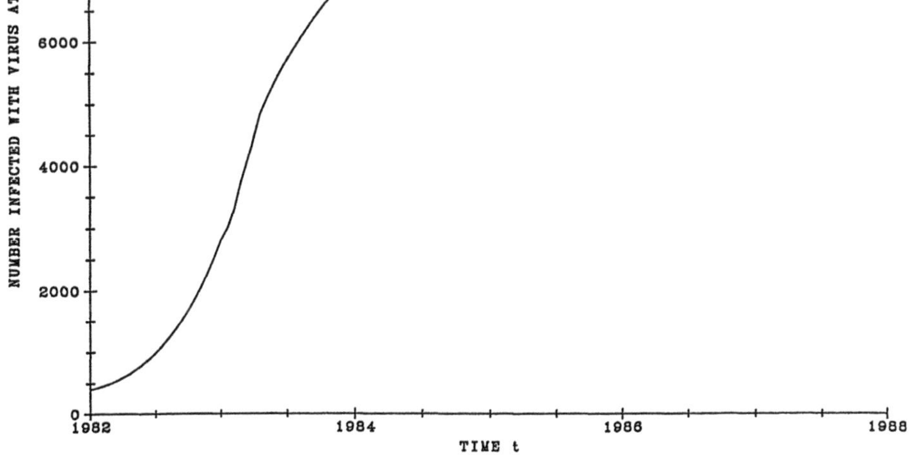

Fig. 3 HIV incidence as a function of t. For details see the text.

NONRANDOM MIXING MODELS OF HIV TRANSMISSION

Edward H. Kaplan, Peter C. Cramton, and A. David Paltiel
Yale School of Organization and Management
Box 1A, New Haven, CT 06520, USA

Abstract

Models of HIV transmission and the AIDS epidemic generally assume random mixing among those infected with HIV and those who are not. For sexually transmitted HIV, this implies that individuals select sex partners without regard to attributes such as familiarity, attractiveness, or risk of infection. This paper formulates a model for examining the impact of nonrandom mixing on HIV transmission. We present threshold conditions that determine when HIV epidemics can occur within the framework of this model. Nonrandom mixing is introduced by assuming that sexually active individuals select sex partners to minimize the risk of infection. In addition to variability in risky sex rates, some versions of our model allow for error (or noise) in information exchanged between prospective partners. We investigate several models including random partner selection (or proportionate mixing), segregation of the population by risky sex rates, a probabilistic combination of segregation and random selection induced by imperfect information (or preferred mixing), and a model of costly search with perfect information. We develop examples which show that nonrandom mixing can lead to epidemics that are more severe or less severe than random mixing. For reasonable parameter choices describing the AIDS epidemic, however, the results suggest that random mixing models overstate the number of HIV infections that will occur.

1. Introduction

The AIDS epidemic has now claimed almost 55,000 lives in the United

States, while the U.S. Centers for Disease Control report roughly 94,000 confirmed cases of AIDS as of April 1989 (CDC, 1989). Though it is now established that risky sex (primarily unprotected receptive anal intercourse with an infected insertive partner) and the sharing of drug injection equipment (e.g. needles) are the major modes of transmitting human immunodeficiency virus (or HIV, the causal virus of AIDS; see Curran et al, 1988), surprisingly little is known about the basic quantities which are driving the AIDS epidemic. Critical facts which have not been firmly established but are thought to be important include the distribution of risky behavior rates across the population (Anderson et al, 1986; May and Anderson, 1987), the manner in which different subpopulations mix (Hyman and Stanley, 1988; Abramson and Rothschild, 1988; Hethcote and Van Ark 1987), the duration of time for which such behaviors are practiced (which is closely linked to the AIDS incubation time; Anderson et al, 1986; May and Anderson, 1987; Kaplan, 1989a; Lui, Darrow and Rutherford, 1988; Brookmeyer and Gail, 1988), and the likelihood of becoming infected given exposure to the HIV virus (Grant, Wiley and Winkelstein, 1987), perhaps adjusting for mode of exposure and variability in infectivity over time and across individuals (Anderson, 1988; May and Anderson, 1988; Wiley, Herschkorn and Padian, 1989).

In two important papers, Anderson et al (1986) and May and Anderson (1987) proposed a simple model of the AIDS epidemic among gay men. Their model incorporates a distribution of risky sex rates across the sexually active gay population. Though their model thus allows for heterogeneity in risky sex rates, they assume that sex partners are selected at random from the population at large. Indeed, the assumption of random partner selection is central to most of the sexually transmitted disease and AIDS models developed to this point (see Anderson et al, 1986; May and Anderson, 1987; Anderson, 1988; Hethcote and Yorke, 1984; Isham, 1988; and Kaplan, 1989a and 1989b for examples). Some researchers have considered departures from random partner selection (Abramson and Rothschild, 1988; Blythe and Castillo-Chavez, 1989; Hethcote and Van Ark 1987; Hyman and Stanley, 1988; Jacquez et al, 1988; Koopman et al, 1988; Nold, 1980). Clearly, random partner selection is not behaviorally realistic, in that attributes such as familiarity, attractiveness and risk of infection are ignored. One might think that random partner selection would produce an epidemic that is worse than what would occur with nonrandom mixing, since random selection would eventually lead to a total mix of the population. This intuition, unfortunately, can be false: random partner selection need not overestimate the size of an epidemic.

In this paper, we consider partner selection alternatives to random mixing. The mixing mechanisms we propose are motivated by behavioral assumptions and represent a broad spectrum of matching methods. Our intention is to determine if the assumption of random mixing is robust over a variety of alternative mixing schemes. We feel this is an important subject to study, given that many policy models of AIDS rely on random mixing formulations (Kaplan 1989a, 1989b; Kaplan and Abramson, 1989). If the results of AIDS models are highly dependent upon random mixing assumptions, then public health strategies which serve to contain an epidemic driven by random mixing might not contain the real epidemic (should random mixing prove false). However, if random mixing models tend to overstate the size of an epidemic, then policies which contain random mixing epidemics should prove robust to more complex mixing behaviors.

Our paper is organized as follows. Section 2 presents our assumptions underlying HIV transmission. Section 3 presents general conditions under which an HIV (and hence AIDS) epidemic can occur in the population under the assumptions of Section 2. The behavioral principle of risk minimizing partner selection is discussed in Section 4. This principle is applied to derive epidemic models corresponding to a variety of partner selection schemes: random partner selection (or proportionate mixing) owing to no information; segregation by risky sex rate owing to perfect information; Bernoulli noise (or preferred mixing) owing to imperfect information; and costly partner search with perfect information. The epidemiological implications of these mixing functions are studied in Section 5. Our concluding remarks appear in Section 6.

2. Assumptions and Model Formulation

The model to be described is similar to the model considered by Hethcote and Van Ark (1987). At time t, the population in question contains n(t) gay men. This population can be divided into m subpopulations, with $n_i(t)$ men in subpopulation i, $\Sigma_{i=1}^{m} n_i(t)=n(t)$. Immigration to subpopulation i occurs at the constant rate of N_i men per year, while the per capita exit rate in all subpopulations (due to death unrelated to HIV or AIDS, or due to emigration) equals μ per man per year. In the absence of HIV infection, then, $n_i(t)$ will approach the steady state value of $n_i=N_i/\mu$.

We assume that HIV infection has been introduced to this population; such infection is assumed to spread via risky sexual contacts. Men in subpopulation i have risky sex with an average of c_i partners per year (c_i is called a risky sex rate). In any risky sexual relationship between an infected member of subgroup i and an uninfected member of subgroup j, the uninfected man becomes infected with probability β_{ij}. The probabilities of HIV transmission (the β_{ij}'s) are assumed to apply per partnership as opposed to per sexual act, an assumption which is gaining empirical support (May and Anderson, 1988; Wiley, Herschkorn and Padian, 1989). We assume that infected men remain sexually active and infectious for an average of D years; the quantity D depends upon both the remaining active sex life from the time of infection, and the AIDS incubation time (see Kaplan, 1989a for a detailed discussion).

When a member of subpopulation i selects a sex partner at time t, the partner selected is a member of subpopulation j with probability $q_{ij}(t)$, $\Sigma_{j=1}^{m} q_{ij}(t)=1$; $i=1,2,...,m$. The probabilities $q_{ij}(t)$ are referred to as the mixing probabilities; they need not reflect random selection among the subpopulations. Unless stated otherwise, we assume that there exists a direct or indirect path of positive mixing probabilities connecting any two subgroups (i.e., all subgroups communicate). This implies that epidemics will either develop in all subgroups, or in no subgroup. Cases where all subgroups do not communicate may be partitioned and analyzed separately. We also assume symmetry in sexual activity: when a man from subpopulation i has risky sex with a man from subpopulation j, the reverse also occurs. This symmetry implies that the mixing probabilities must satisfy the following law of conservation of sex:

$$n_i(t)\ c_i\ q_{ij}(t) = n_j(t)\ c_j\ q_{ji}(t) \qquad \begin{matrix} i=1,2,...,m;\ j=1,2,...,m. \\ t\geq 0 \end{matrix} \qquad (1)$$

Equation (1) simply states that the total rate at which men from subpopulation i have sex with men from subpopulation j balances the total rate at which men from subpopulation j have sex with men from subpopulation i. Any system of mixing probabilities proposed must obey equation (1).

3. Threshold Conditions for HIV Epidemics

There are several basic questions one may ask of epidemic models such as the one just formulated, but the most basic query is this: under what conditions will the number of infected men increase over time following the introduction of HIV infection into the population? To answer this question, assume that the population has reached steady state in the absence of HIV infection (so that $n_i=N_i/\mu$), and that the mixing probabilities $q_{ij}(t)$ have stabilized at q^*_{ij}.

Let Y(t) denote the vector of infected men in the population at time t following the introduction of HIV infection;

$$Y(t) = (Y_1(t), Y_2(t), \ldots, Y_m(t))^T. \qquad (2)$$

We define the nonnegative matrix **A** to contain the elements

$$a_{ij} = c_i \beta_{ij} q^*_{ij} D, \qquad i=1,2,\ldots,m, \qquad (3)$$

where q^*_{ij} denotes the mixing probabilities corresponding to the disease-free steady state. Let **I** be the identity matrix, and **o**(**y**) be a function such that $\lim_{y \to 0} ||o(y)||/||y|| = 0$. With this notation, we assume that

$$\frac{dY(t)}{dt} = \frac{1}{D} (A^T - I)\ Y(t) + o(Y(t)) \qquad (4)$$

early in the epidemic. For time periods close to the origin, this model is a close approximation to many of the AIDS models referred to earlier.

As a first order differential system, it is easy to show that the behavior of $Y(t)$ is governed by the largest eigenvalue of **A** (which equals the largest eigenvalue of A^T, of course). Let $\rho(A)$ denote the largest eigenvalue of **A** (which is guaranteed to be nonnegative, as **A** is a nonnegative matrix; see Strang, 1980). Standard results (e.g. Strang, 1980) then dictate that early in the epidemic, $Y(t)$ will increase exponentially if and only if $\rho(A)>1$; if $\rho(A)\leq 1$, $Y(t)$ remains stable or decreases following an initial transient. A derivation of this threshold via consideration of endemic equilibria was presented by Hethcote and Van Ark (1987) for their model; the rough arguments presented here generalize the approach used by Anderson et al (1986) in their study of random sexual mixing.

To determine when epidemics can occur requires computing eigenvalues under the approach formulated above. However, a much simpler approach which avoids the explicit computation of $\rho(A)$ can be applied providing **I**–**A** is nonsingular. Imagine introducing the infection to an infinite population of susceptibles. Let T_i be the number of ultimate infections (direct and indirect) accounted for by a newly infected type i man, assuming that all risky sex involving infected men occurs with uninfected men (owing to the infinite population of susceptibles). If $T_i<\infty$ for every i, then the infection dies out in the infinite population of susceptibles, implying that no epidemic will materialize in the "real" world. As we will now show, determining the values of T_i is straightforward as long as **I**–**A** is nonsingular.

An infected type i man will remain sexually active on average for time D by assumption. The total number of risky sex partnerships involving this man thus averages $c_i D$. With probability q^*_{ij} (as the total populations of the various subgroups remain in proportion to the values of N_i), the infected type i man has a risky sex partnership with an uninfected type j man. The mean number of ultimate infections generated from such a partnership equals 0 with probability $1-\beta_{ij}$ (that is, the infected type i man did not infect the susceptible type j man), and $1+T_j$ with probability β_{ij} (for if the infection is passed, then the newly infected man counts for one infection, and that same newly infected man will now generate T_j subsequent infections by the definition of T_j). Thus, the T_i's satisfy the following system of equations:

$$T_i = c_i D \sum_{j=1}^{m} q_{ij}^{*} \beta_{ij} (1+T_j), \qquad i=1,2,\ldots,m. \qquad (5)$$

Let $\mathbf{T}=(T_1, T_2, \ldots, T_m)^T$, and $\mathbf{1}=(1, 1, \ldots, 1)^T$. Equation (5) can then be rewritten as the linear system

$$\mathbf{T} = \mathbf{A}\,(\mathbf{1}+\mathbf{T}) \qquad (6)$$

with solution

$$\mathbf{T} = (\mathbf{I}-\mathbf{A})^{-1}\mathbf{A}\,\mathbf{1}, \qquad (7)$$

assuming $\mathbf{I}-\mathbf{A}$ is nonsingular.

Standard results from linear algebra may again be invoked: as $\mathbf{A}$ is a nonnegative matrix, $\mathbf{T}$ is finite and nonnegative if and only if $(\mathbf{I}-\mathbf{A})^{-1}$ is finite and nonnegative, which in turn occurs if and only if $\rho(\mathbf{A})<1$ (Strang, 1980). Thus, if equation (7) results in $0 \le T_i < \infty$ for every i, then $\rho(\mathbf{A})<1$, indicating that an epidemic cannot occur. Alternatively, if $T_i<0$ for some i, the previous discussion implies that $\rho(\mathbf{A})>1$, signalling an epidemic. Of course, only nonnegative values of T_i have physical meaning (for one cannot generate negative infections); thus negative values of T_i should be recognized as characterizing an infinite number of infectious transmissions.

As such, a second approach to determining whether or not an epidemic will occur for a given $\mathbf{A}$ matrix, providing $\mathbf{I}-\mathbf{A}$ is nonsingular, is to evaluate equation (7) and ask whether the resulting T_i's are all nonnegative. If the answer is yes, then an epidemic cannot occur (as $\rho(\mathbf{A})<1$); if the answer is no, an epidemic will occur (as $\rho(\mathbf{A})>1$). Solving equation (7) (or equivalently, the system of equation (5)) can prove much easier than directly evaluating $\rho(\mathbf{A})$, especially if the objective is to obtain closed-form results corresponding to epidemic thresholds for specific mixing functions, as will become clear in Section 5.

4. Behavioral Foundations for the Mixing Probabilities

In this section, we motivate a number of alternative assumptions about partner selection and derive the consequences in terms of the mixing probabilities q_{ij} (we suppress the dependence on time in this section, as our arguments will apply to $q_{ij}(t)$ at all points in time). Our purpose is not so much to realistically model the partner selection process as it is to admit a variety of alternative assumptions which encompass a wide range of mixing possibilities. In later sections, these alternatives are explored to evaluate how sensitive results under the random mixing assumption are to alternative specifications of mixing behavior.

Two important questions motivate our models of partner selection: 1) how much does an individual know about a partner's risky sex rate, and 2) how costly (in time or effort, say) is the search for partners? In the following, we assume that each man is concerned with the risk associated with his sexual contacts. In particular, we assume that a man selects partners to minimize his perceived risk of infection, given the information he has about partners, his pool of available partners, and the rate at which he engages in risky sex. Our alternative models differ in the assumptions they make about the quality of the information individuals have about their partners, and the magnitude of search costs for partners. Given alternative information and cost structures, our models will force mixing among men with different risky sex rates. Such induced mixing can be viewed as an approximation of mixing due to perfect information regarding other attributes such as attractiveness and familiarity.

In all of our models where information plays a role, we assume that the only information signal (perfect or imperfect) is the risky sex rate. Thus, men evaluate the riskiness of a prospective partner in terms of his risky sex rate; the higher the risky sex rate, the higher the perceived risk. Important extensions not considered in this paper include variation in perceived risk due to variability in risky sexual practice (e.g., cognition of the different values of β_{ij}), and variation in perceived risk due to the duration of time for which prospective partners have been sexually active (e.g., a ten-year versus five-year history of sexual activity at the same annual risky sex rate).

In the remainder of this section, we formulate four alternative models of partner selection: (1) random mixing, which is motivated from poorly informed individuals or extremely costly search for partners, (2) segregation, which results from perfect information regarding risky sex rates and negligible search costs, (3) Bernoulli noise, which stems from imperfect information about partners and negligible search costs, and (4) costly search, which is derived from perfect information of risky sex rates, but high searching costs. Each of these models results in specific functions for the mixing probabilities q_{ij}. The epidemiological implications of these models will be examined in Section 5.

4.1 Random Mixing (or Proportionate Mixing)

Random mixing (or proportionate mixing; see Anderson et al, 1986; Hethcote and Van Ark, 1987) across risky sex rates in the population will occur when individuals have no information about prospective partners' risky sex rates, or when search costs are enormous. In either case, a man is unable to influence his perceived risk through careful partner selection; in the case of no information, all partners appear equally risky, while in the case of enormous search costs, a man will choose the first person available for risky sex since it is too costly to search out more desirable partners. Random mixing might also arise if an individual's preferences are such that factors uncorrelated with perceived risk dominate the partner selection decision. Any of these assumptions (no information, enormous search costs, or the dominance of other factors uncorrelated with risk) is sufficient for random mixing to occur, so long as we make the additional assumption that the pool of available partners for members of each subpopulation has the same distribution of risky sex rates as the total population. This assumption would be violated, for example, if men, for social reasons independent of risk minimization, segregate into subpopulations correlated with risky sex rates.

A major virtue of the random mixing model is its simplicity. With random mixing, the pairing mechanism is a random process that depends only on the risky sex rate c_j and the relative proportion $p_j=n_j/\Sigma_{k=1}^{m}n_k$ of types j in the population (where again we have suppressed the time argument in $n_j(t)$ and $p_j(t)$, for these definitions must hold at all points in time). The mixing function is given by (Hethcote and Van Ark, 1987):

$$q_{ij} = q_j \equiv \frac{c_j p_j}{E(c)}, \qquad i,j=1,2,\ldots,m, \qquad (8)$$

where

$$E(c) = \sum_{j=1}^{m} c_j p_j \tag{9}$$

is the mean risky sex rate over the population. Equation (8) states that the likelihood of selecting a member of subpopulation j equals the fraction of all sexual partnerships in the population that involve type j men; note that this probability is independent of i, as one would expect for random mixing. Equation (8) demonstrates a phenomenon known as random incidence. For a detailed discussion of random incidence within the context of AIDS modeling, see Kaplan (1989a).

4.2 Segregation

Again, assume that men are concerned with minimizing their perceived risk of infection. To do so, they attempt to select sex partners with the lowest possible risky sex rates. Segregation of the population by risky sex rate will occur when men have perfect information about prospective partners' risky sex rates, and when search costs are negligible. To see this, note that all men prefer partners with the lowest possible risky sex rate (say type 1). This is true of type 1's as well, however, so type 1's will match exclusively with other type 1's. Type 2's, upon realizing that type 1's are no longer available as sex partners (for type 1's match exclusively with type 1's), can do no better than to match with other type 2's. This segregation continues for all types of individuals. In general, for a type i individual, only type j individuals with the same or higher risky sex rates ($c_j \geq c_i$) are willing to be partners; and from this feasible set of partners, the type i man will prefer another type i, hence segregation by risky sex rate. Recall, however, that although men are assumed to know everyone's risky sex rate, we assume that men do not know how long prospective partners have been sexually active. The mixing function associated with segregation is merely the indicator function, that is

$$q_{ij} = 1_{\{i=j\}} \equiv \begin{cases} 1 & \text{if} \quad i=j \\ 0 & \text{if} \quad i \neq j, \end{cases} \qquad i,j=1,2,\ldots,m. \tag{10}$$

4.3 Bernoulli Noise (or Preferred Mixing)

The preferred mixing formulation to be described was proposed by Nold (1980) and has been employed by Hethcote and Van Ark (1987), Jacquez et al (1988), and Koopman et al (1988), though absent the following derivation. As an intermediate case between random mixing and segregation, imagine a world where all have imperfect information about prospective partners' risky sex rates. Here we consider the simplest model of imperfect information: every man has an apparent risky sex rate which everyone observes perfectly. With probability α, this apparent rate is guaranteed to equal the true rate. With probability $1-\alpha$, the apparent rate is a random incidence pick from the population of risky sex rates (i.e., c_j is observed with probability q_j as defined in equation (8); note that by chance, the random pick could result in the true rate). Hence, with probability α, the information is perfect, while with probability $1-\alpha$, the observed rate contains no information. Again, assume that search costs are negligible. In such a world, individuals will segregate based on observed rates following the reasoning of the segregation model. Both the random mixing model and the segregation model are special cases of Bernoulli noise with $\alpha=0$ and $\alpha=1$, respectively. With $0<\alpha<1$, while individuals still segregate, they do so on the basis of observed rates, allowing mixing among the true risky sex rates. Mixing according to Bernoulli noise can be thought of as an approximation to mixing that results from perfect knowledge of other, unmodeled, attributes such as attractiveness and familiarity.

To determine the mixing probabilities resulting from Bernoulli noise, define s_{ik} as the probability that a man with true risky sex rate c_i signals apparent risky sex rate c_k. In accordance with the assumptions postulated above, it is clear that

$$s_{ik} = \alpha\, 1_{\{i=k\}} + (1-\alpha)\, q_k, \qquad i,k=1,2,\ldots,m. \qquad (11)$$

Now define r_{kj} as the probability that a partner selected with an apparent risky sex rate equal to c_k has a true risky sex rate of c_j. Assuming random incidence within apparent risky sex classes (i.e., sex partners with equal apparent risky sex rates select each other at random), this probability is given by

$$r_{kj} = \frac{c_j p_j s_{jk}}{\sum_{\ell=1}^{m} c_\ell p_\ell s_{\ell k}}, \qquad k,j=1,2,\ldots,m. \qquad (12)$$

The Bernoulli noise mixing probabilities q_{ij} are then given by

$$q_{ij} = \sum_{k=1}^{m} s_{ik}\, r_{kj} = \alpha^2\, 1_{\{i=j\}} + (1-\alpha^2)\, q_j, \quad i,j=1,2,\ldots,m, \qquad (13)$$

with the last result following after tedious but straightforward algebra. Thus, the Bernoulli noise mixing probability function is simply a convex combination of the segregation and random mixing probability functions. Note again that $\alpha=1$ yields segregation while $\alpha=0$ yields random mixing.

4.4 Costly Search

Our final model of the partner selection process allows for mixing among men with different risky sex rates by relaxing the assumption that search costs are negligible. In contrast to the Bernoulli noise model (where information is imperfect and search costs are zero), here information is perfect but search costs are significant (but not large enough to qualify as enormous, which would force random mixing). In this case, an individual, if unsatisfied with a prospective partner due to the partner's high risky sex rate, must consider the high cost of searching for a partner with a lower risky sex rate. In equilibrium, each individual will only be willing to search if the potential partner's risky sex rate is sufficiently higher than his own. For simplicity, we assume that $c_i=i$ for this model, and that individual preferences are such that a type i man will only accept partners with risky sex rates at most k above his own. Thus, a type i man will accept a partner of type j only if $j\le i+k$. Similarly, type j's will only accept type i's if $i\le j+k$. As a consequence, in equilibrium, type i's will only be able to secure type j partners for $i-k \le j \le i+k$. Note that if $k=0$, the costly search model reduces to the segregation model. As k increases, the amount of mixing among individuals of different risky sex rates also increases.

To construct mixing probabilities consistent with these ideas, we first impose symmetry on the q_{ij}'s around the risky sex rate of the searching man, that is

$$q_{ij} = \begin{cases} q_{i,2i-j}, & \max(0,i-k) \le j \le \min(m,i+k) \\ 0 & \text{otherwise} \end{cases} \quad i,j=1,2,\ldots,m. \tag{14}$$

This symmetry is somewhat similar to the use of Gaussian mixing functions by Hyman and Stanley (1988). We next impose $k(k+1)/2$ seed values for the mixing probabilities; the values we specify are the k probabilities q_{12}, q_{13}, ..., $q_{1,k+1}$, the k-1 probabilities q_{24}, q_{25}, ..., $q_{2,k+2}$, ..., and the probability $q_{k,2k}$. The imposition of these seed values, the symmetry of equation (14), the conservation law of equation (1), and the requirement that $\Sigma_{j=1}^{m} q_{ij}=1$ for each j provide a set of linear equations which uniquely determine all of the mixing probabilities. One must be careful in choosing seed values, however, for the solution of the equations just stated could yield values of q_{ij} which are negative; this is especially critical in dynamic simulations of the HIV epidemic, where the values of q_{ij} must be recalculated at each time instant.

5. Epidemiological Implications of the Mixing Probabilities

In this section, we will investigate the sensitivity of our model of HIV epidemics to the alternative mixing probabilities presented. To simplify matters, we will assume that the infectivities β_{ij} all equal the common value β; this is a common assumption in the majority of published work to date (though one could certainly begin to assign differential values of β to different sexual practices such as unprotected or protected insertive versus receptive anal intercourse, for example). We will first present threshold conditions for the random mixing, segregation, and Bernoulli noise models (the costly search model does not yield to more specific treatment than the general conditions Section 2 prescribes). Then we will study some numerical examples of random and nonrandom HIV epidemics generated from common assumptions regarding population immigration and emigration/death rates, AIDS incubation times, infectivity and the distribution of risky sex rates.

5.1 Threshold Condition for Random Mixing

The threshold condition for random mixing was presented by Anderson et al (1986) in terms of the reproductive rate of infection. In our notation, their result may be stated as follows: an HIV epidemic under random mixing occurs if the reproductive rate of infection R_0 exceeds unity, where

$$R_0 \equiv \frac{E(c^2)}{E(c)} \beta D \tag{15}$$

and $E(c^2)=\Sigma_{i=1}^{m} c_i^2 p_i$. To obtain this result from our approach in Section 3, note that the appropriate value of q_{ij}^* to use in equation (5) is

$$q_{ij}^* = q_j^* \equiv \frac{N_j c_j}{\sum_{k=1}^{m} N_k c_k}, \qquad j=1,2,\ldots,m. \tag{16}$$

Inserting (16) into (5), and assuming that $\beta_{ij}=\beta$ for every i,j pair, we obtain the equation

$$T_i = c_i \beta DK, \qquad i=1,2,\ldots,m, \tag{17}$$

where

$$K = \sum_{j=1}^{m} q_j^* \,(1+T_j) = \sum_{j=1}^{m} q_j^* \,(1+c_j \beta DK) = 1/(1-R_0), \tag{18}$$

the last equality following by direct substitution for q_j^*. The theory of Section 2 states that an epidemic occurs if and only if $T_i<0$ for some i; from equations (17) and (18), it is clear that $T_i<0$ for <u>every</u> i if and only if $R_0>1$.

5.2 Thresholds for Segregation

Having derived the epidemic threshold for random mixing, the analysis for segregation is automatic; for any particular segregated subpopulation i can be viewed as a randomly mixing population with mean risky sex rate c_i and zero variance. Thus, an epidemic will occur in subpopulation i if and only if

$$R_{0i} \equiv c_i \beta D > 1, \qquad i=1,2,\ldots,m, \qquad (19)$$

and an epidemic will occur somewhere in the population if and only if $R_{0m}>1$ (assuming c_m is the largest risky sex rate). Already we have the possibility that a particular distribution of risky sex rates might not sustain an HIV epidemic under random mixing (for R_0 of equation (15) might fall below unity), yet this same distribution of risky sex rates could sustain an epidemic under segregation (for R_{0m} could exceed unity even though R_0 does not).

5.3 Threshold for Bernoulli Noise

Recall from equation (16) the definition of the Bernoulli noise mixing probabilities. Given this simple form, one might expect that the threshold condition for a Bernoulli noise epidemic is a simple combination of the thresholds for random mixing and segregation. This is not the case, as we will now show.

First, consider the largest risky sex rate c_m. If $\alpha^2 R_{0m}$ exceeds unity, an epidemic will develop in subgroup m, for men in subgroup m mix among themselves sufficiently to generate a segregated epidemic even after discounting sexual contacts between men in subgroup m and other subgroups. In this instance, an epidemic will develop among all subgroups, as all subgroups communicate for $0<\alpha<1$. Thus, a sufficient condition for a Bernoulli noise epidemic is that $\alpha^2 R_{0m}$ exceeds unity.

Now suppose that $\alpha^2 R_{0m}$ is less than one. To use equation (5), note that the appropriate value of q_{ij}^* equals

$$q_{ij}^* = \alpha^2 \, 1_{\{i=j\}} + (1-\alpha^2)\, q_j^*, \qquad i,j=1,2,\ldots,m, \qquad (20)$$

where q_j^* is given in equation (16). Use of equation (5) then implies that the threshold condition (when $\alpha^2 R_{0m}<1$) for a Bernoulli noise epidemic is crossed when

$$(1-\alpha^2) \sum_{k=1}^{m} q_k^* R_{0k}/(1-\alpha^2 R_{0k}) > 1. \qquad (21)$$

Note that when $\alpha=0$, (21) reduces to $R_0>1$ as expected for random mixing. Also, as the left hand side of (21) exceeds $(1-\alpha^2)R_0$, another sufficient condition for a Bernoulli noise epidemic to occur is $(1-\alpha^2)R_0>1$ (this mirrors the sufficient condition $\alpha^2 R_{0m}>1$ discussed earlier).

The threshold in (21) has an interesting implication. It is entirely possible that a given distribution of risky sex rates could yield $R_0<1$ under random mixing, but for some value of α, the threshold in (21) could be satisfied. As random mixing corresponds to no information about the risky sex rates of prospective partners, while Bernoulli noise implies some information (as measured by α), imperfect information can be worse than no information. Worded differently, a little information can be a dangerous thing. This result differs from our earlier comparison between random mixing and segregation, for if the threshold in (21) is crossed, then all subgroups will experience an HIV epidemic (as opposed to only some of the subgroups as is the case with segregation). Of course, this result is a theoretical possibility; for risky sex distributions which roughly describe the sexual activity of gay men, the severity of HIV epidemics under random mixing is typically harsher than that experienced under any of our nonrandom mixing models, as we will now illustrate.

5.4 Numerical Examples of Nonrandom HIV Epidemics

To simulate HIV epidemics under the various mixing schemes discussed, we make the simplifying assumption that the AIDS incubation time is exponentially distributed with mean $1/\gamma$. Though the exponential is not descriptively accurate, its use simplifies our computations without distorting the impact of the various mixing patterns we consider. Define $X_i(t)$ and $Y_i(t)$ as the number of uninfected and infected men in subpopulation i at time t, $X_i(t)+Y_i(t)=n_i(t)$. Further, define $\pi_i(t)=Y_i(t)/n_i(t)$ as the prevalence of infection in the ith subpopulation. Our assumptions imply the following differential equations:

$$\frac{dX_i(t)}{dt} = N_i - \mu X_i(t) - (1-\pi_i(t)) \sum_{j=1}^{m} c_j Y_j(t) q_{ji}(t) \beta_{ji}, \qquad i=1,2,\ldots,m, \tag{22}$$

and

$$\frac{dY_i(t)}{dt} = (1-\pi_i(t)) \sum_{j=1}^{m} c_j Y_j(t) q_{ji}(t) \beta_{ji} - (\mu + \gamma)\, Y_i(t), \qquad i=1,2,\ldots,m. \tag{23}$$

In the absence of HIV/AIDS, we assume that sex lives average 32 years, thus μ=1/32 per man per year (as assumed by Anderson et al, 1986 and Kaplan, 1989a). The incubation time for AIDS is assumed to average 8 years (see Medley et al, 1987 and Lui, Darrow and Rutherford, 1988) so γ=1/8 per man per year. The infectivity β is set equal to .075 per partnership (this falls within the range of infectivities for receptive anal intercourse estimated by Grant, Wiley and Winkelstein, 1987 and Kaplan, 1989a). Finally, the immigration rates N_i for men with risky sex rates of c_i=i partners per year are assumed to follow

$$N_i = 3125 \frac{11-i}{55}, \qquad i=1,2,\ldots,10. \tag{24}$$

In effect, we are approximating heterogeneity in risky sex rates by dividing the population into 10 different subpopulations. In the absence of HIV, the sexually active population would reach an equibrilibrim of 100,000 men. The mean risky sex rate in the absence of HIV equals 4 partners per year, while the ratio $E(c^2)/E(c)$ equals 5.5 partners per year. Though less variable than the risky sex distributions considered by Anderson et al (1986) and Kaplan (1989a), the mean risky sex rate of 4 is comparable to the average of 5 partners per year employed by these researchers.

To introduce HIV to the population, we establish the following initial conditions:

$$Y_i(0) = n_i(0)\ \theta^{i-10}/\ n_{10}(0) \qquad i=1,2,\ldots,10, \tag{25}$$

where $n_i(0)=N_i/\mu$. Note that $Y_{10}(0)=1$; equation (25) introduces a single infected man into the most active subpopulation and essentially introduces a trace of infection into each of the other subpopulations. Throughout our numerical examples, we set $\theta=5$.

Figure 1 plots the total number of infected men in the population (i.e., $\Sigma_{i=1}^{10}Y_i(t)$) versus time for Bernoulli noise epidemics where the strength of the information signal (as measured by α^2) is varied from 0 (i.e., random mixing) to 1 (i.e., segregation). The reproductive rate of infection for the random mixing case, R_0 (equation (15)), equals 2.64, thus the ensuing epidemic is hardly a surprise. For the parameters of this example, the Bernoulli noise epidemics with α^2=.25,.5 and .75 closely mimic the random mixing epidemic, with the time until peak infection dropping slightly as α increases. However, the segregation epidemic resulting when $\alpha=1$ has a distinctly different pattern. The epidemic moves in waves as each of the subpopulations from 10 through 3 reach their peak levels of infection at different times (after the 100 years simulated here, subpopulations 3 and 4 had yet to reach their peak levels of infection). This is due to two factors: the differences in risky sex rates for the different subpopulations, and the different initial conditions (as stated in equation (25)). The initial conditions in this instance mimic the phased introduction of HIV into the various subpopulations. What is clear from Figure 1, however, is that the random mixing epidemic is the most severe of those considered. These limited simulations suggest that the random mixing model may provide a conservative tool for policy analysts.

It is possible, however, for a nonrandom mixing epidemic to occur when $R_0 \leq 1$. For example, suppose that the infectivity was reduced from .075 to .025 due to some control measure (perhaps due to the sporadic use of condoms). In this case, no random mixing epidemic would ensue, for the reproductive rate R_0 of equation (15) would equal .88, which is less than unity. However, Bernoulli noise epidemics are possible: the threshold condition (21) implies that HIV infection will endure if $\alpha^2>.4427$. The time necessary for such epidemics to develop, however, is long indeed. For example, after a century of HIV infection following the initial conditions of equation (25), about 100 of 99,800 men would be infected with α^2=.75; segregation yields 585 infections out of 98,600 men after the same time period. Utilization of the random mixing model to determine that the control measure would be effective (as $R_0<1$) does not lead to disaster in the event that the population in question really mixes in accordance with Bernoulli noise. The resulting prevalence of infection in this latter case remains low: no higher than 585/98,600=.006 after 100 years. Such low levels of infection over such a long time period cannot be considered serious. Though no hope exists for a rapid medical solution to HIV infection, the same cannot be said for a time frame of a century! Also, behavioral change will surely obviate these results with the passage of time.

Figure 1

Bernoulli Noise HIV Epidemics

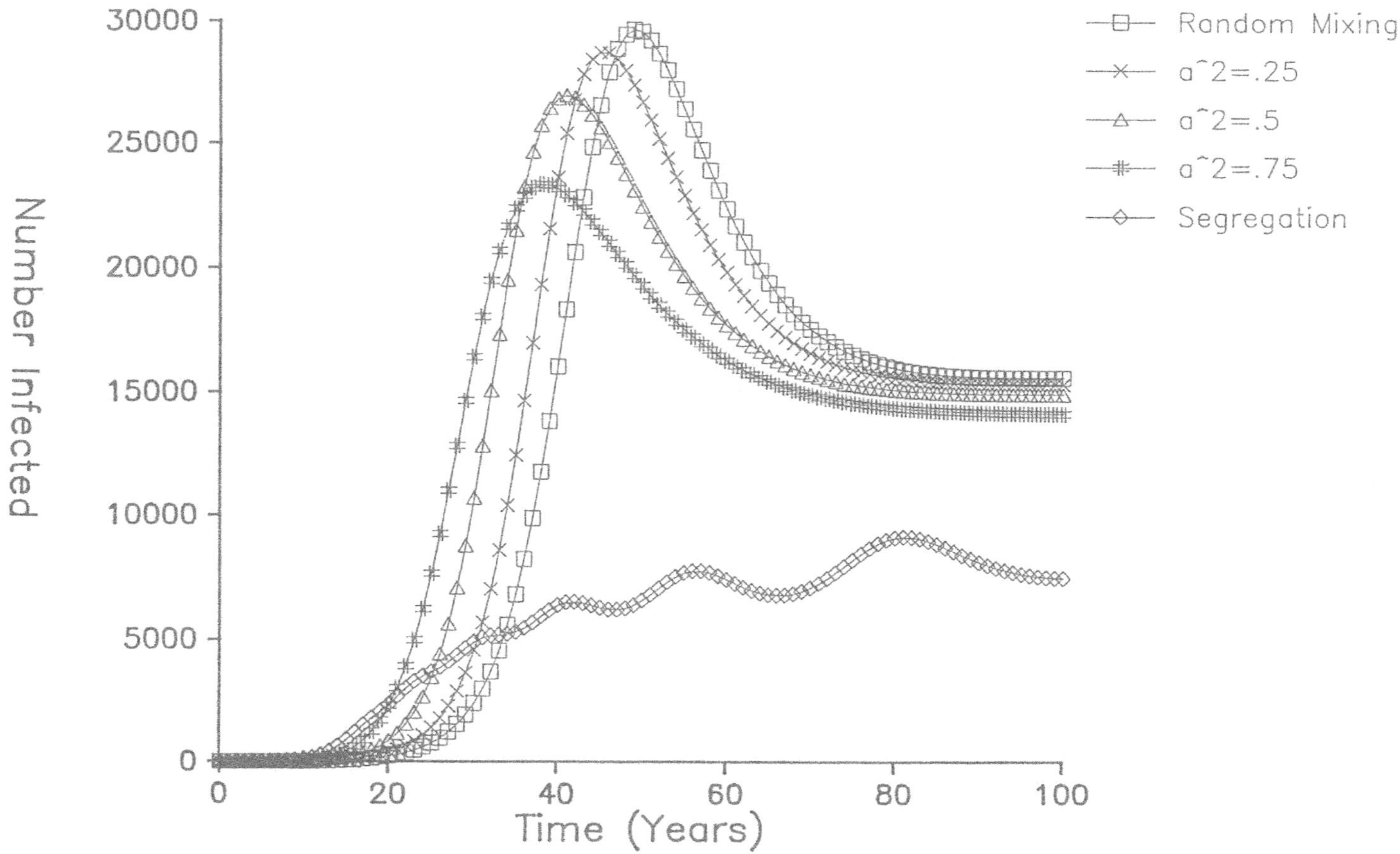

Figure 2 presents three costly search epidemics, along with the segregation epidemic and a Bernoulli noise epidemic with α^2=.9 for comparison. In Case I, $q_{12}(t)$=.1 and $q_{13}(t)=q_{24}(t)$=.05; in Case II, $q_{12}(t)$=.075 and $q_{13}(t)=q_{24}(t)$=.025. In both of these cases, a man is restricted to choosing partners with risky sex rates that differ by, at most, two from his own. Case III is even more stringent; a man is restricted to partners with risky sex rates that differ by, at most, one from his own. In this case, $q_{12}(t)$=.1 Generally speaking, these mixing functions possess modes with probability mass between .5 and .9 at $q_{ii}(t)$ for all time periods and most subpopulations (though $q_{10,10}(t)$ is not modal for subgroup 10 for some time periods in these simulations). Note that the epidemics resulting from the costly search mixing functions have been flattened relatively to Bernoulli noise; there is no rapid rise to peak infection followed by a quick retreat towards steady state. Indeed, the costly search epidemics appear to be smoothed versions of the segregation epidemic, though higher levels of infection are reached. However, the long run levels of HIV infection for the costly search models appear comparable to the Bernoulli noise and random mixing models. Again, random mixing appears to be a worst case.

Figure 2

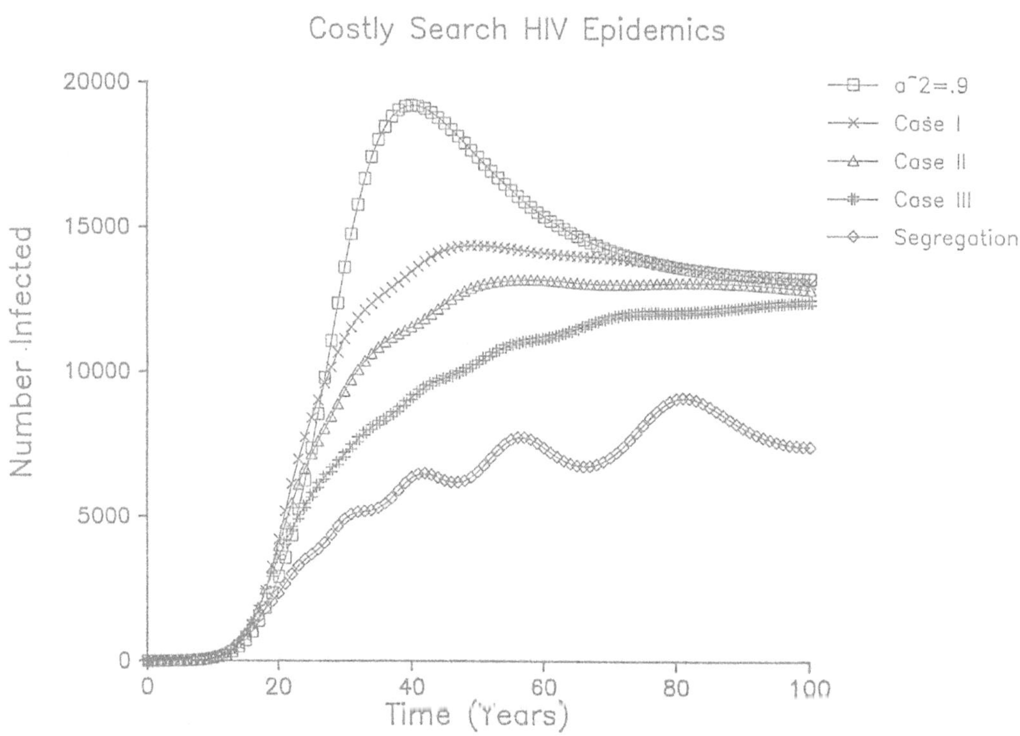

6. Concluding Remarks

This paper has formulated a macromodel of nonrandom mixing, presented two different approaches for deriving threshold conditions for this model, and discussed new approaches to deriving mixing probabilities. Four mixing scenarios were discussed: random mixing, segregation, Bernoulli noise, and costly search. Although it is possible for nonrandom models to produce more serious epidemics than random mixing dictates, we found that epidemiological environments roughly descriptive of the AIDS epidemic produce worse epidemics for random mixing than for the nonrandom models studied.

There is little doubt that, from a purely descriptive point of view, random mixing does not describe human behavior; by implication, some variant of nonrandom mixing does. The important question, however, is whether or not random mixing models of HIV infection can seriously mislead policy analysts working within a fixed epidemiological environment (that is, given a distribution of risky sex rates, immigration and emigration/death rates, infectivities and an incubation time distribution). Our limited experience suggests that for a given epidemiological environment, either random mixing serves as a worst case over nonrandom mixing scenarios (though the bias does not appear to be too extreme), or when random mixing epidemics are not severe, neither are nonrandom epidemics. Thus, having derived a variety of nonrandom mixing models, an important question remains: for a fixed epidemiological environment, can one have a significant nonrandom mixing epidemic (i.e., high prevalence of infection over a short time scale, say 20-30 years) when random mixing does not produce a significant epidemic for the same epidemiological parameters? To our knowledge, this question remains open.

Acknowledgement

We wish to thank Carlos Castillo-Chavez and the six anonymous referees; their suggestions have strengthened this paper.

References

Abramson, P.R. and B. Rothschild (1988). Sex, drugs and matrices: mathematical prediction of HIV infection. J. Sex Res., 25, 106-122.

Anderson, R.M. (1988). The Epidemiology of HIV Infection: Variable incubation plus infectious periods and heterogeneity in sexual activity. J. Roy. Stat. Soc. (Ser. A), 151, 66-93.

Anderson, R.M., G.F. Medley, R.M. May, and A.M. Johnson (1986). A preliminary study of the transmission dynamics of the human immunodeficiency virus (HIV), the causative agent of AIDS. IMA J. Math. Appl. Med. Bio., 3, 229-263.

Blythe, S.P. and C. Castillo-Chavez (1989). Like-with-like preference and sexual mixing models. Math. Biosci. (in press).

Brookmeyer, R. and M., Gail (1988). A method for obtaining short-term projections and lower bounds on the size of the AIDS epidemic. JASA, 83, 301-308.

CDC (1989). HIV/AIDS Surveillance Report. Centers for Disease Control, Public Health Service, U.S. Department of Health and Human Services, May 1989, 1-16.

Curran, J.W., H.W. Jaffe, A.M. Hardy, W. M. Morgan, R.M. Selki, and T.J. Dondero (1988). Epidemiology of HIV infection and AIDS in the United States. Science, 239, 610-616.

Grant, R.M., J.A. Wiley, and W. Winkelstein (1987). Infectivity of the human immunodeficiency virus: estimates from a prospective study of homosexual men. J. Inf. Dis., 156, 189-193.

Hethcote, H.W. and J.W. Van Ark (1987). Epidemiological models for heterogeneous populations: proportionate mixing, parameter estimation, and immunization programs. Math. Biosci., 84, 85-118.

Hethcote, H.W. and J.A. Yorke (1984). Gonorrhea, transmission dynamics, and control. Lecture Notes in Biomathematics 56, Springer-Verlag, Berlin.

Hyman, J.M. and E.A. Stanley (1988). Using mathematical models to understand the AIDS epidemic. Math. Biosci., 90, 415-473.

Isham, V. (1988). Mathematical modeling of the transmission dynamics of HIV infections and AIDS: a review. J. Roy. Stat. Soc. (Ser. A), 151, 5-30.

Jacquez, J.A., C.P. Simon, J. Koopman, L. Sattenspiel, and T. Perry, (1988). Modeling and analyzing HIV transmission: the effect of contact patterns. Math. Biosci., 92, 119-199.

Kaplan, E.H. (1989a). What are the risks of risky sex? Modeling the AIDS epidemic. Op. Res., 37, 198-209.

Kaplan, E.H. (1989b). Needles that kill: modeling human immunodeficiency virus transmission via shared drug injection equipment in shooting galleries. Rev. Inf. Dis., 11, 289-298.

Kaplan, E.H. and P.R. Abramson (1989). So what if the program ain't perfect? A mathematical model of AIDS education. Eval. Rev., 13, 107-122.

Koopman, J., C. Simon, J. Jacquez, J. Joseph, L. Sattenspiel, and T. Park, (1988). Sexual partner selectiveness effects of homosexual HIV transmission dynamics. JAIDS, 1, 486-504.

Lui, K-J, W.W. Darrow, and G.W. Rutherford, III (1988). A model-based estimate of the mean incubation period for AIDS in homosexual men. Science, 240, 1333-1335.

May, R.M. and R.M. Anderson (1987). Transmission dynamics of HIV infection. Nature, 326, 137-142.

May, R.M. and R.M. Anderson (1988). The transmission dynamics of human immunodeficiency virus (HIV). Phil. Trans. Roy. Soc. (in press).

Medley, G.F., R.M. Anderson, D.R. Cox, and L. Billard (1987). Incubation period of AIDS in patients infected via blood transfusion. Nature, 328, 719-721.

Nold, A. (1980). Heterogeneity in diseases-transmission modeling. Math. Biosci., 52, 227-240.

Strang, G. (1980). Linear Algebra and its Applications. Academic Press, New York.

Wiley, J.A., S. Herschkorn, and N. Padian (1989). Heterogeneity in the probability of HIV transmission per sexual contact. Stat. Med., 8, 93-102.

IV. Social Dynamics and AIDS

THE STRUCTURE AND CONTEXT OF SOCIAL INTERACTIONS AND THE SPREAD OF HIV

Lisa Sattenspiel
Department of Anthropology
210 Switzler Hall
University of Missouri
Columbia, MO 65211

Abstract

This study addresses a number of questions associated with the spread of HIV that can be investigated with the use of mathematical models. These include: 1) how to model the patterns of contact among individuals in different risk groups, 2) the effects on the risk of transmission of the social context present at the time of a sexual interaction, and 3) ways to incorporate IV drug use into sexual transmission models. A migration matrix model for disease spread in a subdivided population, originally developed by Sattenspiel (1987) for the spread of hepatitis A in day care centers, is briefly described. The utility of this model for investigating the effects of varying the patterns of contact, the effects of social context, and the multiple modes of transmission of HIV is discussed. The limitations of the model and its applications to diseases other than AIDS and to problems outside the realm of mathematical epidemiology are also described.

1. Introduction

Until the end of the last decade, almost all mathematical models for the spread of disease assumed a constant population of randomly mixing individuals. This is not a reasonable assumption, considering the actual behavior of human populations. Human groups are comprised of a number of different subgroups, within which interactions *may* be random, but among which interactions are certainly not random. An example is the caste system in India, where the degree of social interaction between two individuals from different castes may clearly be limited, especially in certain social contexts. Minturn and Hitchcock (1966) describe a gathering of landowners in a village in India. The men are all sitting together smoking from the same pipe. If a high status Brahman were to join them, he would be given either a different pipe or a different pipe stem every time it was his turn to smoke so that he would not be made unclean by the interaction with the lower status landowners. An Untouchable, on the other hand, would be considered as polluting by the entire group and would not be allowed to join them at all. In the fields, however, the Brahman and the Untouchable could very well work together in close contact.

The assumption of random mixing among the individuals in a population resulted in simpler and more easily analyzed models. As long as mathematical epidemiology was dominated by mathematicians rather than epidemiologists, and as long as there was no attempt to relate the models to data on actual epidemics, the assumption was not seriously questioned, even though there were a few theoretical articles that relaxed the assumption. However, in the late 1970s the rise in the level of sexually transmitted disease in the United States led to the development and application of models for the spread of sexually transmitted diseases which attempted to combine epidemiological data with mathematical modeling (Lajmanovich and Yorke 1976; Yorke, Hethcote, and Nold 1978; Nold 1980; Hethcote, Yorke, and Nold 1982; Hethcote and Yorke 1984). The nature of sexual transmission makes the assumption of one large, randomly mixing population patently unrealistic. At the very minimum, sexually transmitted disease models require a simple structured population divided into two groups: males and females. In the population as a whole, there clearly exists nonrandom mixing, since there is differential contact within and between the sexes.

In almost all recent attempts to combine epidemiological data with mathematical modeling there has been a recognition of the need to consider the structure of social interactions among the individuals in the populations. This has resulted in models which consider the population to be divided into a number of interacting subgroups. In addition to the models for the spread of sexually transmitted disease, structured models have been developed to describe the spread of measles (Haggett 1972,1976; Cliff, et al. 1975), influenza (Baroyan, Rvachev, and Ivannikov 1977; Rvachev and Longini 1985; Longini 1988), smallpox (Travis and Lenhart 1987), and hepatitis A (Sattenspiel 1987; Sattenspiel and Simon 1988). Models for the spread of HIV also fit into this category - both because of the sexual transmission of HIV and because of the present isolation of the infection within fairly well-defined risk groups.

2. Interactions between groups in structured populations

Most models for disease spread in subdivided populations contain an $n \times n$ matrix to describe the interactions among the subpopulations. This matrix has n^2 terms in it, and when more than a few subpopulations are considered, the estimation problems associated with this matrix become insurmountable. Making reasonable simplifying assumptions about the nature of interactions among individuals within and among subgroups is a major concern in the analysis of such models.

The earliest *n*-group model was proposed by Rushton and Mautner (1955) and was a general model without reference to a specific disease. This model considers two infection rates in the population; a_i is the internal infection rate in community *i* and β_{ij} is the rate of infection between communities *i* and *j*. However, this model assumes that there is homogeneous mixing among all individuals in the population - the effect of the subdivision is only to change the probability of infection, not to change the probability of interaction.

Watson (1972) proposed a theoretical model where the transmission rate per capita between groups is a constant fraction of the transmission rate per capita within groups. This does not really lead to heterogeneous mixing since all groups are treated equally. A similar formulation was used by May and Anderson (1984). Travis and Lenhart (1987) assume a constant, equal transmission rate for all groups in most of their analysis. Post, DeAngelis, and Travis (1983) consider a theoretical model with a transmission rate that is either a linear or nonlinear function of the time that two groups spend in contact with each other.

The gonorrhea models of Lajmanovich and Yorke (1976), Yorke, Hethcote, and Nold (1978), Nold (1980), Hethcote, Yorke, and Nold (1982), and Hethcote and Yorke (1984) initially assume that mixing between subgroups (as measured by the number of new sexual encounters between groups) is proportionate to the relative sexual activities of the two groups. Hethcote and Van Ark (1987) also assume proportionate mixing in their model of the effects of immunization on the spread of a non-sexually transmitted disease. This assumption is clearly not realistic for sexually transmitted diseases, since very active individuals tend preferentially to choose other active individuals. The gonorrhea papers thus consider a moderate generalization of the proportionate mixing assumption which defines a mixing matrix in which a fraction, 1 - G, of the population mixes proportionately with individuals from all groups, while the remaining fraction, G, has new sexual encounters distributed in proportion to the fractional activity levels of the opposite sex group within the same activity level. The mixing matrix is thus a combination of proportionate mixing at the population level and selective mixing among individuals with the same rates of sexual activity. G measures the propensity for choosing sexual partners with similar behavior. Hethcote, Yorke, and Nold (1982) and Hethcote and Yorke (1984) compare the results from the proportionate mixing model with those from the more general model in which G is determined in such a way that the prevalence of gonorrhea in women is approximately 3% of the population of women at risk. They find that the proportionate mixing model (G=0) leads to unrealistically high prevalences, but they do not explore the consequences of varying G across a wide range of values. Rather, they choose G to fit observed prevalences given the choices for other parameter values.

Rvachev and Longini (1985) develop a model for the global spread of influenza in which the amount of contact between groups is estimated from data on the number of airline passengers traveling between the cities in a 24-hour period. The elements of the resulting transportation matrix are the average number of individuals that travel from one population to another. In addition, the matrix is assumed to be symmetric.

3. A migration matrix model for disease spread in a structured population

Sattenspiel (1987) developed a variation on the general structured model which incorporates a migration or movement matrix to describe the patterns of contact between individuals from different subgroups. A migration matrix approach was first used by population geneticists (Bodmer and Cavalli-Sforza 1968, Smith 1969) to study the effects of population subdivision on the genetic structure of a population. The genetic models use a backward stochastic migration matrix in which the elements, m_{ik}, give the probabilities of an offspring in population *i* having parents in population *j*. The models are then used to derive the genetic variances and covariances among populations.

In an epidemic model, the migration matrix can be used to describe the probability of two individuals from different subgroups coming into contact. However, this matrix is a forward stochastic matrix whose elements give the probability of an individual from group *i* moving to group *k*. This is similar to the Rvachev and Longini model, but the conceptual basis of this model is an individual's movements rather than the behavior of an entire group.

Social interactions involve at least two individuals. Therefore, a model based on a concept of individual mobility must consider the simultaneous movement of the two or more individuals involved in the social interaction. For example, in an interaction between an individual from group *i* and one from group *j* occurring in group *k*, one individual moves from group *i* to group *k* and the second individual moves from group *j* to group *k*. The total probability of contact between these two individuals is the sum of the probabilities that interactions occur in each neighborhood *k*, or

$$\sum_{k=1}^{n} m_{ik} m_{jk}.$$

This term also gives the *ij* -th element of the matrix mm^T; the migration matrix model will henceforth be called the mm^T model.

In addition to the different formulation for the probability of contact between individuals from different subpopulations, the mm^T model considered a hierarchical subdivision of the population. The entire population was divided into *n* discrete subpopulations. Each subpopulation was further divided into two groups of individuals: social and nonsocial. Nonsocial individuals stayed at home and interacted only with other individuals (both social and nonsocial) from within the local neighborhood. Social individuals, on the other hand, were able to travel to other neighborhoods for the purpose of social activities. Therefore, they had two independent risks for infection - risk from within the neighborhood as a consequence of local interactions and risk as a consequence of social activities in their own and other neighborhoods. The movement matrix then describes the probability of interaction between two social individuals as a consequence of their social activities.

The social/nonsocial structure combined with the movement matrix approach leads to the following system of equations to describe the epidemic process (see Sattenspiel (1987) for a complete derivation):

$$\frac{dx_{oi}}{dt} = b_iN_{oi} - b_ix_{oi} - \beta s_i(x_{oi}y_{oi} + x_{oi}y_{si}),$$

$$\frac{dx_{si}}{dt} = b_iN_{si} - b_ix_{si} - \beta s_i(x_{si}y_{oi} + x_{si}y_{si}) - \beta x_{si}\sum_{j=1}^{n}\sum_{k=1}^{n} m_{ik}m_{jk}y_j,$$

$$\frac{dy_{oi}}{dt} = \beta s_i(x_{oi}y_{oi} + x_{oi}y_{si}) - g_iy_{oi} - b_iy_{oi},$$

$$\frac{dy_{si}}{dt} = \beta s_i(x_{si}y_{oi} + x_{si}y_{si}) + \beta x_{si}\sum_{j=1}^{n}\sum_{k=1}^{n} m_{ik}m_{jk}y_j - g_iy_{si} - b_iy_{si},$$

$$\frac{dz_{oi}}{dt} = g_iy_{oi} - b_iz_{oi},$$

$$\frac{dz_{si}}{dt} = g_iy_{si} - b_iz_{si},$$

where x_{oi}, y_{oi}, and z_{oi} are the numbers of susceptible, infective, and recovered individuals, respectively, in nonsocial subgroup oi; and x_{si}, y_{si}, and z_{si} are the corresponding numbers for social subgroup si. The birth and death rates are given by b_i. g_i is the recovery rate in subpopulation i, ß is the transmission rate per unit contact, and s_i is a neighborhood-specific adjustment of the transmission rate. All individuals entering the population through birth are susceptible, but deaths occur in all classes. Note the additional term in the equations for socially susceptible and infective individuals — this term reflects the between-group interaction of these individuals.

As Hethcote, Yorke, and Nold did in the gonorrhea models, Sattenspiel (1987) discussed the effects of heterogeneity in the amount of contact among subpopulations. This was done by varying the structure of the movement matrix. Three distinct patterns were analyzed: 1) total isolation of all subpopulations (represented by the identity matrix), 2) completely random mixing (represented by a matrix with each element equal to 1/n), and 3) division of the population into a small locally mixing cluster of subpopulations and a larger randomly mixing cluster of subpopulations. In the third pattern, individuals living in one of the subpopulations making up the locally mixing cluster could only move to one of the other local groups for their social activities, while an individual from one of the randomly mixing subpopulations could move to any one of the subpopulations, including those within the local cluster. Results of the analysis showed that when there was a mixture of subpopulation types (as in the third example), there were significant effects on the pattern and rate of spread of the infection throughout the population. More specifically, results showed that those individuals who came from a local group were at much higher risk of infection, because they had intense local interactions due to the relative isolation of the group; and in addition, they had a significant rate of introduction to the infection due to the lack of total isolation. Therefore, the infection was likely to be introduced into the groups, and then, once established, it prospered due to the intense local interactions.

The analysis of this model was later refined and extended, and it was shown analytically that a critical factor in this behavior is the asymmetry of the mixing matrix (Sattenspiel and Simon 1988). A logical explanation for this is that when the mixing matrix is asymmetric, the subgroups receiving a disproportionate number of "migrants" have a larger effective population size. Because of this, actual neighborhood sizes can be smaller and still support the disease at an endemic level. However, the analytical results have only been proven for a 2 x 2 movement matrix, and consequently, it is not clear whether the results observed are a general consequence of the symmetry properties or whether they are a consequence of assuming a stochastic movement matrix.

The theoretical results of this model were also compared to data on the incidence of hepatitis A among day care centers in Albuquerque, New Mexico. There was a large city-wide epidemic throughout most of 1979, with over 700 cases, 28% of which were clearly associated with day care centers. These cases involved 36 different day care centers and one bowling alley with nursery facilities. Hadler, et al. (1980) have defined an outbreak of hepatitis A in day care centers as the appearance of the disease in three or more families over a three month interval. Using this definition, fifteen centers in Albuquerque and the bowling alley had outbreaks of the disease.

Analysis of these data supports the hypothesis that local clusters are at higher risk for epidemics. Six of the fifteen centers reporting cases of hepatitis A had 10 or more cases of the disease. Four of these centers were owned and operated by the same family, one of the remaining centers was located within the geographic region bounded by the family-operated centers (which included a fifth center with only one case of hepatitis A), and the sixth center was located on the local Air Force base and had a direct link with another center located very near one of the family-owned centers. The family-run centers were not particularly localized geographically, although it is probable that there were several social contacts between the centers, both among children and among staff members. Close social ties link up these centers in a small local cluster which helps to explain the disproportionate number of cases of the disease associated with these centers.

Both the movement matrix formulation and the hierarchical structure of the mm^T model have important applications to the problem of modeling the spread of AIDS. These applications will be discussed further below.

4. Heterogeneity in contact patterns and the spread of AIDS

The presence of well-defined risk groups for AIDS, clear evidence for non-random mixing among groups, and the public health emergency resulting from the spread of the disease have resulted in the proliferation of mathematical models of the spread of disease in structured populations. Most of the existing models consider only the sexual transmission of the disease, largely because there are better data available for this problem for historical reasons. Although there are several aspects of the natural history of the disease which models can address, the bulk of modeling efforts are concerned with the consequences of one or more of three factors: 1) the effect that variability in infectivity throughout the course of the disease in an individual has on the spread of the infection throughout the population, 2) the effect of level of sexual activity on an individual's risk for disease, and 3) the effect that assumptions about mixing between groups have on both individual risk and transmission throughout a population.

Hyman and Stanley (1988, 1989) and Jacquez, et al. (1988) demonstrate that variations in the shape of the infectivity curve over the course of infection can markedly influence the outcome of the epidemic. Hyman and Stanley use an infectivity curve that peaks sharply early in the infectious period, followed by a low level of infectivity that rises gradually with the time since infection. Results show that, in a model in which all individuals have the same risk behavior, the rate at which the susceptible population is infected changes dramatically when the infectivity curve is altered. These effects are most marked when the alterations change the early peak in infectivity.

The effect of level of sexual activity has been studied by Anderson, et al. (1986), Kießling, et al. (1986), Knox (1986), May and Anderson (1987), Blythe and Anderson (1988), and De Grutolla and Mayer (1988). These studies clearly show that the level of sexual activity is a critical factor influencing the rate of spread and the intensity of the epidemic in each subgroup. However, these models usually assume proportionate mixing of individuals within the population - assumptions which the previous studies on gonorrhea and hepatitis A demonstrated to be unrealistic.

Jacquez, et al. (1988), Koopman, et al. (1988), Sattenspiel, et al. (1989), Hyman and Stanley (1988, 1989), and Blythe and Castillo-Chavez (manuscript) have explored the effects of varying the patterns of sexual activity as well as the levels of activity. They show conclusively that lack of randomness in the choice of sexual partner can profoundly affect the course of the epidemic and is an important confounding factor to the levels of sexual activity.

The Michigan HIV modeling group uses a mixing pattern called "preferred mixing" (Jacquez, et al. 1988; Koopman, et al. 1988; Sattenspiel, et al. 1989; see also Hyman and Stanley 1988). This pattern is similar to the pattern used in the gonorrhea models in that a fraction of the population selects partners from any activity level with a probability proportionate to the total number of contacts of that group, while the remaining fraction of the population select partners preferentially from within their own activity level. These studies show that the degree of preference for within-group mixing markedly affects the initial stages of the epidemic. Intermediate levels of restriction lead to the most severe outbreaks, probably because of elevated individual risk due to intense within-group contact combined with a high probability of spread between groups as a consequence of the mixing. These results are analogous to those found for the mm^T model developed and analyzed by Sattenspiel (1987) and Sattenspiel and Simon (1988) discussed above. In addition, the epidemic curves for models with severely restricted mixing (99% and 99.999% within-group mixing) show a bimodal distribution which reflects an initial epidemic in high activity groups followed by delayed spread and a later epidemic in lower activity groups.

Although preferred mixing gives more realistic results than total proportionate mixing, it still may be an unrealistic assumption. Preferred mixing assumes that, of all the individuals making up a group, a certain proportion of them choose partners from within the group in a given time period and the remainder choose partners from any group, with the probability of choosing a particular group proportional to the activity of that group. Other models may be just as likely. For example, it may be that monogamous individuals have a bias towards either other monogamous individuals or towards prostitutes, the two extremes of the activity distribution, rather than randomly choosing individuals from any group, while individuals with intermediate levels of activity do tend to follow proportional mixing.

Little exploration of other possible mixing patterns has been done. Hyman and Stanley (1989) relax the strict assumptions of preferred mixing somewhat by considering a continuous model for partnership choice. Although all individuals are assigned to a specific risk group, they choose their partners on the basis of a function that describes those partners that are both acceptable and available. They analyze a situation where people choose partners from similar, but not necessarily identical risk groups. The function they use peaks at like activity levels and falls off with distance. Analyses of other possible patterns have not yet been done.

Blythe and Castillo-Chavez (manuscript, 1989) generalize the preferred mixing model of the gonorrhea models and the Michigan AIDS models. Their "generalized preferred mixing" allows preferences for partners with activities which are arbitrary multiples of one's own activity. Like Hyman and Stanley (1989), they consider a formulation which uses "neighborhood" functions to express preference as a continuous function that has a peak at like activity levels for partners and then falls off to either side.

Although all of these models are a step in the right direction in that they go beyond proportional mixing, there is a critical need for more theoretical analysis of the sensitivity of model outcomes to variations in the mixing patterns. Given the variability in patterns of actual sexual activity in a population, what is the simplest model that can be used to capture the nature of this behavior? This question cannot be answered without further research.

5. The context of social interactions and the spread of AIDS

One question that is not addressed in any of the models described above is the effect of the social context of the sexual interactions on the likelihood of transmission of the infection. These models assume that the only factors influencing the transmission are characteristics associated with the specific groups i and j of the individuals involved in an interaction. However, this is probably not a reasonable assumption to make. Behaviors are dynamic and plastic and tend to change when the environmental conditions change. The risks for transmission of a disease depend on the behaviors that are occurring at the time of contact, not on the behaviors that normally occur.

Consider the following example: interaction between a homosexual male who has one new partner a month and a second homosexual who has two new partners a month. If these two individuals meet for an anonymous encounter in a rest room, they will likely engage in different risk behaviors than if they spend an entire evening together in more intimate surroundings. These behaviors may or may not depend on the amount of time actually spent in overt sexual activities — they may have more to do with the degree of comfort the two individuals have with each other and their willingness to overcome or overlook inhibitions that might be present. This could work either way — some people may be more willing to engage in highly risky behaviors with a stranger, others may require more knowledge of the person involved. In any case, the important point is that the likelihood of transmission is a function of the risk behaviors present at the time of contact, which may very well be dependent upon the social context at that time rather than upon the behaviors that usually characterize the individuals involved. Consequently, realistic models must be able to incorporate the effects of the social context present at the time of the interactions.

One approach that may work in modeling the effects of social context is the mm^T model described above. As previously mentioned, the conceptual basis of this model is an individual's movements, not the behavior of a whole class of individuals. The mm^T formulation resulted from a consideration of all the ways a susceptible individual and an infective individual could come together for a social interaction. There are four possible ways for this to happen: 1) a susceptible from neighborhood i becomes infected by an infective from neighborhood j (any j, including $j = i$) in neighborhood i, 2) a susceptible from neighborhood i becomes infected by an infective from neighborhood j in neighborhood j, 3) both the individuals are from the same neighborhood i, but interact in a different neighborhood k, and 4) a susceptible from neighborhood i and an infective from neighborhood j interact in neighborhood k. The key to this formulation is that although the individuals involved are always from either neighborhood i or j, the interaction can take place in a setting removed from their homes. This allows for factors operating at the location of the social interaction to be easily incorporated into the model even if they are not characteristic of the normal environments of the individuals involved.

Although the mm^T model was originally conceived as a model for geographic subdivisions of a population, it can also be used for models such as the HIV models that divide the population into behavioral classes. However, in these models, the interpretation of the matrix, m, is a little more difficult. The behavioral classes must be defined on the basis of a set of normative behaviors shown by the members of the group. For example, group 1 may consist of individuals who engage only in oral sex, do not use drugs and prefer encounters with a known individual in intimate surroundings. Group 2 individuals may prefer oral sex and drugs, but will occasionally engage in anal sex and prefer encounters with a known individual in intimate surroundings. Group 3 individuals may enjoy all types of sex and drugs in a free environment with group sex among strangers or near-strangers. The term m_{13} in this situation then corresponds to the probability that an individual who normally engages in behaviors characteristic of group 1 takes on behaviors characteristic of group 3. The term $m_{13}m_{23}$ describes the probability that an individual whose normal behaviors are characteristic of group 1 interacts with an individual whose normal behaviors are characteristic of group 2, but that the interaction involves a different set of behaviors that are characteristic of group 3. The existing AIDS transmission models would consider an interaction between an individual from group 1 and an individual from group 2 to be of low risk, because neither individual regularly engages in anal sex and both prefer intimate surroundings with more knowledge of their partner. However, consider the case where both individuals went to a meeting in San Francisco in 1980 and decided that they wanted to try out one of the gay bathhouses. Within that environment, they may have succumbed to peer pressure and taken on behaviors that are characteristic of group 3 rather than their usual behaviors. This encounter in San Francisco could well have had a substantially higher risk of disease transmission as a consequence of the contact between the two individuals, because they may have been more likely to engage in the highest risk behaviors in the unusual social context of the bathhouse.

The behavioral mobility discussed above is an example of temporary mobility, where individuals take on new behaviors on the spur of the moment. A similar kind of movement matrix is appropriate for formulating the effects of permanent behavior change in the population. In this case, the terms of the matrix describe the probability that an individual who behaves according to the defined norms of group i permanently adopts behaviors characteristic of group j. This individual then becomes a new resident of group j.

6. Hierarchical structuring of AIDS models

One of the major limitations of most existing AIDS models is that they only look at one mode of transmission of the disease, usually homosexual activities, heterosexual activities, or use of intravenous drugs. However, the disease is spread by all of these activities simultaneously, and there are complex interactions between sexual activity and IV-drug use that are not accounted for in the existing models. The hierarchical structuring of the mm^T model is one approach that may be valuable in developing models for both sexual and IV transmission.

As mentioned above, the mm^T model considered a population that was divided into n discrete neighborhoods. Each of these neighborhoods was further divided into two subneighborhoods. One of these subneighborhoods consisted of all individuals who engaged in social activities that might take them to other neighborhoods and the other consisted of nonsocial individuals who did not interact with individuals from other neighborhoods. This concept of population structure has surfaced in a number of fields, most notably in the study of social mobility. Models for social mobility which consider these two types of individuals are known as mover-stayer models, with the stayers corresponding to nonsocial individuals and the movers corresponding to social individuals. The mover-stayer model was originally developed by Blumen, Kogan, and McCarthy (1955) and was later élaborated by Spilerman (1972a,b) and Singer and Spilerman (1974,1979).

A key advantage of the social/nonsocial formulation of the mm^T model is that with this formulation it is possible to consider simultaneously independent forms of risk. The total risk for social individuals in the hepatitis model was a combination of within-neighborhood interactions with both social and non-social local individuals and additional between-neighborhood interactions with social individuals from other neighborhoods.

A similar hierarchical population structure could be used to consider the joint effects of IV-drug use and sexual activity. The population could be divided into groups on the basis of sexual activity and sex and then each group could be subdivided on the basis of use of IV-drugs. The social individuals in this model would be IV-drug users, while nonsocial individuals would not use drugs. The risk to non-drug-users would be from sexual activity only, while the risk to IV-drug users would be a combination of sexual activity and IV-drug use.

Consider a population of males and females with five sexual activity levels and only heterosexual transmission. When drug use is taken into account, the mixing (or contact) matrix will be of dimension 20 x 20. Many of the elements of this matrix will be zero, since there is no possibility for certain kinds of transmission to occur, for example transmission from a female drug user to a female non-drug user. The matrix indicates when there is contact between individuals from different groups. Differences in the transmission rates for different types of contact can then be incorporated within each term in the matrix. For example, the term in the first row and second column of the matrix represents the likelihood of contact between an IV-drug-using monogamous male and an IV-drug-using monogamous female. This term would be multiplied by the probability of transmission for that type of contact, which would be a combination of risks due to drugs and to sexual activity. This transmission probability is likely to be higher than the probability of transmission when there is contact between a non-drug-using female from activity level 1 and a non-drug-using male from activity level 1, especially since this latter transmission rate would derive only from sexual activity. An illustration of this matrix is shown in Figure 1. Note that individuals who use drugs have an excessive number of positive elements in the matrix relative to those who do not use drugs because of the multiple modes of transmission of the disease.

7. Limitations of the mm^T model

Although the mm^T model allows for the incorporation of context effects, changes in behavior, and simultaneous consideration of IV-drug use and sexual activity, there are several limitations associated with it. One limitation is that the number of groups quickly becomes so large that even the most powerful computers are unable to handle the model. This limitation is present for all discrete models for the spread of disease in subdivided populations and is difficult or impossible to overcome with the present state of technology. It is partly for this reason that existing models are limited to one mode of transmission only. This remains an unsolved problem for epidemiological modeling and seriously limits the utility of such models for accurate prediction of future trends.

		Drug User										Non-drug user									
		m1	f1	m2	f2	m3	f3	m4	f4	m5	f5	m1	f1	m2	f2	m3	f3	m4	f4	m5	f5
	m1	+	+	+	+	+	+	+	+	+	+	O	+	O	+	O	+	O	+	O	+
	f1	+	+	+	+	+	+	+	+	+	+	+	O	+	O	+	O	+	O	+	O
	m2	+	+	+	+	+	+	+	+	+	+	O	+	O	+	O	+	O	+	O	+
D	f2	+	+	+	+	+	+	+	+	+	+	+	O	+	O	+	O	+	O	+	O
r	m3	+	+	+	+	+	+	+	+	+	+	O	+	O	+	O	+	O	+	O	+
u	f3	+	+	+	+	+	+	+	+	+	+	+	O	+	O	+	O	+	O	+	O
g	m4	+	+	+	+	+	+	+	+	+	+	O	+	O	+	O	+	O	+	O	+
s	f4	+	+	+	+	+	+	+	+	+	+	+	O	+	O	+	O	+	O	+	O
	m5	+	+	+	+	+	+	+	+	+	+	O	+	O	+	O	+	O	+	O	+
	f5	+	+	+	+	+	+	+	+	+	+	+	O	+	O	+	O	+	O	+	O
	m1	O	+	O	+	O	+	O	+	O	+	O	+	O	+	O	+	O	+	O	+
N	f1	+	O	+	O	+	O	+	O	+	O	+	O	+	O	+	O	+	O	+	O
o	m2	O	+	O	+	O	+	O	+	O	+	O	+	O	+	O	+	O	+	O	+
	f2	+	O	+	O	+	O	+	O	+	O	+	O	+	O	+	O	+	O	+	O
D	m3	O	+	O	+	O	+	O	+	O	+	O	+	O	+	O	+	O	+	O	+
r	f3	+	O	+	O	+	O	+	O	+	O	+	O	+	O	+	O	+	O	+	O
u	m4	O	+	O	+	O	+	O	+	O	+	O	+	O	+	O	+	O	+	O	+
g	f4	+	O	+	O	+	O	+	O	+	O	+	O	+	O	+	O	+	O	+	O
s	m5	O	+	O	+	O	+	O	+	O	+	O	+	O	+	O	+	O	+	O	+
	f5	+	O	+	O	+	O	+	O	+	O	+	O	+	O	+	O	+	O	+	O

Figure 1. The mixing matrix for a heterosexual population with five sexual activity levels and IV-drug use. + indicates a positive probability of contact between individuals of the given types. These values are generally not all equal. 0 indicates no contact between individuals of the given types.

The use of a discrete movement matrix also has limitations with regard to its representation of actual human behavior. The original mm^T model considered a matrix, m, that represented the actual daily mobility of individuals. An analogous AIDS model would have a matrix that represented the propensity of individuals to temporarily take on behaviors other than their normal behaviors. The stochastic matrix used to represent these types of mobility is based on a Markov process and depends upon the assumption that all individuals have the capability of changing state at each time period (although they may stay in the same state), and that the probability of moving from one state to another depends only on the present state, not on any past history. Both of these assumptions are unrealistic for real human behavior. All people do not spend a constant and equal amount of time in any one state - some people go to another location for a couple of hours, some go for several days or longer, and the longer individuals stay in any one place, the less likely they are to leave it. Some people have sexual liaisons that last for less than an hour, others have them lasting several hours or more. Also, with both physical mobility and behavioral mobility, the probability of returning to the prior state is not random - if the duration of stay in a new state is short, the probability of return is much higher than would be expected. For longer durations of stay, there is probably some nonlinear functional relationship between the length of stay and the probability of return to the state of origin. This is a problem of biased return to the state of origin.

These same problems have been addressed in the sociological literature on social mobility. The original mover-stayer models also assumed that all individuals changed states at the same time and they assumed that the probability of moving from one state to another depended only on the present state. More recent models have been developed to overcome these problems. Models which deal with duration-of-stay effects are based on semi-Markov processes rather than Markov processes. A semi-Markov process is one in which the changes in state remain discrete and do not depend on the history of an individual's movements, but where the length of time spent in any state is not constant. Semi-Markov models for social mobility include those of McGinnis (1968), Henry, McGinnis, and Tegtmeyer (1971), Ginsberg (1971, 1972a,b), and Gilbert (1973). This approach may prove useful in modeling the duration effects for the sexual partnerships themselves as well as the duration effects with behavioral mobility. However, although this body of theory looks appealing for the modeling of epidemics, it appears to have somewhat limited support from the sociological community due to the sophistication of mathematical analysis required with semi-Markov processes.

The problem of biased return has not been addressed either in the sociological literature. There have been a number of studies analyzing migration data which show that there is biased return of migrants to their place of birth (Ledent 1981; Lee 1974; Long and Hansen 1975; Miller 1977). However, there have not been many attempts to develop models to describe biased return; although Philipov and Rogers (1981) did introduce higher transition probabilities for return migrants into a multiregional population projection model. It may be possible to build in a functional form for the transition probabilities that depends on duration of stay in a location: for example, one that has a high rate of return to origin shortly after moving, followed by a decline in the probability of return after an adjustment period, and then with a second rise later on. Since the semi-Markov processes have been used precisely to deal with non-constant duration of stay effects, it may be possible to link the return rates with these variable durations.

8. Applicability of the mm^T model to other problems

The spread of an epidemic is only one example of a contagion process. Such a process occurs whenever some kind of "information" is transmitted when two people interact. For example, changes in opinions, political parties, etc. do not usually arise spontaneously in an individual; they are the consequence of interactions with other individuals with different ideas. A person comes into contact with someone and exchanges information with them. As a consequence of this exchange of information, the person may or may not change his/her ideas. In the case of diseases, a susceptible individual comes into contact with an infected person and, depending upon numerous environmental factors, the disease may be transmitted from the infected person to the susceptible person. Because these processes are analogous, the same basic models are appropriate for describing them. The mm^T model is quite general and can apply to diseases and to other kinds of contagion processes with only minor modifications.

One logical extension of this model is to the geographic spread of diseases with other modes of transmission, such as host-vector diseases. One such model has already been developed (Sattenspiel (in preparation)). In this model, as in the hepatitis model, a population is assumed to be divided into n neighborhoods, each of which consist of a population of humans and a population of mosquitoes. The mosquitoes are assumed to have a very small home range and to stay within the neighborhood, so that all transmission between neighborhoods is due to human movement. The model is completely analogous to the mm^T hepatitis model, with the exception that the transmission rate must vary across neighborhoods and is specific to the neighborhood in which the human social interaction occurs, not to the neighborhood from which the humans derive. This is because of the intervening mosquitoes.

In this model an infective individual from neighborhood i travels to neighborhood k and gets bitten by a mosquito. Subsequently a susceptible individual travels from neighborhood j to neighborhood k and gets bitten by the now-infective mosquito. This individual returns home to neighborhood j and becomes ill with the disease. The infection has now passed from neighborhood i to neighborhood j. However, the contextual effects influencing the transmission of this disease were specific to neighborhood k and were dependent upon the characteristics of the risk factors relative to mosquito density, biting rate, and survival in that neighborhood, not in neighborhoods i and j.

This model can also easily be extended to deal with changes in political orientation or with the spread of other ideas. Brown and Sattenspiel (in preparation) have been developing models to examine how the context of social interactions affects political behavior. They have been considering the process by which individuals from different groups come together and change personal political orientations and behaviors. This process can be represented by a modification of the hepatitis mm^T model. The model allows one to distinguish the effects of a Democrat debating with a Republican the week before an election at a gathering of staunch Republicans from the effects of debating with the Republican at a gathering of staunch Democrats. [It is interesting to note that at least one eminent mathematical epidemiologist has also worked on the subject of contagion models for voting behavior (May and Martin 1975).]

The quantitative tradition in the social sciences holds a wealth of untapped information for mathematical epidemiologists. In particular, the literature on social mobility is a valuable source of insight on ways to approach the modeling of social and behavioral factors influencing the spread of AIDS. However, there is a major difference between the process of social mobility and the spread of information or diseases. Social mobility is an individual phenomenon, and although the likelihood of actually changing status is affected by environmental variables which may involve interactions with others, these interactions are not an integral part of the phenomenon. Contagion models, on the other hand, must include these interactions. This necessity influences the appropriate formulation of the contact matrix.

Because social mobility models consider only a single individual it is sufficient to describe the process with a single matrix giving the probability that an individual from any group i moves to a group j . However, because contagion processes involve two individuals, and because the environment under which the transmission occurs can be different from the normal environment of both individuals, the mm^T model or some analogous formulation must be used. Conlisk (1976), Smallwood and Conlisk (1979), and Bartholomew (1982, 1984) develop models with interactive Markov chains, where the likelihood of an individual changing states depends upon how other individuals in a population are distributed. These models have been used to describe the distribution of grant monies among universities, the use of medical clinics by families in a town, the results of certain kinds of psychological experiments, the diffusion of a news item through a large population, the use of products by consumers, the process of migration, and the cycling of fashions. The basic Markov process in these models becomes a nonlinear process. Therefore, these models may prove more valuable to mathematical epidemiologists than other models for social and occupational mobility.

Great strides have been made in the field of mathematical epidemiology since the beginning of the AIDS epidemic. However, there is still much work to be done: i.e. increasing the sophistication and realism of the models themselves and continuing to try to develop models that are compatible with data that have been or can be collected. Some of the approaches outlined in this paper may be of use in the development of better models.

Acknowledgements

The following people provided helpful discussions on the ideas presented in this paper: Steven Tanner, Thad Brown, Ann Stanley, Carl Simon, John Jacquez, and Jim Koopman. This work has been partially supported by a Summer Research Fellowship from the University of Missouri Faculty Research Council.

References

Anderson, R.M., R.M. May, G.F. Medley, and A. Johnson. (1986). A preliminary study of the transmission dynamics of the human immunodeficiency virus (HIV), the causative agent of AIDS. *IMA J. Math. Appl. Med. Biol.* 3, 229-263.

Baroyan, O.V., L.A. Rvachev, and L.A. Ivannikov. (1977). Modeling and forecasting of influenza epidemics for the territory of the USSR. *Gameleya I nstitute of Epidemiology and Microbiology, Moscow* (In Russian).

Bartholomew, D.J. (1982). *Stochastic Models for Social Processes, Third Edition.* Wiley, Chichester.

Bartholomew, D.J. (1984). Recent developments in nonlinear stochastic modeling of social processes. *Canad. J. Stat .* 12, 39-52.

Blumen, I., M. Kogan, and P.J. McCarthy. (1955). *The Industrial Mobility of Labor as a Probability Process.* Cornell Studies of Industrial and Labor Relations, no. 6. Cornell University Press, Ithaca.

Blythe, S.P. and R.M. Anderson. (1988). Heterogeneous sexual activity models of HIV transmission in male homosexual population. *IMA J. Math. Appl. Med. Biol.* 5, 237-260.

Blythe, S.P. and C. Castillo-Chavez. (1989). Like-with-like preference and sexual mixing models (manuscript).

Bodmer, W.B. and L.L. Cavalli-Sforza. (1968). A migration matrix model for the study of random genetic drift. *Genetics* 59, 565-592.

Cliff, A.D., P. Haggett, J.K. Ord, K. Bassett, and R.B. Davies. (1975). *Elements of Spatial Structure: A Quantitative Approach.* Cambridge University Press, Cambridge.

Conlisk, J. (1976). Interactive Markov chains. *J. Math. Sociol.* 4, 157-185.

De Grutolla, V. and K.H. Mayer. (1988). Assessing and modeling heterosexual spread of the Human Immunodeficiency Virus in the United States. *Rev. Infect. Dis.* 10, 138-150.

Gilbert, G. (1973). Semi-Markov processes and mobility: A note. *J. Math. Sociol.* 3, 139-145.

Ginsberg, R.B. (1971). Semi-Markov processes and mobility. *J. Math. Sociol.* 1, 233-262.

Ginsberg, R.B. (1972a). Critique of probabilistic models: Application of the semi-Markov model to migration. *J. Math. Sociol.* 2, 63-82.

Ginsberg, R.B. (1972b). Incorporating causal structure and exogenous information with probabilistic models: With special reference to choice, gravity, migration, and Markov chains. *J. Math. Sociol.* 2, 83-103.

Haggett, P. (1972). Contagious processes in a planar graph: An epidemiological application. In *Medical Geography* . N.D. McGlashan (ed.), pp. 307-324. Methuen, London.

Haggett, P. (1976). Hybridizing alternative models of an epidemic diffusion process. *Econ. Geog.* 52, 136-146.

Henry, N.W., R. McGinnis, and H.W Tegtmeyer. (1971). A finite model of mobility. *J. Math. Sociol.* 1, 107-118.

Hethcote, H.W. and J.W. Van Ark. (1987). Epidemiological models for heterogeneous populations: Proportionate mixing, parameter estimation, and immunization programs. *Math. Biosc.* 84, 85-117.

Hethcote, H.W. and J.A. Yorke. (1984). *Gonorrhea Transmission and Control.* Lecture Notes in Biomathematics, No. 56, Springer-Verlag, New York.

Hethcote, H.W., J.A. Yorke, and A. Nold. (1982). Gonorrhea modeling: A comparison of control methods. *Math. Biosc.* 58, 93-109.

Hyman, J.M. and E.A. Stanley. (1988). Using mathematical models to understand the AIDS epidemic. *Math. Biosc.* 90, 415-474.

Hyman, J.M. and E.A. Stanley. (1989). The effect of social mixing patterns on the spread of AIDS. In *Mathematical Approaches to Ecological and Environmental Problem Solving.* Lecture Notes in Biomathematics, C. Castillo-Chavez, S.A. Levin, and C. Shoemaker (eds.). Springer-Verlag (in press).

Jacquez, J.A., C.P. Simon, J. Koopman, L. Sattenspiel, and T. Perry. (1988). Modeling and analyzing HIV transmission: The effect of contact patterns. *Math. Biosc.* 92, 119-199.

Kießling, D., S. Stannat, I. Schedel, and H. Deicher. (1986). Überlegungen und hochrechnungen zur epidemiologie des "acquired immunodeficiency syndrome" in der Bundesrepublik Deutschland. *Infection* 14, 217-221.

Knox, E.G. (1986). A transmission model for AIDS. *Eur. J. Epidemiol.* 2, 165-177.

Koopman, J., C. Simon, J. Jacquez, J. Joseph, L. Sattenspiel, and T. Park. (1988). Sexual partner selectiveness effects on homosexual HIV transmission dynamics. *JAIDS* 1, 486-504.

Lajmanovich, A. and J.A. Yorke. (1976). A deterministic model for gonorrhea in a nonhomogeneous population. *Math. Biosc.* 28, 221-236.

Ledent, J. (1981). Constructing multiregional life tables using place-of-birth-specific migration data. In *Advances in Multiregional Demography,* A. Rogers (ed.), RR-81-6. International Institute for Applied Systems Analysis, Laxenburg, Austria.

Lee, A.S. (1974). Return migration in the United States. *Int. Migr. Rev.* 8, 283-300.

Long, L.H., and K.A. Hansen. (1975). Trends in return migration to the South. *Demography* 12, 601-614.

Longini, I.M., Jr. (1988). A mathematical model for predicting the geographic spread of new infectious agents. *Math. Biosc.* 90, 367-383.

May, R.M. and R.M. Anderson. (1984). Spatial heterogeneity and the design of immunization programs. *Math. Biosc.* 72, 83-111.

May, R.M. and R.M. Anderson. (1987). Transmission dynamics of HIV infection. *Nature* 326, 137-142.

May, R.M. and B. Martin. (1975). Voting models incorporating interactions between voters. *Public Choice,* Vol. XXII, Summer 1975, 37-53.

McGinnis, R. (1968). A stochastic model of social mobility. *Am. Sociol. Rev.* 33, 712-722.

Miller, A.R. (1977). Interstate migrants in the United States: Some social-economic differences by type of move. *Demography* 14, 1-17.

Minturn, L. and J.T. Hitchcock. (1966). *The Rajputs of Khalapur, India..* John Wiley and Sons, Inc., New York.
Nold, A. (1980). Heterogeneity in disease-transmission modeling. *Math. Biosc..* 52, 227-240.
Philipov, D. and A. Rogers. (1981). Multistate population projections. In *Advances in Multiregional Demography,* A. Rogers (ed.), RR-81-6. International Institute for Applied Systems Analysis, Laxenburg, Austria.
Post, W.M., D.L. DeAngelis, and C.C. Travis. (1983). Endemic disease in environments with spatially heterogeneous host populations. *Math. Biosc.* 63, 289-302.
Rushton, S. and A.J. Mautner. (1955). The deterministic model of a simple epidemic for more than one community. *Biometrika* 42, 126-132.
Rvachev, L.A. and I.M. Longini. (1985). A mathematical model for the global spread of influenza. *Math. Biosc.* 75, 3-22.
Sattenspiel, L. (1987). Population structure and the spread of disease. *Hum. Biol.* 59, 411-438.
Sattenspiel, L., J. Koopman, C. Simon, and J. Jacquez. (1989). The effects of population structure on the spread of the HIV infection. *Am. J. Phys. Anth.* (in press).
Sattenspiel, L., and C.P. Simon. (1988). The spread and persistence of infectious diseases in structured populations. *Math. Biosc..* 90, 341-366.
Singer, B., and S. Spilerman. (1974). Social mobility models for heterogeneous populations. In *Sociological Methodology 1973-1974* . H. Costner (ed.), pp. 356-401. Jossey-Bass, San Francisco.
Singer, B., and S. Spilerman. (1979). Clustering on the main diagonal in mobility matrices. In *Sociological Methodology,* K.F. Schuessler (ed.), pp. 172-208. Jossey-Bass, San Francisco.
Smallwood, D.E. and J. Conlisk. (1979). Product quality in markets where consumers are imperfectly informed. *Quart. J. Econ.* 93, 1-23.
Smith, C.A.B. (1969). Local fluctuations in gene frequencies. *Ann. Hum. Genet.* 32, 251-260.
Spilerman, S. (1972a). The analysis of mobility processes by the introduction of independent variables into a Markov chain. *Amer. Sociol. Rev.* 37, 277-294.
Spilerman, S. (1972b). Extensions of the mover-stayer model. *Amer. J. Sociol.* 78, 599-627.
Travis, C.C. and S.M. Lenhart. (1987). Eradication of infectious diseases in heterogeneous populations. *Math. Biosc..* 83, 191-198.
Watson, R.K. (1972). On an epidemic in a stratified population. *J. Appl. Prob.* 9, 659-666.
Yorke, J.A., H.W. Hethcote, and A. Nold. (1978). Dynamics and control of the transmission of gonorrhea. *Sex. Trans. Dis.* 5, 51-56.

PAIR FORMATION IN SEXUALLY-TRANSMITTED DISEASES

Roland Waldstätter
Dept. of Biomathematics
Auf der Morgenstelle 10
D-7400 Tübingen 1
West Germany

Abstract

Most epidemiological models of sexually-transmitted diseases (STD's) consider populations of single individuals. These models assume that every encounter by a susceptible possibly involves a different partner and such individuals get infected, with a constant probability per encounter, by infected partners. In order to match the model with data it is assumed that the probability of infection per "encounter" sums over all sexual contacts during a partnership. Although in reality the majority of individuals live in steady partnerships, it is usually assumed that these models are good approximations.

Models that use a different approach show other results. This paper presents a brief overview of recent models that take into account pair formation and explicitly follow pairs in the equations. The effect of prostitution on the Dietz/Hadeler model is investigated. Some results are compared with those from the usual "single" models without pairs. Simulations show that the disease can spread up to three times more slowly in pair formation models than in the approximated models without pairs.

1. Pair Formation and Mixing

Population structure determines the pattern of the spread of a disease. In the AIDS epidemic, for example, there appear to be several risk groups with nonproportional mixing among them. Mixing behavior recently has received a great deal of attention (see for example Jacquez et al. (1988), Sattenspiel and Simon (1988), Hyman and Stanley (1988,1989), Blythe and Castillo-Chavez (1989)). However, most of the studies of sexually-transmitted diseases (STD's) concentrate on homosexual populations and have not dealt with the heterogeneities introduced by two sexes and pair formation. Although the majority of individuals live in steady partnerships, these models do not follow pairs in the equations. They implicitly assume that the duration of partnerships is zero and that all sexual contacts happen instantaneously. This approximation may be justified in highly sexually active subgroups, but otherwise one has to take into account the fact that pairs of susceptibles are practically immune and that pairs with at least one infected partner do not spread the disease outside the pairs as long as they remain together and do not have other partners. This can strongly influence the initial phase of an epidemic because the majority of existing pairs consists of susceptible individuals.

It is therefore important in the modelling of sexually transmitted diseases, as in human demography, to have a mathematical description of the formation and dissolution of pairs. Mixing behavior of individuals produces one constraint on pair formation. Before the formation of a pair, there must be an encounter between possible partners. A first approach to pair formation is thus the "encounter-mating" model, in which pair formation involves two steps: the encounter of a possible partner and the decision whether to "mate". The mixing pattern determines the encounter step. The decision to mate is often treated as instantaneous step but this may not be true. Individual preferences are often not easily recognizable at the first encounter (Gimelfarb (1988a,b)). The two terms "mixing" and "preference" are often confused. The terms refer to different phenomena: mixing describes which individuals are met, preference describes which individuals are likely to be chosen (for instance as partners). Whereas mixing between subgroups must be symmetric, i.e. subgroup i mixes as many times with subgroup j as subgroup j mixes with subgroup i, preferences need not be symmetric. In models to describe mixing patterns in AIDS, preferences often are not considered.

Until about 1947, all population models considered only one sex. They typically focused on the female population because births are more easily attributable to the mother. But the same models were also applied to the male sex. Kuczynski (1932) calculated the female and male net reproduction numbers for France 1920-3 (the average number of daughters (sons) that will be born to a female (male)) and he found the female rate to be 0.977 and the male rate to be 1.194. One-sex models would therefore predict either a decrease or an increase of the population, depending on the sex. Kuczynski at that time explained these differences in the rates as being due to wars.

As a first attempt to overcome the inconsistencies in one-sex population models, A. H. Pollard (1948) artificially attributed the number of male births to females and the number of female births to males. Kendall (1949) suggested some different deterministic approaches to this so-called "two-sex problem". First he considered the simplest one-sex model

$$x' = (\lambda - \mu)\, x, \tag{1}$$

where x(t) is the number of females at time t, λ the birth rate and μ the death rate. Then he generalized this equation to two sexes:

$$\begin{aligned} x' &= -\mu x + 1/2\, \Lambda(x,y), \\ y' &= -\mu y + 1/2\, \Lambda(x,y), \end{aligned} \tag{2}$$

where the term $\Lambda(x,y)$ is symmetric in x and y and describes the births due to males and females. It is easy to see by subtracting one equation from the other, that an initial excess of one sex will disappear in time in this model. Later, Kendall considered a model that explicitly followed single females x, single males y and couples p:

$$\begin{aligned} x' &= -\mu x + (\lambda+\mu)p - \varphi(x,y), \\ y' &= -\mu y + (\lambda+\mu)p - \varphi(x,y), \\ p' &= -2\mu p + \varphi(x,y), \end{aligned} \tag{3}$$

where the birth and death rates λ and μ are the same for males and females. $\varphi(x,y)$ describes the number of new pairs. Kendall assumed $\varphi(x,y)$ to be $\rho \min(x,y)$, $\rho = \text{const}$. Although this model is quite realistic, it has the disadvantage of assuming that male and female birth and death rates are equal, which is often a poor approximation.

Since 1949 numerous authors have worked on the two sex problem. Keyfitz (1972), Parlett (1972) and J.H.Pollard (1973) designed and discussed models with different mating functions and understood that a realistic mating function is definitely nonlinear. Fredrickson (1971) and McFarland (1972) specified some conditions that had to be satisfied by a mating function:

(i) Definiteness:
In the absence of males and females there should be no pair formation,

$$\varphi(0,y) = \varphi(x,0) = 0. \tag{4}$$

(ii) Homogeneity:
If the sex ratio remains constant, the pair formation increases proportionally to the total population size,

$$\varphi(\alpha x,\alpha y) = \alpha\varphi(x,y) \quad \text{for all } \alpha,x,y \geq 0. \tag{5}$$

(iii) Monotonicity:
The pair formation increases if the number of males or females increases

$$u \geq 0,\ v \geq 0 \quad \text{then} \quad \varphi(x+u,y+v) \geq \varphi(x,y) \quad \text{for all } x,y \geq 0. \tag{6}$$

A consequence of the second condition is that all mating functions can be written in the form

$$\varphi(x,y) = x\, g(y/x) = y\, h(x/y) \tag{7}$$

where g and h are functions for $x,y > 0$ of one variable. Hence we can interpret the number of formed pairs per unit time as the number of females times a function of the number of males per female describing the availability of males (or the number of males times another function describing the availability of females). The most common examples in the literature are the minimum function

$$\varphi(x,y) = \rho \min(x,y), \tag{8}$$

the geometric mean

$$\varphi(x,y) = \rho \sqrt{xy}, \tag{9}$$

and the harmonic mean

$$\varphi(x,y) = 2\rho\, xy/(x+y). \tag{10}$$

These demographic models based on Kendall's model assume that the birth rate is linear in the number of pairs. To study the behavior, J. H. Pollard (1973) looked for exponential solutions. Hadeler et al.(1988) confirmed this approach with the theory of homogeneous evolution equations. This theory has also the potential of being applicable to a wider class of population models and epidemiological models (e.g. Nold (1980), Busenberg and van den Driessche (1989), Busenberg et. al. (1989)). Hadeler et al. (1988) used this technique to investigate the qualitative behavior of a general two-sex model of the Kendall type. They added a break-up rate for pairs with a general pair-formation law and showed that, if the mortalities of males and females do not differ very much there is a globally attractive two-sex exponential solution with constant sex ratio (see also Yellin and Samuelson (1974)). Instead of birth rates depending linearly on the number of pairs, one can also consider a constant recruitment rate κ in demographic models:

$$\begin{aligned} x' &= \kappa - \mu x + (\sigma+\mu)p - \varphi(x,y), \\ y' &= \kappa - \mu y + (\sigma+\mu)p - \varphi(x,y), \\ p' &= -(\sigma+2\mu)p + \varphi(x,y), \end{aligned} \tag{11}$$

where σ is a constant break-up rate, μ the death rate (independent of sex, for simplicity) and φ satisfies the conditions (i)-(iii). In this model, exponential solutions do not play an essential role because the equations are not homogenous. There is always a globally stationary solution (x,y,p), where p is determined by the equation

$$\varphi(\kappa/\mu - p, \kappa/\mu - p) = (\sigma+2\mu)p. \tag{12}$$

If one assumes that the numbers of both sexes are approximately equal, then the mating functions (8)-(10) are essentially indistinguishable. What then is the value of discrimination among the mating functions? One area where the distinction becomes important is that of age-structured models. Pair formation clearly depends strongly on the ages of the individuals and the numbers in different age classes can be very different.

Several papers about mating models (e.g. Goodman (1967), Fredrickson (1971), Keyfitz (1972), Hoppensteadt (1975), Staroverov (1977), Hadeler (1989a,b), and several others) have treated age structure, which I do not consider further in this paper. Goodman (1953) considers stochastic rather than deterministic models; other papers investigated mating functions in models of population genetics (e.g. Wilson (1973), Wagener (1976) or Karlin (1979)). An application of preferred or assortative mating in one-sex models is presented in Levin and Segel (1982).

2. Two-Sex Models in Sexually Transmitted Diseases

Dietz (1987, 1988) and Dietz and Hadeler (1988) presented a two-sex model for diseases spread through sexual contacts among heterosexuals. They assumed that a pair begins with the first sexual contact and that an individual can be a member of only one pair at a time. The population is divided into eight disjunct classes:

- x_0 single females, noninfected;
- x_1 single females, infected;
- y_0 single males, noninfected;
- y_1 single males, infected;
- p_{00} pairs, both partners noninfected;
- p_{01} pairs, only male infected;
- p_{10} pairs, only female infected;
- p_{11} pairs, both partners infected.

Individuals are only recruited into the noninfected single classes with a constant rate κ. Single females and males are removed with constant death rates μ_0 (uninfected) or μ_1 (infected) and by forming a pair. Pairs end by breaking up or by death of one partner. The break-up rate is a constant σ. Furthermore it is assumed that the probability of infection in one sexual contact is a constant h and that the average number of sexual contacts within a pair is β. Then the model equations read:

$$
\begin{aligned}
dx_0/dt &= \kappa - \mu_0 x_0 + (\mu_0+\sigma)p_{00} + (\mu_1+\sigma)p_{01} - \varphi_{00} - \varphi_{01};\\
dy_0/dt &= \kappa - \mu_0 y_0 + (\mu_0+\sigma)p_{00} + (\mu_1+\sigma)p_{10} - \varphi_{00} - \varphi_{10};\\
dx_1/dt &= - \mu_1 x_1 + (\mu_0+\sigma)p_{10} + (\mu_1+\sigma)p_{11} - \varphi_{10} - \varphi_{11};\\
dy_1/dt &= - \mu_1 y_1 + (\mu_0+\sigma)p_{01} + (\mu_1+\sigma)p_{11} - \varphi_{01} - \varphi_{11};\\
dp_{00}/dt &= -(2\mu_0+\sigma)p_{00} + \varphi_{00};\\
dp_{01}/dt &= -(\mu_0+\mu_1+\sigma+h\beta)p_{01} + (1-h)\varphi_{01};\\
dp_{10}/dt &= -(\mu_1+\mu_0+\sigma+h\beta)p_{10} + (1-h)\varphi_{10};\\
dp_{11}/dt &= -(2\mu_1+\sigma)p_{11} + h\beta p_{01} + h\beta p_{10} + h\varphi_{01} + h\varphi_{10} + \varphi_{11}.
\end{aligned}
\tag{13}
$$

This model contains the demographic model (11) if there is no infection in the population and I will call it the Dietz/Hadeler or PSI-model (Pair formation - SI - model). The pair formation φ is defined by

$$
\varphi_{ij}(x_0, x_1, y_0, y_1) = \rho_{ij}\, y_j\, x_i / (x_0+x_1) \tag{14}
$$

which is derived from a model where males of type j meet females of type i with fraction $x_i/(x_0+x_1)$ and mate with a constant rate ρ_{ij} without competition (male dominance). Although this function satisfies the conditions (i), (ii), (iii) it has the effect that for very small numbers of females there are a larger number of pairs formed than the total number of females. To avoid this problem, the authors assume in their paper that the number of females is greater than or equal to the number of males.

Alternatively, assume that females of type i will encounter males of types 0 and 1 in the proportions $\alpha_{i0} : \alpha_{i1}$ and that males of type j will encounter females of types 0 and 1 in the proportions $\beta_{0j} : \beta_{1j}$, $\alpha_{i0}+\alpha_{i1}=1$ and $\beta_{0j}+\beta_{1j}=1$. Assume that α_{ij} and β_{ij} are density dependent, i.e.

$$\alpha_{ij} = \alpha_{ij}(y_0,y_1), \quad \beta_{ij} = \beta_{ij}(x_0,x_1). \tag{15}$$

Furthermore, again let be ρ_{ij} be the probability that a female of type i forms a pair with a male of type j, given a meeting. Then

$$\varphi_{ij}(x_0,x_1,y_0,y_1) = 2\rho_{ij}\, \alpha_{ij}\, x_i\, \beta_{ij}\, y_j \,/\, (\alpha_{ij}\, x_i + \beta_{ij}\, y_j). \tag{16}$$

This function is a generalization of the harmonic mean (10) and of the preferential mating in Levin and Segel (1982). If we assume random mixing,

$$\alpha_{ij} = y_j /(y_0+y_1), \quad \beta_{ij} = x_i /(x_0+x_1), \tag{17}$$

the mating function (16) simplifies to (see also Hadeler and Ngoma (1989))

$$\varphi_{ij}(x_0,x_1,y_0,y_1) = 2\rho_{ij}\, x_i\, y_j \,/\, (x_0 + x_1 + y_0 + y_1). \tag{18}$$

If, furthermore, $x_i = y_i$ for $i=0,1$, (18) is exactly the same function as (14). Dietz and Hadeler (1988) showed that there is always a trivial noninfected stationary solution $(x_0,x_0,0,0,p_{00},0,0,0)$. They derived a threshold condition for existence of another stationary solution which is determined by the sign of D, where

$$D = h\rho_{01}\,[2\mu_1(\mu_1+\sigma) + \sigma(\mu_0+\sigma+\beta)] - \mu_1(2\mu_1+\sigma)(\rho_{01}+\sigma+\mu_0+\mu_1+h\beta). \tag{19}$$

Stability analysis is carried out for the special case with symmetric assumptions and no disease-induced mortality.

Dietz (1988) compares these results to those of a simplified model which does not explicitly follow pairs. He matches the probability of infection appropriately by adjusting the parameters of the simplified model. Even so, with realistic parameters, the PSI-model reaches its equilibrium about three times more slowly than the approximate model. Also, the equilibrium prevalence of the disease is significantly lower in the original model.

The Dietz/Hadeler model presents an initial step towards the development of more general models of disease transmission. A realistic approach to AIDS must take into account more complex social and sexual behavior. For instance the use of an average number of sexual contacts within a pair is doubtful. Furthermore, individuals can also get infected through sexual partners other than their "social" partner, such as prostitutes or steady liasons. One should also build both homosexual pairing and needle sharing by IV drug users into the model. Another idea is to extend the model to variable infectivity over time (see Castillo-Chavez (1989)).

Hadeler and Ngoma (1988) considered a model similar to the PSI-model where they considered vertical transmission. In some diseases, the time scales of the recruitment rate and of the demographic process are roughly equal. In this case, it may be appropriate to define the recruitment to be linear in the numbers of pairs. Mathematically, the model contains Kendall's model (3) if there is no infection. In this case, exponential solutions play an important role, and the authors use the stability analysis in Hadeler et. al. (1988).

3. Pair Formation Models with Female Prostitutes

Models omitting pair formation and the PSI-model may be seen as two extreme approximations to describe STD's. The former may best describe individuals with many different partners, and the latter may best describe individuals who do not have more than one steady partnership at a time. Dietz (1988) showed in simulations that, in the PSI-model, the virus is spread much more slowly, even if, in models without pairs, the rate of encounters and the infection rate per encounter are matched appropriately. If individuals have more than one steady partner at a time, i.e. if they have liasons or visit prostitutes, it is expected that the disease will spread faster than in the PSI-model. But how much does this aspect influence the disease? Do pair formation models with more heterogeneities, such as short-term liasons, still show that the disease is spread more slowly and that the prevalence of infectives is lower than in models without pairs? In order to investigate these questions, let us introduce two additional classes of female prostitutes, F_0 and F_1. Again, 0 means noninfected, 1 infected. For simplicity, assume that the interaction of prostitutes and males consists of a single sexual contact with duration zero. Prostitutes become infected through males and transmit the virus into the male population but have no interaction with females (see Fig.2). Let $\psi_s dt$ and $\psi_c dt$ be the number of sexual contacts per unit time with prostitutes by single men and paired men respectively. One can assume that ψ_s and ψ_c are linear in the male variable,

$$\psi_s(F_i,y_j) := \theta y_j F_i/(F_0+F_1), \tag{20}$$

$$\psi_c(F_i,p_{kj}) := \xi p_{kj} F_i/(F_0+F_1). \tag{21}$$

Let κ_F be the constant recruitment rate of noninfected prostitutes and ν_0,ν_1 the rates at which noninfected and infected prostitutes retire from their business. Let the "social" pair formation be described by the harmonic mean function (16). Since my interest is to look at the possible effects of prostitutes in the dynamics of a STD, we start by random mixing (17,18). The new model reads:

$$dx_0/dt = \kappa - \mu_0 x_0 + (\mu_0+\sigma)p_{00} + (\mu_1+\sigma)p_{01} - \varphi_{00} - \varphi_{01};$$
$$dy_0/dt = \kappa - \mu_0 y_0 + (\mu_0+\sigma)p_{00} + (\mu_1+\sigma)p_{10} - \varphi_{00} - \varphi_{10} - h\psi_s(F_1,y_0);$$
$$dx_1/dt = - \mu_1 x_1 + (\mu_0+\sigma)p_{10} + (\mu_1+\sigma)p_{11} - \varphi_{10} - \varphi_{11};$$
$$dy_1/dt = - \mu_1 y_1 + (\mu_0+\sigma)p_{01} + (\mu_1+\sigma)p_{11} - \varphi_{01} - \varphi_{11} + h\psi_s(F_1,y_0);$$

$$dp_{00}/dt = -(2\mu_0+\sigma)p_{00} + \varphi_{00} - h\psi_c(F_1,p_{00});$$
$$dp_{01}/dt = -(\mu_0+\mu_1+\sigma+h\beta)p_{01} + (1-h)\varphi_{01} + h\psi_c(F_1,p_{00}); \tag{22}$$
$$dp_{10}/dt = -(\mu_1+\mu_0+\sigma+h\beta)p_{10} + (1-h)\varphi_{10} - h\psi_c(F_1,p_{10});$$
$$dp_{11}/dt = -(2\mu_1+\sigma)p_{11} + h\beta p_{01} + h\beta p_{10} + h\varphi_{01} + h\varphi_{10} + \varphi_{11} + h\psi_c(F_1,p_{10});$$

$$dF_0/dt = \kappa_F - \nu_0 F_0 - h\psi_s(F_0,y_1) - h\psi_c(F_0,p_{01}) - h\psi_c(F_0,p_{11});$$
$$dF_1/dt = -\nu_1 F_1 + h\psi_s(F_0,y_1) + h\psi_c(F_0,p_{01}) + h\psi_c(F_0,p_{11}).$$

I will call this model the PSI+P model.

Again, there is always a noninfected state $(x_0,x_0,0,0,p_{00},0,0,0,F_0,0)$. Assume that the rate of pair formation does not depend on the infection

$$\rho_{00} = \rho_{01} = \rho_{10} = \rho_{11} = \rho\,, \tag{23}$$

and furthermore, that the pair formation rate with prostitutes is the same for single and coupled men,

$$\theta = \xi. \tag{24}$$

The Jacobian of the system in the noninfected state shows the stability behavior in this infection-free state. After some cumbersome calculations, one gets the threshold condition

$$D_1 = \nu_0\kappa h^2[(d_1\rho^2+d_2\rho+d_3)(2\mu_0+\sigma) + (f_1\rho^2+f_2\rho+d_3)\rho]\theta^2 + (l_1\rho^2+l_2\rho+l_3)\kappa_F\mu_0(\rho+2\mu_0+\sigma_{11}) \tag{25}$$

for the noninfected state to be locally asymptotically stable. Here

$$d_1 = -[\mu_1 a(1-h)^2 + b^2] < 0,$$
$$d_2 = -2\mu_1 c_1[(1-h)a + b] < 0,$$
$$d_3 = -\mu_1 c_1^2(2\mu_1+\sigma) < 0,$$
$$f_1 = d_1 + h^2 a c_2 < 0,$$
$$f_2 = -[c_1\{a(2\mu_1(1-h)+h^2\beta)+2\mu_1 b\} + h^2\beta^2(1-h)a] < 0,$$
$$l_1 = \nu_1 b[(1-h)\mu_1(2\mu_1+\sigma)-h\sigma c_2],$$
$$l_2 = 2\nu_1\mu_1^2 c_1[(1-h)a+b] > 0,$$
$$l_3 = \nu_1(2\mu_1+\sigma)\mu_1^2 c_1^2 > 0,$$

and $a = \mu_1+\sigma$, $b = h(\mu_0+\sigma+\beta)+\mu_1$, $c_1 = \mu_0+\mu_1+\sigma+h\beta$, $c_2 = \mu_0+\mu_1+\sigma+\beta$.

If there is no pair formation with prostitutes ($\theta = \xi = 0$), then the threshold condition is identical to that in the Dietz/Hadeler model. Fix $h, \mu_0, \mu_1, \sigma, \beta, \nu_0, \nu_1, \kappa, \kappa_F$ and vary ρ, θ. Then we have the two cases:

Case 1 ($l_1 < 0$)

If the average number β of sexual contacts within a pair or the infection probability h is "high", then $l_1 < 0$, and we get the following domain of stability:

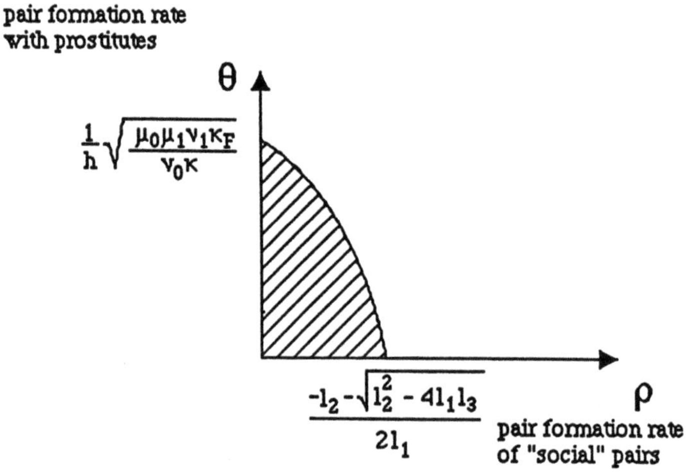

Case 2 ($l_1 > 0$)

If β or h is "low" then $l_1 > 0$. In that case the "social" pair formation does not play an important role in the spread of the disease. For every ρ there is an interval $[0,\theta_0]$ where the disease-free equilibrium is still stable.

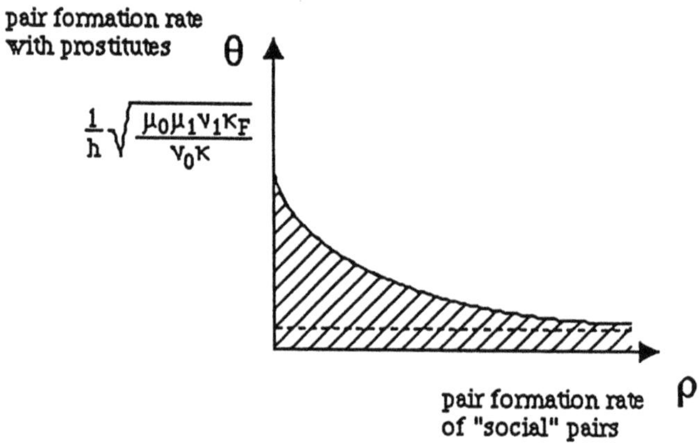

In order to understand the effect of considering a class of female prostitutes in pair formation models, let us approximate another model. If the break-up rate σ tends to infinity in the PSI+P model, we arrive at the following model which neglects pairs:

$$\begin{aligned}
dx_0/dt &= \kappa - \mu_0 x_0 - 2kqx_0y_1/(x_0+x_1+y_0+y_1);\\
dy_0/dt &= \kappa - \mu_0 y_0 - 2kqx_1y_0/(x_0+x_1+y_0+y_1) - h\theta y_0F_1/(F_0+F_1);\\
dx_1/dt &= -\mu_1 x_1 + 2kqx_0y_1/(x_0+x_1+y_0+y_1);\\
dy_1/dt &= -\mu_1 y_1 + 2kqx_1y_0/(x_0+x_1+y_0+y_1) + h\theta y_0F_1/(F_0+F_1);\\
dF_0/dt &= \kappa_F - \nu_0 F_0 - h\theta y_1F_0/(F_0+F_1);\\
dF_1/dt &= -\nu_1 F_1 + h\theta y_1F_0/(F_0+F_1).
\end{aligned} \tag{26}$$

Here k is the number of partners per unit time, and q is the probability of getting infected from one partner. This model assumes that all sexual contacts with one partner occur at the same time. k and q take the place of the parameters ρ, σ, β and h in the original model. For this model the threshold (compare with (25)) is

$$D_2 = \nu_1\mu_0\kappa_F(kq)^2 + \mu_1h^2\kappa\nu_0\theta^2 - \nu_1\mu_0\mu_1{}^2\kappa_F. \tag{27}$$

To get a sense of the difference between these models, with and without pairs, let us assume some realistic values for the parameters. In the noninfected state, the total number of (single and coupled) females and males must each be κ/μ_0. Let κ be 200,000 per year and μ_0 = 0.02 per year, so that the number of individuals at risk in the infection-free state is 20 million (Hethcote and Yorke (1984)). Let us further assume that κ_F is 16,667, $\nu_0 = 0.067$ and ν_1 = 0.125 per year. Then, in the infection-free equilibrium, we have about 250,000 prostitutes. Let ρ be 4.5 per year, θ be 1 and σ be 0.46 per year, $\mu_1 = 0.1$, h = 0.002 and β =100 per year. To match the probability of infection and the pair formation rate in both models, we use the formulas

$$k = (\mu_0 + \sigma)^{-1} + \rho^{-1}$$

and (28)

$$q = 1 - (1-h)^c, \quad \text{where} \quad c = 1 + \beta/(\mu_0 + \sigma)$$

as in Dietz (1988). We then calculate k = 0.43 and q = 0.342 per year.

These parameters yield case 1 in the pair formation model (22). For both models PSI+P and (26), the infection free state is unstable. The models differ in the time to approach the equilibrium. Simulations show that, if the noninfected state is unstable, there is always an endemic equilibrium. The model without pairs reaches its equilibrium more than twice as fast as the original model with pairs. The infection prevalence in the endemic equilibrium is significantly lower in the pair formation model (see Fig. 1).

4. Discussion

A brief overview of pair formation and two-sex models in epidemics has been presented. The model of Dietz and Hadeler has been extended by considering an additional class of female prostitutes in order to look at the effects of female prostitution on the dynamics of pair formation models. It was assumed that prostitutes interact only with the male population. Social structure other than sex has still been ignored.

Simulations indicate that only high values of θ, the rate at which males visit prostitutes, alter the course of the disease significantly. This result depends strongly on the transmission probability per sexual contact. As in the Dietz/Hadeler model, a comparison to a model not explicitly considering pairs shows that the prevalence of the disease in the pair formation model is much lower than in the model without pairs, even if prostitution is considered. Whereas in the model without pairs, the equilibrium prevalence for certain realistic parameters is about 30%, the pair formation model with female prostitutes shows a prevalence of about 15%. Simulations also indicate that the equilibrium is reached twice as fast in the model without pairs (see Fig.1).

	Maximum		**Equilibrium**	
	after	**% infected**	**after**	**% infected**
Model without pairs (26) $\theta=0$	148.5 years	31.4 %	348.5 years	31.1 %
PSI+P model $\theta=0$	513.5 years	14.8 %	689 years	14.8 %
Model without pairs (26) $\theta=1$	148 years	32.1 %	349.5 years	31.5 %
PSI+P model $\theta=1$	488 years	15.3 %	665.5 years	15.3 %

Fig. 1: Comparison of simulations of the PSI+P model and model (23). The time to equilibrium is measured when the distance of the trajectory and the equilibrium is for the last time more than 1000 individuals.

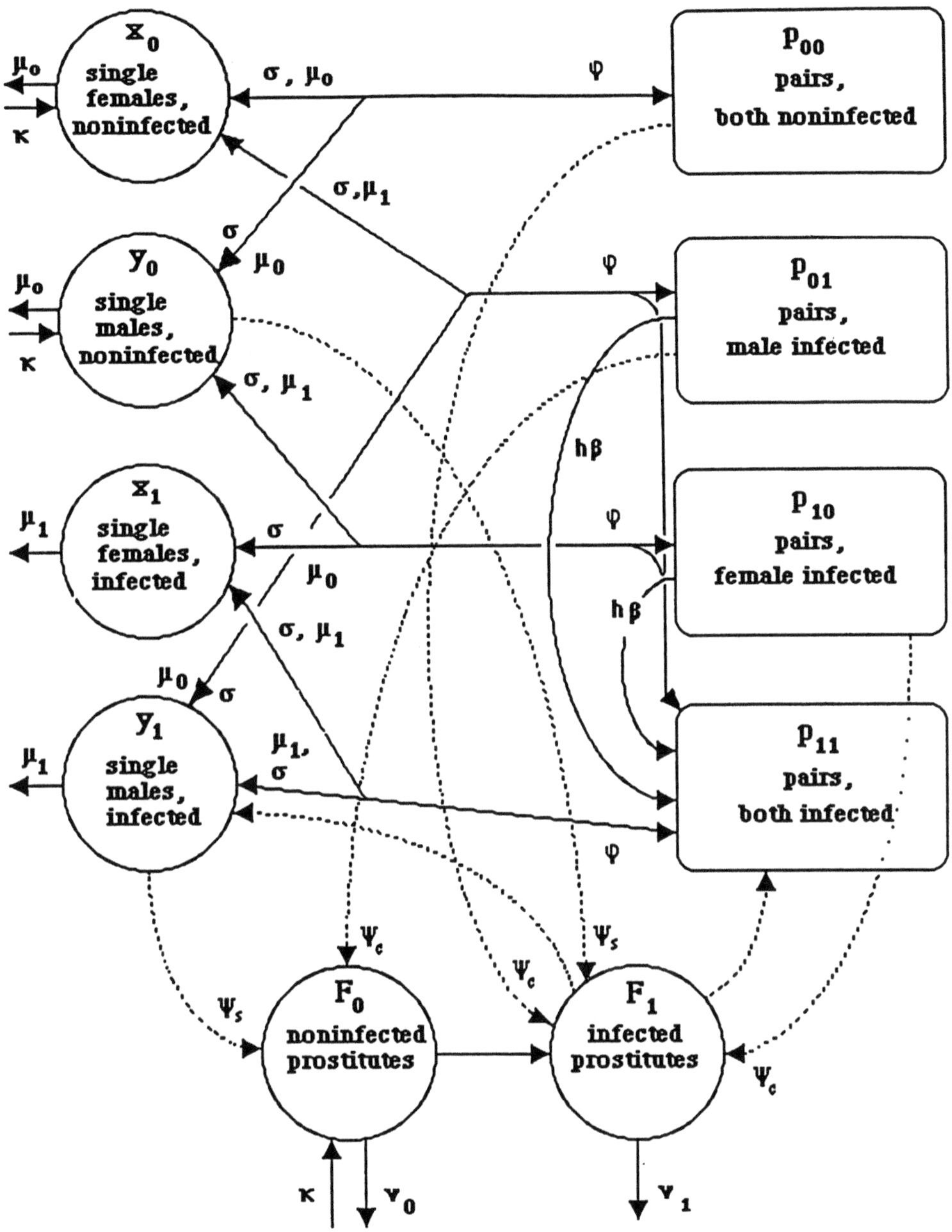

Fig. 2: Possible interactions in a two-sex model of heterosexuals with prostitution.

In reality, prostitutes are not a social class "outside of society"; their mixing behavior is much more complex. In models with prostitution, there are a lot of uncertainties. Estimates of the number of prostitutes in the United States lie inbetween 80,000 and 800,000 (Castillo-Chavez, personal communication). It is also difficult to get an idea of the magnitude of θ.

Unfortunately, pair formation models are very cumbersome to analyze, and the number of parameters that have to be estimated is very large. Although simulations cannot replace analytical treatment, one may get some useful insights into the behavior of these models.

ACKNOWLEDGEMENTS

I would like to thank Carlos Castillo-Chavez and Simon A. Levin whose ideas and suggestions made this work possible. This work was partially supported by the German Exchange Program (DAAD) 315/402/690/9 and by Hatch Project NYC 151-409, USDA, to Carlos Castillo-Chavez. I also wish to thank Fred Adler and Dan Grünbaum for reading and correcting the text and Karl P. Hadeler for his valuable comments on the paper, as well as the Center for Applied Mathematics, Cornell University, for supporting my work.

REFERENCES

Blythe, S.P. and C. Castillo-Chavez (1989). Like-with-like preference and sexual mixing models. *Math. Biosci.* (in press).

Busenberg, S. and P. van den Driessche (1989). Analysis of a disease transmission model in a population with varying size. *J. Math. Biol.* (submitted).

Busenberg, S., K. L. Cooke and H. Thieme (1989). Investigation of the transmission and persistence of HIV/AIDS in a heterogeneous population (Preprint).

Castillo-Chavez, C. (1989). Review of recent models of HIV/AIDS transmission. In Levin, S.A., T. G. Hallam and L. J. Gross,(eds.): *Applied Mathematical Ecology*. Biomathematics 18, Springer Verlag.

Dietz, K. (1987). Epidemiological models for sexually transmitted infections. *Proc. First World Congress Bernoulli Soc.*, Tashkent 1986, VNU Science Press, Utrecht

Dietz, K. (1988). On the transmission dynamics of HIV. *Math. Biosci.* 90: 397-414.

Dietz, K. and K. P. Hadeler (1988). Epidemiological models for sexually transmitted diseases. *J. Math. Biol.* 26, 1-25.

Fredrickson, A. G. (1971). A mathematical theory of age structure in sexual populations: Random mating and monogamous marriage models. *Math. Biosci.* 10, 117-143.

Gimelfarb, A. (1988a). Processes of pair formation leading to assortative mating in biological populations: encounter-mating model. *Americ. Natur.* 131, No. 6, 865-884.

Gimelfarb, A. (1988b). Processes of pair formation leading to assortative mating in biological populations: dynamic interaction model. *Theor. Pop. Biol.* 34, 1-23.

Goodman, L. A. (1953). Population growth of the sexes. *Biometrics* 9, 212- 225.

Goodman, L. A. (1967). On the age-sex composition of the population that would result from given fertility and mortality conditions. *Demography* 4, 423-441.

Hadeler, K. P. (1989a). Pair formation in age-structured populations. *Acta Applic. Math.* 14, 91-102.

Hadeler, K. P. (1989b). Modeling AIDS in structured populations. Invited paper of the 47th Biennial Session of the International Statistical Institute, Paris 1989.

Hadeler, K. P., R. Waldstätter and A. Wörz-Busekros (1988). Models for pair formation in bisexual populations. *J. Math. Biol.* 26: 635-649.

Hadeler, K. P. and K. Ngoma (1988). Homogeneous models for sexually transmitted diseases. Proc. G. Butler Memorial Conference, Edmonton 1988, *Rocky Mtn. Math. Journal* to appear.

Hethcote, H.W. and J. A. Yorke (1984). *Gonorrhea transmission dynamics and control.* Lecture Notes in Biomathematics, No. 56, Springer Verlag, New York.

Hoppensteadt, F. C. (1975). *Mathematical theories of populations: demographics, genetics and epidemics.* CBMS, vol. 20, SIAM, Philadelphia.

Hyman J. M. and E. A. Stanley (1988). A risk base model for the spread of the AIDS virus. *Math. Biosci.* 90, 415-473.

Hyman J. M. and E. A. Stanley (1989). The effect of social mixing patterns on the spread of AIDS. In C. Castillo-Chavez, S.A. Levin and C. Shoemaker (eds.), *Matheematical approaches to problems in resource management.* Lecture Notes in Biomathematics, Springer Verlag (in press).

Jacquez, J. A., C. P. Simon, J. Koopman, L. Sattenspiel and T. Perry (1988). Modeling and analyzing HIV transmission: The effect of contact patterns. *Math. Biosci.* 92: 119-199.

Karlin, S. (1979). Models of multifactorial inheritance: I. Multivariate formulations and basic convergence results. *Theor. Pop. Biol.* 15, 308-355.

Kendall, D. G. (1949). Stochastic processes and population growth. *Roy. Statist. Soc.*, Ser B2, 230-264.

Keyfitz, N. (1972). The mathematics of sex and marriage. *Proceedings of the Sixth Berkeley Symposium on Mathematical Statistics and Probability*. Vol. IV: Biology and Health, pp. 89-108.

Kuczynski, R. R. (1932). *Fertility and reproduction*. New York: Falcon Press 36-38.

Levin, S.A. and L.A. Segel (1982). Models of the influence of predation on aspect diversity in prey populations. *J. Math. Biol.* 14: 253-284.

McFarland, D. D. (1972). Comparison of alternative marriage models. In Greville, T.N.E. (ed.), *Population Dynamics*, pp.89-106, New York London, Academic Press.

Nold A. (1980). Heterogeneity in disease-transmission modeling. *Math. Biosci.* 52, 227-240.

Parlett, B. (1972). Can there be a marriage function? In Greville, T.N.E.,(ed.), *Population Dynamics*, pp.107-135, New York London, Academic Press.

Pollard, A. H. (1948). The measurement of reproductivity. *J. Inst. Actuaries* 74, 288-318.

Pollard, J. H. (1973). *Mathematical models for the growth of human populations*, Chap.7: The two sex problem. Cambridge University Press.

Sattenspiel, L. and C. P. Simon (1988). The spread and persistence of infectious diseases in structured populations. *Math. Biosci.* 90, 341-366.

Staroverov. O. V. (1977). Reproduction of the structure of the population and marriages. (Russian) *Ekonomika i matematiceskije metody* 13, 72-82.

Wagener D. K. (1976). Preferential mating. Nonrandom mating of a continuous phenotype. *Theor. Pop. Biol.* 10, 185-204.

Wilson, S. R. (1973). The correlation between relatives under the multifactorial models with assortative mating: I. The multifactorial model with assortative mating. *Ann. Human. Genetics* 37, 289-304.

Yellin J. and P.A. Samuelson (1974). A dynamical model for human population. *Proc. Nat. Acad. Sci. USA* 71, No.7, 2813-2817.

MIXING FRAMEWORK FOR SOCIAL/SEXUAL BEHAVIOR

Carlos Castillo-Chavez
Biometrics Unit and
Center for Applied Mathematics
341 Warren Hall
Cornell University
Ithaca, NY 14853-7801
U. S. A.

Stephen P. Blythe
Dept. of Physics and
Applied Physics
John Anderson Building
University of Strathclyde
107 Rottenrow, Glasgow
G4 ONG Scotland

Abstract

In this paper, we continue the numerical and analytical investigation of our recently developed method for incorporating preference into one-sex mixing models with continuously distributed characteristics. Preference is incorporated through a mixing function which determines the proportion of partnerships (sexual or social) formed by individuals of specified sexual/social activity with individuals of all other sexual/social activities. Our method allows for the specification of preference through an arbitrary preference function with well-understood properties. Our illustrations concentrate on the effects that the mean sexual activity of the population, the variance in the preference function (which affects partner selectivity), and the distribution of sexual activity have on the shape of the mixing function.

1. Introduction

Determining who is mixing with whom is an important theoretical question in the study of social dynamics, and it has become a central question in the study of the dynamics of the HIV (human immunodeficiency virus). It is important because a better knowledge of the heterogeneities involved in human interactions is crucial to an understanding of transmission and to the evaluation of preventive measures. We need to determine the mixing function, that is, the function that specifies, for each activity level (new partners per unit time), the fraction of the partners corresponding to all other activity levels. Knowledge of this function will help determine the effects of social/sexual mixing on the relative rates of spread of HIV, and therefore will also help in the construction of a qualitative picture of the spread of HIV in highly heterogeneous populations. Furthermore, estimates of the mixing function can be fed into dynamic models to reduce the level of uncertainty of mid- and long-term predictions of HIV and AIDS incidence. Dynamic models not only provide us with a reasonable approach to evaluating the effects of behavioral changes on these predictions, but also with a systematic approach to studying the effects of possible intervention plans on different subpopulations. We also note that the alternative to general theories such as the one provided in this article and recently extended in Busenberg and Castillo-Chavez (1989a, b) is to plug huge numbers of data points into complicated models. This last approach, however, usually violates the constraints inherent in mixing, particularly that of partnership conservation (see condition 2, below).

The absence of a fully-developed theory of mathematical epidemiology for non-randomly mixing populations capable of generating testable hypotheses, and the lack of empirical studies that challenge the reliability of current theories has, in our opinion, seriously limited the scientific study of social/sexual interactions and their relationship to disease dynamics. This is quite surprising, particularly given the example of population genetics (see Crow and Kimura 1970; Nagylaki 1977) where there has always been a strong emphasis on the study of the effects of heterogeneity in gene flow dynamics and hence in the heterogeneities induced by mating systems. A glance at the literature in mathematical epidemiology, however, shows that most models for the spread of infectious diseases have assumed that populations mix at random (proportionate mixing). Nold (1980) modified this assumption and introduced a form of biased mixing. Hethcote and Yorke (1984) also introduced this type of mixing in their important work on gonorrhea and were able to obtain a good fit to data on gonorrhea incidence.

Sattenspiel (1987a), motivated by her background in sociology and anthropology and her interest in the spread of hepatitis A in day care centers in New Mexico, was one of the first researchers to seriously question the use of proportionate mixing in epidemiological models of disease transmission. She emphasized the importance of non-homogeneous mixing both within and between subpopulations while concentrating on the effects of social and nonsocial behaviors on the dynamics of disease. Although her formulation was motivated by a specific disease and a specific spatial distribution, she has always been aware (see Sattenspiel 1987a,1989; Sattenspiel and Simon 1988) that her framework can be applied to other situations, in particular to the study of the spread of sexually-transmitted diseases (STD's). Hyman and Stanley (1988,1989), partially motivated by Sattenspiel's work, have used a general type of biased mixing that fits into the framework of this paper. Their simulations of a model for a single population with heterogeneously distributed sexual activity allow them to contrast the effects of biased mixing vs. random mixing on the initial dynamics of HIV. Their simulations clearly point out the dangers of using proportionate mixing. Jacquez et al. (1988) have also shown the dangers of using proportionate mixing on models for the spread of HIV/AIDS.

In this paper, we illustrate the role of preference and show, through numerical simulations, the effects of several factors on the shape of the mixing function. These factors include: the mean sexual activity of the population under consideration, the shape of the preference function (more specifically its width or variance), and the distribution of sexual activity of the population. Although the mixing function described in this article does not provide us with the general solution to the mixing problem, it comes very close to doing so (see Section 4 and Busenberg and Castillo-Chavez 1989a, b). The main body of this paper consists of two sections. Section 2 introduces our mixing framework and illustrates a method of constructing very general mixing functions. Section 3 provides a specific example for which an approximate expression for the mixing function can be calculated and offers a series of numerical simulations for a variety of like-with-like preference functions. We conclude this paper, in Section 4, with some general remarks regarding our results. We also indicate some future directions for research.

2. One-sex mixing framework

For one-sex models with heterogeneous social/sexual activity, the interactions between individuals of different activity levels are partially described by the mixing function. The *mixing function* $\rho(s, r,t)$ (Blythe and Castillo-Chavez 1989) is such that

$$\int_{r}^{r+\Delta r} \rho(s,u,t)du$$

denotes the fraction of partnerships that a person with activity level s (s new partners per unit time) has with persons with activity levels in the interval $(r,r+\Delta r)$ at time t. It therefore satisfies the following constraints for all s, r, and t:

$$\rho(s, r,t) \geq 0, \quad (1)$$

$$\int_0^\infty \rho(s, r,t)dr= 1, \quad (2)$$

$$\rho(s, r,t)sT(s,t) = \rho(r, s,t)rT(r,t), \quad (3)$$

where $T(r,t)\Delta r$ denotes the number of individuals in the population with activities in the interval $(r,r+\Delta r)$. Conditions (1) and (2) are obvious and allow us to interpret $\rho(s,r,t)$ as a probability density function. Condition (3) represents a conservation law as it expresses the principle that the total number of partnerships of s-people with r-people must equal the total number of partnerships of r-people with s-people. Since properties (1)-(3) have to be satisfied for all positive time, in the remainder of this paper we omit the variable t. We further note that there is no loss of generality in looking for solutions of the form $rT(r)B(s,r)$, and that condition (3) implies that $B(s,r) = B(r,s)$.

During the completion of this volume, Busenberg and Castillo-Chavez (1989a,b) found an expression for the general solution (also in the presence of age-structure) of the above functional relationships (1-3). This representation formula is given in terms of the preference function described in Blythe and Castillo-Chavez (1989a) and is motivated by the general family of solutions generated in Blythe and Castillo-Chavez (1989) and by the fact (shown in Busenberg and Castillo-Chavez 1989a) that proportionate mixing is the only separable solution of system (1)-(3). In the framework described in this article, the standard mixing model for proportionate mixing is given by

$$\rho(s, r) = \frac{rT(r)}{\int_0^\infty uT(u)du} \quad . \tag{4}$$

We note that $\rho(s,r)$ is independent of s. Proportionate mixing corresponds to a situation where the fraction of partnerships formed by any individual in the population with individuals of activity r is proportional to the total number of partnerships formed by all r-people. It is obvious that (4) satisfies conditions (1)-(3).

An example of a biased additive solution, that is, a solution for which individuals mix in a biased form but where this bias is additive, is given by the so-called preferred or biased mixing function, namely:

$$\rho(s, r) = (1-\alpha) \frac{rT(r)}{\int_0^\infty uT(u)du} + \alpha\, \delta(s-r), \tag{5}$$

where $\delta(s-r)$ is a Dirac delta function and the constant α represents the bias or preference towards partners of the same activity level. A discrete version of this model can be found in the work of Jacquez *et al.* (1988). In general, we note that any convex linear combination of mixing functions is a mixing function, that is, if $\delta_i(s,r)$ are mixing functions $(i = 1,\cdots,N)$ and the constants $\alpha_i > 0$ $(i = 1,\cdots,N)$ are such that $\Sigma_{i=1}^N \alpha_i = 1$, then $\delta(s,r) = \Sigma_{i=1}^N \alpha_i \delta_i(s,r)$ is also a mixing function.

A general example of a biased multiplicative solution, a solution for which individuals mix in a biased form (as determined by a preference function) but where the bias is multiplicative, is given by the following mixing function:

$$\rho(s, r) = f(r)\left\{ \frac{P(r)P(s)}{\int_0^\infty f(u)P(u)du} + \frac{\phi(s-r)}{A} \right\}, \tag{6}$$

where

$$f(r) = rT(r), \tag{7}$$

the preference function ϕ is such that $\phi(s-r) = \phi(r-s)$ and

$$\int_\omega^{+\infty} \phi(y)dy = 1, \tag{8}$$

and

$$P(x) = 1 - \frac{1}{A}\int_0^\infty f(u)\phi(x-u)du. \tag{9}$$

A is an appropriately chosen constant guaranteeing that P(x) is strictly positive. It is now trivial to show that the mixing function defined by (6) satisfies conditions (1)-(3). We note that the general solution to the mixing constraints, Equations (1)-(3), consists of multiplicative perturbations similar to those described by Equation (6) (for more details see Section 4). In the next section, we proceed to look numerically at the effects of the preference function in the shape of the mixing function. We observe that the mixing function determines the nonlinearity in the dynamics of classical epidemiological models for the spread of sexually transmitted diseases (see Castillo-Chavez *et al.* 1989).

3. Like-with-like preference mixing functions

This section provides some specific examples of mixing functions of the multiplicative type. Below, a simple example is computed directly, and some numerical examples are provided using three preference functions.

To compute a mixing function directly, we choose a family of preference functions given by a delta sequence. Since $\phi(x)$ is a non-negative, locally integrable function for which

$$\int_{-\infty}^{\infty} \phi(x)dx = 1, \tag{10}$$

then with $\alpha > 0$, the family

$$\phi_\alpha(x) \equiv \frac{1}{\alpha}\, \phi(\tfrac{x}{\alpha}) \tag{11}$$

generates a sequence of delta functions. This family of functions $\{\phi_\alpha$: α a positive parameter$\}$ satisfies the following properties:

$$\int_{-\infty}^{\infty} \phi_\alpha(x)dx = 1, \tag{12}$$

$$\lim_{\alpha\to 0} \int_{|x|>A} \phi_\alpha(x)dx = 0 \quad \text{for each } A > 0, \text{ and} \tag{13}$$

$$\lim_{\alpha\to 0} \int_{|x|<A} \phi_\alpha(x)dx = 1 \quad \text{for each } A > 0. \tag{14}$$

Hence, for small positive α, $\phi_\alpha(x)$ is highly concentrated about $x = 0$ in such a way that the total strength of this distributed source is one. Families of this type are potentially useful for modeling like-with-like preference. It can then be easily shown for very general functions $\pi(x)$ that

$$\lim_{\alpha\to 0} \int_{-\infty}^{\infty} \phi_\alpha(x)\pi(x)dx = \pi(0). \tag{15}$$

In this case (and for some of the expressions below), convergence means convergence in distribution, as defined in the study of generalized functions (see Stakgold 1979).

If we substitute a delta sequence of this type into Equation (6), we get

$$\rho(s, r) = f(r)\left\{ \frac{P(r)P(s)}{\int_0^\infty f(u)P(u)du} + \frac{\phi_\alpha(s-r)}{A} \right\} \tag{16}$$

with

$$P(x) = 1 - \frac{1}{A}\int_0^\infty f(u)\phi_\alpha(x - u)du \ . \tag{17}$$

If we now let $\alpha \to 0$, we get the following explicit expression for the mixing function:

$$\rho(s, r) = f(r)\left\{ \frac{(1 - \frac{f(r)}{A})(1 - \frac{f(s)}{A})}{\int_0^\infty f(u)(1 - \frac{f(u)}{A})du} + \frac{\delta(s-r)}{A} \right\}. \tag{18}$$

If we take

$$\phi_\alpha(s-r) = \begin{cases} 0 & \text{if} \quad |s - r| > \frac{1}{2h} \\ k & \text{if} \quad |s - r| < \frac{1}{2h} \end{cases} , \tag{19}$$

where $\alpha = 1/2h$, then for sufficiently small α, we can compute the following expression for the mixing function:

$$\rho(s, r) \simeq f(r)\left[\frac{(1 - 2\alpha\,\frac{f(r) + f(s)}{A})}{\int_0^\infty f(u)du - 2\alpha\,\frac{\int_0^\infty [f(u)]^2 du}{\int_0^\infty f(u)du}} + \frac{f(r)}{h\int_0^\infty f(u)du} \right]. \tag{20}$$

A further approximation (which is justified if α is sufficiently small) is given by

$$\rho(s, r) \simeq \frac{f(r)}{\int_0^\infty f(u)du}\left\{1 - \frac{2\alpha}{\int_0^\infty f(u)du}\left[f(s) + f(r) - \frac{\int_0^\infty [f(u)]^2 du}{\int_0^\infty f(u)du} \right] + z(s,r)\right\}, \tag{21}$$

where

$$z(s,r) = \begin{cases} \dfrac{f(r)}{\int_0^\infty f(u)du} & \text{if} \quad s - \alpha < r < s + \alpha \\ 0 & \text{elsewhere} \end{cases} \tag{22}$$

We note that the above expressions have only been derived for the purpose of illustrating our mixing framework, and hence, we do not suggest that real populations have such simple functional forms. If, furthermore, we let (as in Blythe and Castillo-Chavez 1989) $T(s) = Lke^{-ks}$, where T(s) is the distribution of sexual activity in the population, L is the total population size and 1/k is the mean sexual activity; we find that

$$\rho(s,r) \simeq k^2 re^{-kr}\Big[1 - 2k\alpha\{kse^{-ks} + kre^{-kr}\}\Big] + \sigma(s,r), \tag{23}$$

where

$$\sigma(s,r) = \begin{cases} k^2 re^{-kr} & \text{if} \quad s - \alpha < r < s + \alpha \\ 0 & \text{elsewhere} \end{cases} \tag{24}$$

All the following numerical examples use the above distribution of sexual activity. This distribution was used in Blythe and Castillo-Chavez (1989) where it was fitted to the data of Carne and Weller (partners per month of homosexual men attending STD clinics in London) as reported by Hyman and Stanley (1989). Figure 1 illustrates the proportionate mixing case: here ρ is in fact independent of s. Figure 2 illustrates the case where the preference function $\phi(s,r)$ is a narrow rectangular with width 2α; $\alpha = 0.1$. The approximate form is a ridge along s=r superimposed on a proportionate mixing surface. We note that, as the width of the preference function α increases, the shape of the mixing function becomes closer to that of proportionate mixing.

This example can be easily generalized to include preference functions of the form

$$\phi(s,r) = \beta_{m+1}\delta(s - r) + \sum_{i=1}^{m} \beta_i[\delta(s - a_i r) + \delta(sa_i - r)], \tag{25}$$

where the β_i's are properly chosen (for details see Blythe and Castillo-Chavez 1989). This function describes the preference of individuals with activity s for individuals with activities $s/a_1,\ldots,s/a_{2m+1}$. If, for example, we let

(a) $\Lambda = \sup_x f(x), \quad \Lambda < \infty$ and

(b) $Q(s) = \int_0^\infty \phi(s,r)f(r)dr,$

then $\rho(s,r)$ is given by the expression

$$\rho(s, r) = f(r)\left\{ \frac{(1 - \frac{Q(r)}{\Lambda})(1 - \frac{Q(s)}{\Lambda})}{\int_0^\infty f(u)(1 - \frac{Q(u)}{\Lambda})du} + \frac{f(r)}{\Lambda}\phi(s,r) \right\} \tag{26}$$

which can almost be "read" off Equation (18).

The following set of simulations use a Gaussian preference function; specifically,

$$\phi(s,r) = \frac{1}{\sigma(2\pi)^2} e^{-\left[\frac{(s-r)^2}{2\sigma^2}\right]}, \tag{27}$$

$$P(x) = 1 - \frac{k}{(2\pi)^2} e^{-\frac{x^2}{2\sigma^2}} e^{\left[\frac{\sigma^2}{4}\{k - \frac{x}{\sigma^2}\}\right]} D_{-1}\left[(k - \frac{x}{\sigma^2})2\sigma\right], \tag{28}$$

where

$$D_{-1}(z) = e^{-\frac{z^2}{4}} \int_0^\infty e^{-zx - \frac{x^2}{2}} x \, dx, \quad \text{(a parabolic function)}. \tag{29}$$

In our set of simulations, we used the parameters $\sigma = 0.25$ (Figure 3), $\sigma = 1.0$ (Figure 4) and $\sigma = 4.0$ (Figure 5). We then used a population with mean sexual activity $1/k = 2$ (new partners per month). In Figure 3, the preference function $\phi(s,r)$ is a Gaussian distribution with mean s=r. Since the variance is small, there is a well defined narrow ridge along the line s=r (compare with Figure 2). The background is essentially proportionate mixing. In Figure 4, we have kept the same preference function but have increased the variance. For intermediate variance, there is a significant deviation from the underlying (approximately) proportionate mixing surface, mainly in the vicinity of the line s=n r, and for r close to zero. In Figure 5, the variance of the Gaussian preference function is now significantly increased. For large variance, the surface is very similar to that of proportionate mixing. We note that significant increases or decreases in the mean sexual activity of the population $1/k$ can have a substantial effect on the shape of the mixing function. For further details, see Blythe and Castillo-Chavez (1989).

4. Conclusion

In this article, we have explored numerically and through some analytical approximations the effects of the preference function in the shape of the mixing function. Since our mixing functions have been generated through Equation 6, we have concentrated on the effects of like-with-like mixing. As pointed out in our earlier simulations (Blythe and Castillo-Chavez 1989), the fidelity of the transformation $\rho(s,r)$ to the underlying preference (neighborhood) function $\phi(s,r)$ depends upon the width of ϕ, the mean activity $1/k$, and (not explored in this paper) the value of s in relation to $1/k$. These results support some of the numerical experiments of Hyman and Stanley (1988,1989) regarding the width of the neighborhood preference function and its relationship to proportionate mixing. If, in addition, we assume that $rT(r)sT(s) = 0$

$\Rightarrow \rho(s,r) = 0$, then the general solution to the mixing problem is given by the following result:

Representation Theorem (Busenberg and Castillo-Chavez 1989a, b):

Let $\phi:\Re_+^2 \rightarrow \Re^+$ be a measurable and jointly symmetric function, and suppose that

$$\int_0^\infty \bar{\rho}(r)\phi(s,r)dr \leq 1 \text{ and}$$

$$\int_0^\infty \bar{\rho}(r)\left\{\int_0^\infty \bar{\rho}(u)\phi(u)du\right\}dr < 1.$$

Defining $\rho_1(s)$ by

$$\rho_1(s) = 1 - \int_0^\infty \bar{\rho}(u)\phi(s,u)du, \tag{30}$$

we arrive at the following fundamental representation formula for a mixing function:

$$\rho(s,r) = \bar{\rho}(r)\left[\frac{\rho_1(s)\rho_1(r)}{\int_0^\infty \bar{\rho}(r)\rho_1(r)dr} + \phi(s,r)\right], \tag{31}$$

where

$$\bar{\rho}(r) = \frac{rT(r)}{\int_0^\infty r\,T(r)dr}\ . \tag{32}$$

The converse also holds; that is, for every mixing function ρ, there exists a preference function ϕ satisfying the hypotheses of the theorem such that ρ is given by (31) with ρ_1 defined by (32). A similar result holds when we allow ρ to be a generalized function, i.e., when we include the possibility of delta functions or other distributions. The above theorem can be also extended to deal with age-structured populations. For more details see Busenberg and Castillo-Chavez (1989a and this volume).

This theorem allows us to look at situations other than like-with-like mixing. The mixing function plays a key role in disease dynamics as it determines the incidence rate ("force" of infection). A glance at the literature shows that several authors have used very different expressions for the "force" of infection. Our framework makes it clear that all of them were "correct," in the sense that they assumed (implicitly or explicitly) different types of mixing. This re-interpretation can be accomplished through the determination of all possible mixings, and this is what the above representation theorem is all about. The above framework (as was pointed out to us by Andrea Pugliese) is very general in the sense that it could easily incorporate a spatial distribution. All we have to do is consider the mixing of different types at a specific location (i.e., a localized mixing function) and then superimpose a movement/migration matrix like those of Sattenspiel (1987a,b and 1989) and Sattenspiel and

Simon (1988). Although the use of a general framework of this type could be very useful in theoretical considerations, its applicability to specific situations is probably quite limited due to the tremendous number of parameters involved.

Some possible future directions for research involve the analytical and numerical explorations of more general mixings (i.e., other than like-with-like), the expansion of the above framework to include two sexes (see Castillo-Chavez and Busenberg 1989), and the incorporation of the above framework into dynamic models for the spread of sexually transmitted diseases with and without age-structure (see Busenberg and Castillo-Chavez 1989a and this volume). We finally note that the above formulation allows an alternative approach to that of Dietz and Hadeler (1988) and hence to the study of models that follow pairs (see Castillo-Chavez and Busenberg 1989).

ACKNOWLEDGMENTS

This research has been partially supported by NSF grant DMS-8906580, NIAID grant R01 A129178-01, and Hatch project grant NYC 151-409, USDA awarded to Carlos Castillo-Chavez. The authors thank them for their generous support.

REFERENCES

Blythe, S.P. and C. Castillo-Chavez. (1989). Like-with-like preference and sexual mixing models. *Math. Biosci.* 96, 221-238.

Busenberg, S. and C. Castillo-Chavez. (1989a). Interaction, pair formation and force of infection terms in sexually transmitted diseases. (Submitted.)

Busenberg, S. and C. Castillo-Chavez. (1989b). Risk and age-dependent mixing functions and force of infection terms in sexually transmitted diseases. (This volume.)

Castillo-Chavez, C. and S. Busenberg. (1989). Pair formation in age- and risk-structured populations. (Manuscript in preparation.)

Huang, W., C. Castillo-Chavez, K. Cooke, and S.A. Levin. (1989). On the role of long incubation periods in the dynamics of acquired immunodeficiency syndrome (AIDS). Part 2. Multiple group models. (This volume.)

Crow, J.F. and M. Kimura. (1970). An introduction to population genetics theory. Harper and Row, New York.

Dietz, K. and K.P. Hadeler. (1988). Epidemiological models for sexually transmitted diseases. *J. Math. Biol.* 26, 1–25.

Hethcote, H.W. and J.A. Yorke. (1984). *Gonorrhea Transmission Dynamics and Control.* Lecture Notes in Biomathematics 56, Springer-Verlag, New York.

Hyman, J.M. and E.A. Stanley. (1988). Using mathematical models to understand the AIDS epidemic. *Math.Biosci.* 90, 415-473.

Hyman, J.M. and E.A. Stanley. (1989). The effect of social mixing patterns on the spread of AIDS. In *Mathematical Approaches to Problems in Resource Management and Epidemiology.* C. Castillo-Chavez, S.A. Levin and C. Shoemaker (eds.). Lecture Notes in Biomathematics 81, Springer-Verlag, Berlin, Heidelberg, New York, Tokyo.

Jacquez, J.A., C.P. Simon, J. Koopman, L. Sattenspiel and T. Perry. (1988). Modeling and analyzing HIV transmission: the effects of contact patterns. *Math. Biosci.* 92, 119-199.

Nagylaki, T. (1977). *Selection in One- and Two-Locus Systems.* Lecture Notes in Biomathematics 15, Springer-Verlag, Berlin, Heidelberg, New York, Tokyo.

Nold, A. (1980). Heterogeneity in disease transmission modelling. *Math. Biosci.* 52, 227-250.

Sattenspiel, L. (1987a). Population structure and the spread of disease. *Human Biol.* 59, 411-438.

Sattenspiel, L. (1987b). Epidemics in nonrandomly mixing populations: a simulation. *Am. J. Phy. Anthropol.* 73, 251-265.

Sattenspiel, L. and C.P. Simon (1988). The spread and persistence of infectious diseases in structured populations. *Math. Biosci.* 90, 341-366.

Sattenspiel, L. (1989). The structure and context of social interactions and the spread of HIV. (This volume.)

Stakgold, I. (1979). *Green's Functions and Boundary Value Problems.* John Wiley & Sons, New York.

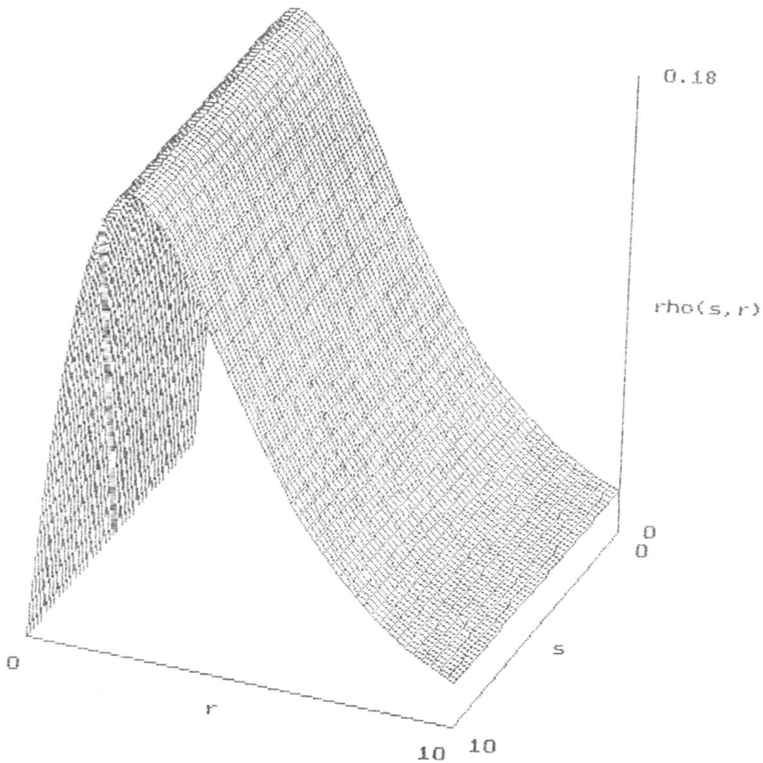

Fig. 1 Proportionate mixing with mean s = 2.0. The mixing function $\rho(s,r)$ is independent of s..

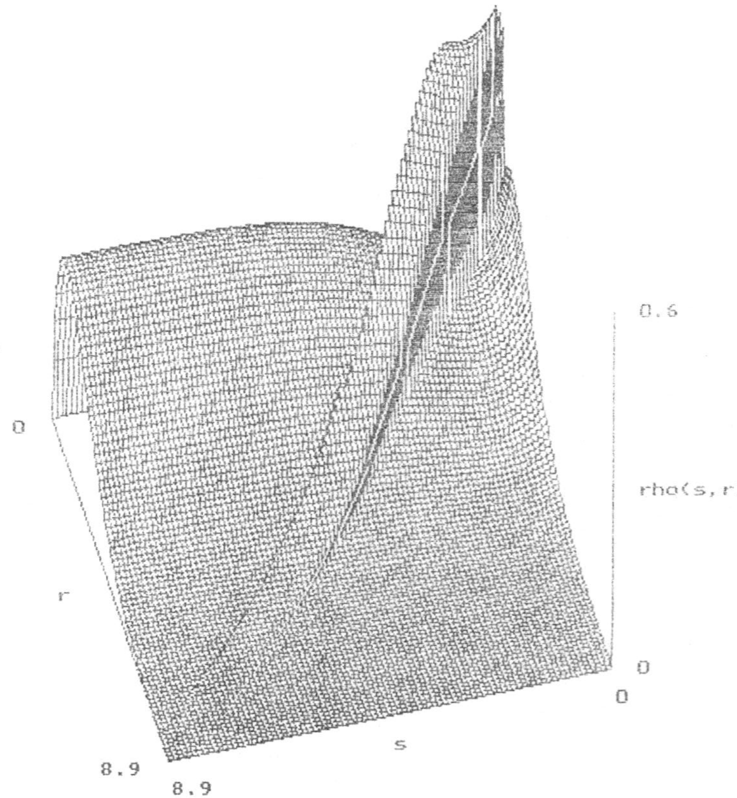

Fig. 2 Graph of the mixing function $\rho(s,r)$ for a narrow rectangular preference function ϕ with mean s = 2 and $\alpha = 0.1$.

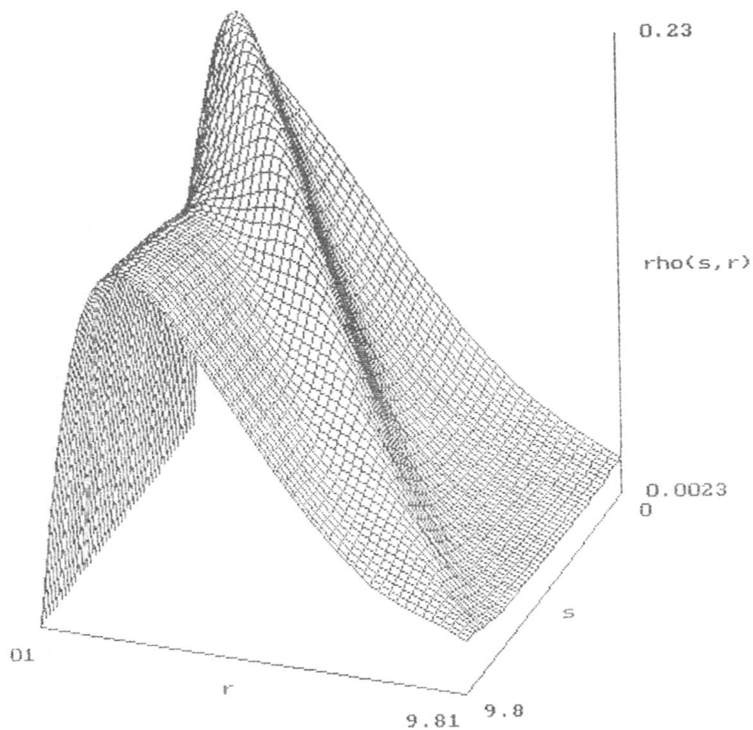

Fig. 3 Graph of the mixing function ρ(s,r) for a gaussian preference function ϕ with $\sigma =$ 0.25.

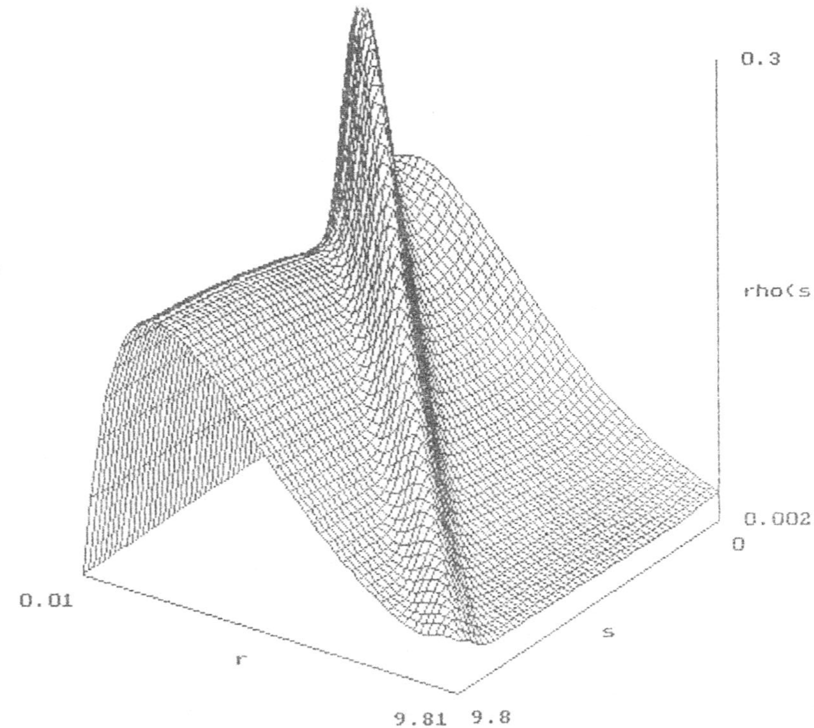

Fig. 4 Graph of the mixing function ρ(s,r) for a gaussian preference function ϕ with $\sigma =$ 1.0.

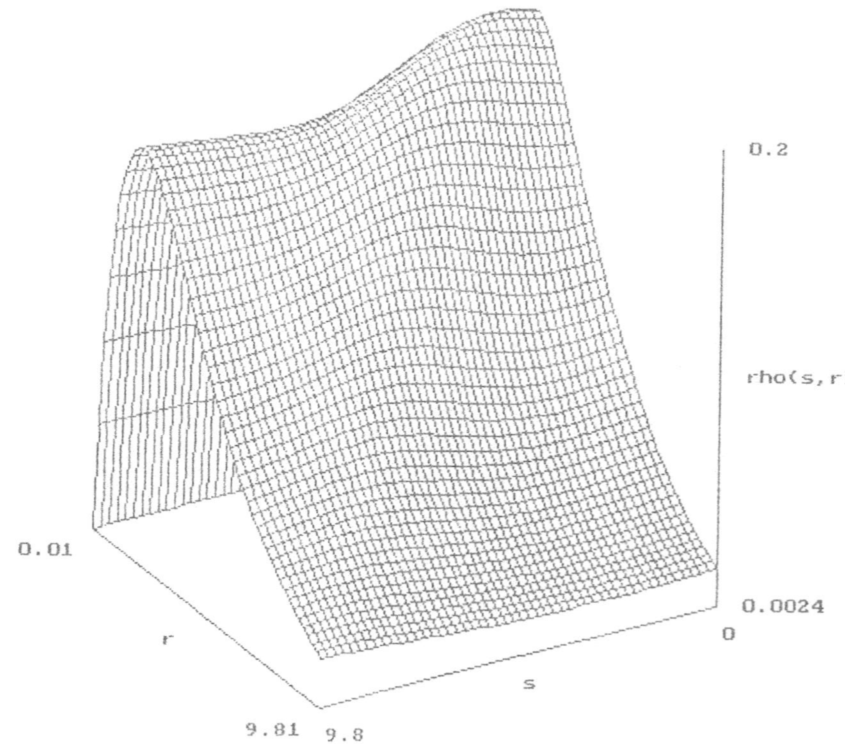

Fig. 5 Graph of the mixing function $\rho(s,r)$ for a gaussian preference function ϕ with $\sigma =$ 4.0.

INTERACTION, PAIR FORMATION AND FORCE OF INFECTION TERMS IN SEXUALLY TRANSMITTED DISEASES

Stavros Busenberg
Department of Mathematics
Harvey Mudd College
Claremont, California 91711
U. S.

Carlos Castillo-Chavez
Biometrics Unit/ Center for Applied Math.
341 Warren Hall
Cornell University
Ithaca, NY 14853-7801
U.S.

Abstract

A central question in the study of the dynamics of sexually-transmitted diseases — one emphasized by the AIDS epidemic — is that of mixing. In this note we formulate a generalization of the Blythe and Castillo-Chavez social/sexual framework for human interactions through the incorporation of age-structure, and derive an explicit expression for the general solution to this formulation. An age-structured epidemic model for a single sexually-active homosexual population, stratified by risk and age, with arbitrary risk and age-dependent mixing and variable infectivity is formulated. In the special case of proportionate mixing in age and risk, an explicit expression for the basic reproductive number is given.

1. Introduction

Theoretical models have shown that the key factors, given the present information, determining the dynamics of HIV (human immunodeficiency virus, the etiological agent for AIDS) are variable infectivity and mixing. In this article, we formulate a general framework for age- and risk- (average number of sexual partners per unit time) dependent mixing. This framework generalizes those currently found in the literature and hence many specific forms of mixing presently used fit within our framework (for a more detailed discussion see the final section). In addition, we state a representation theorem that includes all possible solutions to this framework. If preference (like-with-like, etc.) is a central, and measurable, determinant of social/sexual dynamics, then our representation theorem solves the mixing problem for a homosexual population.

The mathematical literature on age-dependent models (see Castillo-Chavez *et al.* 1988, 1989a; Castillo-Chavez 1989) shows that mixing determines one of the nonlinear terms.

Further, in the absence of nonlinear per capita birth and death rates, mixing is the only source of nonlinear phenomena. Biologically realistic mixing terms are provided by the "mass-action" law and proportionate mixing. Models for the AIDS epidemic have shown that other types of mixing have to be explored (see Jacquez *et al.* 1988; Hyman and Stanley 1988). Our representation theorem provides all possible nonlinear expressions for the "force" of infection (new cases per unit time) and hence, opens the possibility of evaluating past and current model assumptions.

The local dynamics of many epidemiological models are generally governed by the basic reproductive number R_0, which is usually defined as the number of secondary infections generated by a typical infectious individual in a population of susceptibles (see Diekmann *et al.* 1989 for a recent discussion). Usually the maintenance of the disease at endemic levels can occur only if $R_0 > 1$, and this fact allows one to consider strategies that can reduce R_0 below its critical value. Approaches of this type have long been valuable in disease management, for example in the development of vaccination strategies for other diseases, or in educational programs for reducing transmission. In this article, we note that the reproductive number is given implicitly by a nonlinear function of the mixing and the infectivity. Hence, it is not possible to find an explicit expression for the reproductive number, except in very special situations such as proportionate mixing. However, a formula for the reproductive number in the case of proportionate mixing may be very useful in order to study the relative effects of distinct control measures.

In this paper, a formula for the reproductive number that involves risk, age, and variable infectivity is presented. Since our main objective is to make these results available to those researchers interested in modelling the AIDS epidemic we concentrate on presenting some key ideas. Further results, more detailed examples, and the mathematical details will be published elsewhere (see Busenberg and Castillo-Chavez 1989).

2. Mixing framework

We consider a single group of sexually-active homosexual individuals who are structured according to the following variables: a = age ; τ = time since infection ; r = activity or risk level. In addition, we let $N(r,a,\tau,t)$ denote the total population density per unit age, activity, and time since infection, at time t. This population is divided into the following epidemiological classes: S = susceptible, I = asymptomatic infective, A = symptomatic infective. Note that the I class can include the traditional exposed but not infective class E, by taking simply the infectivity of an I individual to be zero when τ is less than a given threshold τ_0, or by employing some probability measure on the τ variable. We assume that τ is a hidden internal variable that does not distinguish individuals other than through their level of infectivity, and perhaps their mortality. For the case of AIDS, we let $T = S + \int_0^\infty I(r,a,\tau,t)d\tau =$ total age and activity-level density of the population active in disease transmission contacts; i.e., we assume that A-individuals ("full-blown" AIDS) are sexually inactive. Sexual mixing is defined through the mixing function:

$\rho(r,a,r',a',t) =$ proportion of partners of an (r,a) individual (i.e., a person of activity level r at age a) who are (r′,a′) individuals at time t,

and we let

$C(r,a,T(r,a,t)) =$ expected or average number of partners per unit time; of an (r,a) individual, given that the sexually-active population density is T(r,a,t). We assume that $C \geq 0$.

The following natural conditions characterize the mixing function:

(i) $\rho \geq 0$,

(ii) $\int_0^\infty \int_0^\infty \rho(r, a, r', a', t)dr'da' = 1$,

(iii) $\rho(r,a,r',a', t)C(r,a, T(r, a, t))T(r,a,t) = \rho(r',a',r,a)C(r',a', T(r',a',t))T(r',a',t)$,

(iv) $C(r,a, T(r, a, t))T(r,a,t)C(r',a', T(r',a',t))T(r',a',t) = 0 \Rightarrow \rho(r,a,r',a') = 0$,

Condition (ii) is due to the fact that ρ is a proportion. Condition (iii) simply states that the total number of pairs of (r,a) individuals with (r′,a′) individuals equals the total number of pairs of (r′,a′) individuals with (r,a) individuals (all this is per unit time, age, and time since infection). Condition (iv) says that there is no mixing in the age and activity levels where there are no active individuals; i.e., on the set $S = \{(r,a,r',a'): C(r,a,T(r,a,t))T(r,a,t)C(r',a',T(r',a',t))T(r',a',t) = 0\}$.

Since the above properties hold for all $t \geq 0$, we omit t; to further simplify the discussion we often assume that $C = C(r,a)$.

There are situations when it is necessary to consider mixing functions ρ which are Dirac delta functions (see Nold 1980, Jacquez *et al.* 1988, Blythe and Castillo-Chavez 1989, Castillo-Chavez and Blythe 1989), or, more generally, distributions or generalized functions. The above conditions (i)-(iv) also characterize these mixing distributions, provided that they are interpreted appropriately. Explicitly, two modifications to the interpretation of conditions (i) and (iv) are necessary:

(i′) $\rho \geq 0$ in the sense of distributions, i.e.,

$$\int_0^{\infty}\int_0^{\infty} \rho(r,a,r',a')f(r',a')dr'da' \geq 0 \quad \text{for all } f\geq 0, \text{ and}$$

(iv′) $\rho(r,a,r',a') = 0$ on a set S, means

$$\iint_S \rho(r,a,r',a')f(r,a')drda' = 0 \text{ for all f.}$$

In writing the conditions characterizing ρ we have exhibited their functional dependence on (r,a,r',a') and, for notational convenience, suppressed their dependence on t and T.

Pair formations can involve selectivity (according to age or activity level) by individuals, they can be random pairings without regard to these variables, or they can be any combination or mixture of the two extremes. A detailed discussion of these possibilities and of the restrictions they place on the mixing function ρ can be found in Busenberg and Castillo-Chavez (1989).

The effects of mixing on disease transmission can be modelled through the incidence rate (new infected cases per unit time) or "force" of infection. We begin by letting $\beta(r,a,\tau,r',a')$ = the probability that a pairing between a (r',a',τ) infective individual and an (r,a) susceptible will lead to the passing of the infection to the susceptible. The force of infection term B takes the form:

$$B(r,a,t) = S(r,a,t)C(r,a,T(r,a,t))\int_0^{\infty}\int_0^{\infty}\int_0^{\infty} \beta(r,a,\tau,r',a')\rho(r,a,r',a')\,\frac{I(r',a',\tau,t)}{T(r',a',t)}\,dr'da'd\tau,. \quad (1)$$

since a proportion I/T of the contacts of a susceptible individuals is with infectives.

The implied dynamics for the susceptible class are governed by

$$\frac{\partial S}{\partial t}(r,a,t) + \frac{\partial S}{\partial a}(r,a,t) + \mu(r,a,t)S(r,a,t) = \Lambda(r,a,t,T(a,r,t)) - B(r,a,t), \quad (2)$$

where Λ denotes the "recruitment" rate into the susceptible class, and μ denotes the natural per capita mortality rate. We observe that there are several constitutive forms of the interaction term ρ; examples without age structure can be found in Blythe and Castillo-Chavez (1989) and Castillo-Chavez and Blythe (1989). A table that considers several possibilities, for age and activity dependent mixing, can be found in Busenberg and Castillo-Chavez (1989), where the nine general cases discussed in detail include proportionate mixing in the age variable only, proportionate mixing in the activity variable only, and proportionate mixing in both age and partner variables. One of the simplest forms of mixing is that of proportionate or random mixing, and in our present framework, this includes both variables (age and activity level) and is given by a generalization of that used for situations without age-structure by Anderson and May (1987) and May and Anderson (1989):

$$\bar{p}(r,a,r',a') = \frac{C(r',a',T(r',a',t))T(r',a',t)}{\int_0^{\infty}\int_0^{\infty} C(r',a',\, T(r',a',\, t))T(r',a',t)da'dr'}\ . \quad (3)$$

In (3), as well as in similar formulas that follow, $\bar{p}(r,a,r',a')$ is defined to be identically equal to zero whenever $C(r,a,T(r,a,t))$ vanishes identically, of course, in order to satisfy (ii) we must have a set of positive measure for which C and T are strictly positive. This solution plays an important role in the determination of all possible solutions to the mixing framework (i)-(ii)-(iii)-(iv). Busenberg and Castillo-Chavez (1989) have established the following results:

(I) The only separable mixing function, i.e. $\rho(r,a,r',a') = \rho_1(r,a)\rho_2(r',a')$, satisfying conditions (i)-(ii)-(iii)-(iv) is the total proportionate mixing $\bar{p}$ given by (3).

(II) If we let

$$h(r,a,t) = C(r,a,T(r,a,t))T(r,a,t), \tag{4}$$

then the general solution of (i)-(ii)-(iii) has the form (omitting time)

$$\rho(r,a,r',a') = \bar{p}(r',a') + \psi(r,a,r',a'), \tag{5}$$

where ψ satisfies:

$$\psi \geq -\bar{p}, \int_0^\infty\int_0^\infty \psi(r,a,r',a')dr'da' = 0, \int_0^\infty\int_0^\infty \psi(r,a,r',a')h(r',a')dr'da' = 0, \text{ and} \tag{6}$$

$$\psi(r,a,r',a')h(r,a) = \psi(r',a',r,a)h(r',a'). \tag{7}$$

(III) If we let $\phi(r,a,r',a')$, be jointly symmetric in the (r,a) and (r',a') variables- - i.e., $\phi(r,a,r',a') = \phi(r',a',r,a)$, and assume that $\int_0^\infty\int_0^\infty \bar{p}(r',a')\phi(r,a,r',a')dr'da' = 1$ – then we have the following general representation form for the mixing function satisfying (i)-(ii)-(iii)-(iv):

$$\rho(r,a,r',a') = \bar{p}(r',a')\phi(r',a',r,a). \tag{8}$$

Conversely, every mixing function ρ that satisfies (i)-(ii)-(iii)-(iv) is given by the form (8), where ϕ is symmetric and satisfies the hypothesis of the theorem.

Using the above results and condition (iv) we derive a explicit representation formula for the construction of arbitrary mixing functions. This representation is based on perturbations of a particularly convenient special form.

Representation Theorem. To describe the representation formula given by this theorem, we let $\phi:\Re^4_+ \rightarrow \Re^+_+$ be a measurable and jointly symmetric function which satisfies

$$\int_0^\infty\int_0^\infty \bar{p}(r',a')\phi(r,a,r',a')dr'da' \leq 1 \text{ and}$$

$$\int_0^\infty\int_0^\infty \bar{p}(r,a)\left\{\int_0^\infty\int_0^\infty \bar{p}(r',a')\phi(r,a,r',a')dr'da'\right\}drda < 1.$$

Defining $\rho_1(r,a)$ by

$$\rho_1(r,a) = 1 - \int_0^\infty\int_0^\infty \bar{\rho}(r',a')\phi(r',a',r,a)dr'da', \tag{9}$$

then the following representation formula yields a mixing function

$$\rho(r,a, r',a') = \bar{\rho}(r',a') \left[\!\left[\frac{\rho_1(r,a)\rho_1(r',a')}{\int_0^\infty\int_0^\infty \bar{\rho}(r',a')\rho_1(r',a')dr'da'} + \phi(r,a,r',a') \right]\!\right]. \tag{10}$$

The converse also holds; that is, for every mixing function ρ there exists ϕ satisfying the hypotheses of the theorem such that ρ is given by (10) with ρ_1 defined by (9). We note that condition (iv) is needed in order to prove the uniqueness of this representation. A similar result holds when we allow ρ to be a generalized function and include the possibility of delta functions or other distributions.

An elementary but important result is that a convex combination of mixing functions is also a mixing function. Specifically, if $\alpha_1,...\alpha_N$ are positive constants such that $\sum_{i=1}^{N}\alpha_i = 1$, and $\rho_1,...,\rho_N$ are mixing functions, then $\sum_{i=1}^{N}\alpha_i\rho_i$ is a mixing function.

Here we include only the proof of (I). The proof of (II)-(III) and the representation theorem, as well as the proofs of further results for specific cases can be found in Busenberg and Castillo-Chavez (1989).

The proportionate mixing (in age and risk) $\bar{\rho}$ is the only separable solution that satisfies the mixing axioms (i)-(iv).

Proof:

A mixing function ρ is called separable if it can be written in the form

$$\rho(r,a,r',a') = \rho_1(r,a)\rho_2(r',a') \ .$$

Note that the total proportionate mixing function $\bar{\rho}$ is separable.

Suppose that ρ is separable; then a direct substitution of this separable solution in (ii) leads to

$$\rho_1(r,a) = \frac{1}{\iint_0^\infty \rho_2(r',a')dr'da'} = k \ \text{(a constant)}.$$

Hence it follows that $\rho(r,a,r',a') = k\rho_2(r',a')$.

We next note a useful relation obtained by integrating (iii) over the variables r′ and a′ and using condition (ii),

$$C(r,a, T(r,a))T(r,a) = \iint_0^\infty \rho(r',a',r,a)C(r',a', T(r',a'))T(r',a')dr'da' \tag{*}$$

mixing function ρ^* but that always has the property that $M(0,r,a,r',a') = 0$. We observe that $k^*(r,a) \equiv 0$ is always a solution of (15) and it corresponds to the infection-free state. Any other nonnegative solutions to (15) correspond to an endemic equilibrium. In the special case where $\rho = \bar{\rho}$, C and Λ are independent of the active population density T, and $\beta=\beta(\tau,r',a')$, we find the that the existence of an endemic state is dependent on the value of the basic reproductive number given by

$$R_0 = \int_0^\infty \int_0^\infty C(r',a') \left\{ \int_0^{a'} e^{-\int_x^{a'} \mu(y)dy} \Lambda(r',x)dx \right\} \int_0^\infty \Big[\beta(\tau,r',a')C(r',a'-\tau) \times e^{-\int_0^\tau [\mu(a'+\sigma-\tau)+\xi(a'+\sigma-\tau,\sigma)+\gamma(a'+\sigma-\tau,\sigma)]d\sigma} d\tau\Big] da'dr', \qquad (16)$$

which follows directly from (15).

The basic reproductive number is a threshold of critical importance in the study of disease dynamics. It allows us to study the effects of demographic and epidemiological parameters in disease transmission. For example, we note that R_0 is given by three types of risk- and age- dependent expressions: those involving death-adjusted “recruitment”, those involving time spent in the infectious state – appropriately weighted by infectivity, and those involving average sexual activity. Furthermore, we observe that any uniform increase in these expressions; i.e., an increase in the incubation period, in the mean number of sexual partners, or in the recruitment of susceptibles will generate an increase in the reproductive number. However, a change in any of these parameters, which represents an average increase over old age and activity classes, need not lead to an increase in R_0, and in fact, may cause R_0 to decrease due to the close coupling between these epidemiological parameters and the age- and activity level- dependent demographic parameters. The results concerning uniform increases agree in principle with those found for reproductive numbers for age-independent homogeneously mixing models, in which the reproductive number is given as the product of three factors: the mean infectious period, the mean number of sexual partners per unit time, and the average infectivity (see Anderson and May 1987). In addition, for models in which the mean number of sexual partners depends on the “recruitment” rate, we observe that the reproductive number is a nondecreasing function of this rate (see Busenberg *et al.* 1989, Castillo-Chavez *et al.* 1989b, c, d and Thieme and Castillo-Chavez 1989a, b). However, the lack of age- and activity-level structure makes it impossible to use these simpler age- and activity-independent models in the fine tuning and testing of specific control measures. The expression for R_0, given by Equation (16), allows us to look at the effects of potential control measures that are targeted to individuals of specific age and activity levels.

which we can also write using (4) as

$$h(r,a) = \iint_0^{\infty} \rho(r',a',r,a)h(r',a')dr'da' \quad . \tag{**}$$

Substituting the expression for ρ in (**), we obtain

$$h(r,a) = k\rho_2(r,a)\iint_0^{\infty} h(r',a')dr'da'.$$

Hence,

$$k\rho_2(r,a) = \frac{h(r,a)}{\iint_0^{\infty} h((r',a')dr'da'} \quad ;$$

that is, $\rho = \bar{\rho}$. Since $\bar{\rho}$ satisfies (i)–(ii)–(iii)-(iv) the proof is complete.

Age and risk based model with variable infectivity

We now use some of the above observations to formulate a specific model. A dynamic model for the sexual spread of HIV/AIDS in a single sexually-active homosexual population is given by the following set of equations for $S(r,a,t)$, $I(r,a,\tau,t)$, and $A(r,a,\tau,t)$:

$$\frac{\partial S}{\partial t} + \frac{\partial S}{\partial a} + \mu(a)S = \Lambda(r,a,t,T(a,r,t)) - B(r,a,t), \tag{11}$$

$$\frac{\partial I}{\partial t} + \frac{\partial I}{\partial a} + \frac{\partial I}{\partial \tau} + \{\mu(a) + \xi(a,\tau) + \gamma(a,\tau)\}I = 0, \tag{12}$$

$$\frac{\partial A}{\partial t} + \frac{\partial A}{\partial a} + \frac{\partial A}{\partial \tau} + \{\mu(a) + \eta(a,\tau)\}A = \gamma(a,\tau)I, \tag{13}$$

where

$$S(r,0,t) = I(r,0,\tau,t) = A(r,0,\tau,t) = 0,\ I(r,a,0,t) = B(r,a,t), \tag{14}$$

ξ and η denote the disease-induced mortalities, and γ is the rate of entry into the AIDS class. The other parameters are as previously defined, and $(t,a,\tau) \in \Re^3_+$.

For this model, we have obtained a general expression, which characterizes the reproductive number R_0 of the disease. This expression is obtained by formally substituting the expression for the endemic equilibrium, $(S^*(r,a), I^*(r,a,\tau))$, calculated through the method of characteristics, into the force of infection, $B^*(r,a)=k^*(r,a,\rho^*)C(r,a)S^*(r,a)$, where ρ^* denotes the mixing at equilibrium. This substitution lead us to a relationship of the form

$$k^*(r,a) = \iint_0^{\infty} [\![\int_0^{a'} \beta(r,a,\ \tau,r',a')M(k^*,r,a,r',a')d\tau]\!] dr'da', \tag{15}$$

where a $M \equiv M(k^*,r,a,r',a')$ denotes a nonlinear functional which depends on the particular

4. Conclusion

In this note we have extended the mixing framework of Blythe and Castillo-Chavez (1989) through the incorporation of age-structure, and have found the general solution to the mixing problem for a homosexual population. This general solution, as well as a number of other results, are new even in the simpler contest with no age-dependence. We have further clarified the role of proportionate mixing by showing that it is the only separable solution. We have formulated a general epidemic model for a single, age-dependent, sexually active, homosexual population with distributed activity levels, and have obtained an explicit expression for the reproductive number for the special case of proportionate mixing.

Our work (Busenberg and Castillo-Chavez, 1989) shows that the reproductive number is a complex nonlinear function of the mixing. Future work should be devoted to the clarification of the role of the mixing function on the reproductive number. This may be partially accomplished by the systematic study of special cases, such as that of preferred mixing (see Nold 1980, Jacquez *et al.* 1988, Blythe and Castillo-Chavez 1989, Castillo-Chavez and Blythe 1989, and Busenberg and Castillo-Chavez 1989, Castillo-Chavez *et al.* 1989d, Huang *et al.* 1989).

We note (Andrea Pugliese's remark) that our mixing framework can be easily generalized to include geographical variability by assuming that each community has its own mixing function, $\rho^j(r,a,r',a')$, which denotes the proportion of partners of an (r,a) individual who are (r',a') individuals and that take place at location j. Each of these mixing functions satisfy the mixing axioms, and hence can be expressed through our representation theorem. To complete the model, the specification of a migration matrix such as that of Sattenspiel (1987a, b) and Sattenspiel and Simon (1988) is needed to model the movement of individuals between communities. Although the use of a general framework of this type could be very useful in theoretical consideration, its applicability to specific situations is probably quite limited due to the tremendous number of parameters involved.

Finally, we note that the extension of the above framework to two-sex populations is quite simple and specific solutions can be found. We are presently working to determine the general solution to this two-sex framework. We note that the formulation of a two-sex framework along the lines of the one-sex framework described in this article provides an alternative formulation to that of Dietz and Hadeler (1988). Models that consider pairs and follow the dynamics of pairs have been studied by Kendall (1949), Fredrickson (1971), Dietz and Hadeler (1988), Dietz (1988), Hadeler (1989a, b), and Waldstätter (1989). Analogous models can be formulated using solutions to a two-sex framework similar to the one described in this article. Our approach (one- and two-sex formulations) has perhaps the added advantage that it allows us to compare the results of models with pairs and without pairs (i.e., the duration of each partnership is zero) from frameworks derived under the same basic assumptions. A manuscript discussing a model with pairs that incorporates this approach for specific mixing functions is under preparation (see Castillo-Chavez and Busenberg 1989).

ACKNOWLEDGMENTS

We thank John Jacquez for his comments. This research has been partially supported by the Center for Applied Mathematics at Cornell University and NSF grant DMS-8703631 to Stavros Busenberg, and NSF grant DMS-8906580, NIAID Grant R01 A129178-01, and Hatch project grant NYC 151-409, USDA to Carlos Castillo-Chavez.

REFERENCES

Anderson, R.M. and R.M. May. (1987). Transmission dynamics of HIV infection. *Nature* 326, 137-142.

Blythe, S.P. and C. Castillo-Chavez. (1989). Like-with-like preference and sexual mixing models. *Math. Biosci.* 96, 221-238.

Busenberg, S. and C. Castillo-Chavez. (1989). Risk and age-dependent mixing functions and force of infection terms in STD's. (Submitted.)

Busenberg, S., K. Cooke, and H. Thieme. (1989). Transmission and persistence of AIDS in a heterogeneous population. (Manuscript.)

Castillo-Chavez, C. (1989). Some applications of structured models in population dynamics. In *Applied Mathematical Ecology*, Biomathematics 18, Springer-Verlag, Berlin, Heidelberg, New York, Tokyo. (In press.)

Castillo-Chavez, C. and S.P. Blythe. (1989). Mixing framework for social/sexual behavior. (This volume.)

Castillo-Chavez, C. and S. Busenberg. (1989). Pair formation in age- and risk-structured populations. (Manuscript in preparation.)

Castillo-Chavez, C., H.W. Hethcote, V. Andreasen, S.A. Levin, and W.M. Liu. (1989a). Epidemiological models with age structure, proportionate mixing, and cross-immunity. *J. Math. Biol.* 27, 233-258.

Castillo-Chavez, C., K. Cooke, W. Huang, and S.A. Levin. (1989b). On the role of long periods of infectiousness in the dynamics of acquired immunodeficiency syndrom (AIDS). In *Mathematical Approaches to Problems in Resource Management and Epidemiology*. C. Castillo-Chavez, S.A. Levin, and C. Shoemaker (eds.). Lecture Notes in Biomathematics 81, Springer-Verlag, Berlin, Heidelberg, New York, Tokyo. (In press.)

Castillo-Chavez, C., K. Cooke, W. Huang, and S.A. Levin. (1989c). On the role of long incubation periods in the dynamics of acquired immunodeficiency syndrome (AIDS), Part 1. Single population models. *J. Math. Biol.* 27, 373-398.

Castillo-Chavez, C., K. Cooke, W. Huang, and S.A. Levin. (1989d). Results on the dynamics for models for the sexual transmission of the human immodeficiency virus. *Applied Mathematics Letter.* (In press.)

Castillo-Chavez, C., K. Cooke, W. Huang, and S.A. Levin. (1989e). On the role of long incubation periods in the dynamics of acquired immunodeficiency syndrome (AIDS), Part 2. Multiple group models. (This volume.)

Castillo-Chavez, C., H.W. Hethcote, V. Andreasen, S.A. Levin, and W.M. Liu. (1988). Cross-immunity in the dynamics of homogeneous and heterogeneous populations. In *Mathematical Ecology,* L. Gross, T.G. Hallam, and S.A. Levin (eds.). Proceedings, Autumn Course Research Seminars, Trieste 1986, pp. 303-316. World Scientific Publishing Co., Singapore.

Diekmann, O., J.A.P. Heesterbeek, and J.A.J. Metz. (1989). On the definition of R_0 in models for infectious diseases in heterogeneous populations. (Manuscript.)

Dietz, K. (1988). On the transmission dynamics of HIV. *Math. Biosci.* 90, 397-414.

Dietz, K. and K.P. Hadeler. (1988). Epidemiological models for sexually transmitted diseases. *J. Math. Biol.* 26, 1-25.

Frederickson, A.G. (1971). A mathematical theory of age structure in sexual populations: Random mating and monogamous marriage models. *Math. Biosci.* 20, 117-143.

Hadeler, K.P. (1989a). Pair formation in age-structured populations. *Acta Applicandae Mathematicae* 14, 91-102.

Hadeler, K.P. (1989b). Modeling AIDS in structured populations. (Manuscript.)

Huang, W., K. Cooke, and C. Castillo-Chavez. (1989). Stability and befurcation for a multiple group model for the dynamics of HIV/AIDS transmission. (Manuscript.)

Hyman, J.M. and E.A. Stanley. (1988). A risk-based model for the spread of the AIDS virus. *Math. Biosci.* 90, 415-473.

Jacquez, J.A., C.P. Simon, J. Koopman, L. Sattenspiel, and T. Perry. (1988). Modelling and analyzing HIV transmission: the effect of contact patterns. *Math. Biosci.* 92, 119-199.

Kendall, D.G. (1949). Stochastic processes and population growth. *Roy. Statist. Soc., Ser. B* 2, 230-264.

May, R.M. and R.M. Anderson. (1989). The transmission dynamics of human immunodeficiency virus (HIV). *Phil. Trans. R. Soc. London B* 321, 565-607.

Nold, A. (1980). Heterogeneity in disease-transmission modeling. *Math. Biosci.* 52, 227-240.

Sattenspiel, L. and C.P. Simon. (1988). The spread and persistence of infectious diseases in structured populations. *Math. Biosci.* 90, 341-366.

Sattenspiel, L. (1987a). Population structure and the spread of disease. *Human Biology* 59,

411-438.

Sattenspiel, L. (1987b). Epidemics in nonrandomly mixing populations: a simulation. *American Journal of Physical Anthropology,* 73, 251-265.

Thieme, H.R. and C. Castillo-Chavez. (1989a). On the role of variable infectivity in the dynamics of the human immunodeficiency virus. (This volume.)

Thieme, H.R. and C. Castillo-Chavez. (1989b). On the possible effects of infection-age-dependent infectivity in the dynamics of HIV/AIDS. (Manuscript.)

Waldstätter, R. (1989). Pair formation in sexually transmitted diseases. (This volume.)

STRUCTURED MIXING:
HETEROGENEOUS MIXING BY THE DEFINITION OF ACTIVITY GROUPS.

John A. Jacquez
Departments of Physiology and Biostatistics
University of Michigan
Ann Arbor, MI 48109

Carl P. Simon
Departments of Mathematics and Economics
University of Michigan
Ann Arbor, MI 48109

James Koopman
Department of Epidemiology
University of Michigan
Ann Arbor, MI 48109

Abstract

Motivated by the needs of our models of spread of HIV, we have devised a way of specifying non-random contacts between subgroups in a population. Population heterogeneity is characterized by dividing the population into disjoint subgroups, the population subgroups. The contacts of the population subgroups are then partitioned into activity groups. The activity groups are defined in terms of processes that drive the contacts or in terms of the arenas where contacts are made by specifying the allocations of the contacts of the population subgroups to activity groups. All mixing is within activity groups and may, in general, be by any mechanism that gives a symmetric contact matrix. This method handles heterogeneity in mixing in a simple manner while automatically satisfying the inherent constraints on contact matrices.

1. Introduction

One of the basic problems of epidemiology is to relate the patterns of disease spread to the mechanisms of spread of the disease agent (Taylor and Knowelden 1964; Fox et al. 1970). Indeed, for diseases that require close personal contact for transmission, such as the sexually transmitted diseases, there is a tradition of case study and contact tracing that focuses on the particularities of transmission on a case-by-case basis.

In the early attempts to model the spread of disease (Ross 1911; Kermack and McKendrick 1927; Soper 1929; Serfling 1952; Dietz 1988a; Dietz and Schenzle 1985), the population at risk was treated as homogeneous with a fixed constant probability of a contact effective in transmission between two individuals. This hypothesis of homogeneous mixing characterizes the first or classical phase of epidemiological modeling.

Nonetheless, it was recognized right from the start that populations are made up of subgroups and that heterogeneity must affect the process of disease transmission. Some early attempts were made to introduce specific types of heterogeneity, but contacts between individuals were still modeled as random. Random contacts in a heterogeneous population lead to proportional mixing (Barbour 1978; Nold 1980) between the groups. The hypothesis of proportional mixing characterizes the second phase of epidemiological modeling.

We are now in a third phase in which we are concerned with the modeling of "non-random" mixing. Our goal in this paper is first to review the work on the specification of contact patterns for a population divided into discrete subgroups. Then we introduce a general method of specifying mixing between discrete subgroups that can be used to specify contacts between age groups, contacts between geographically defined subgroups, contacts between socially defined subgroups, and overlaps. In short, it handles heterogeneity in a simple and rational manner while automatically satisfying the natural constraints on contact matrices.

2. Modeling Contact Patterns

Populations are heterogeneous in many ways that affect disease transmission. For example, age, geographical separation and population density effects are obvious sources of heterogeneity. In addition, members of ethnic and some social groups often tend to mix more with members of their own groups than with outsiders, leading to further sources of heterogeneity.

At the outset, we need to distinguish between three types of matrices that have been used in the modeling of heterogeneity: contact matrices, mixing or contact fraction matrices and transmission parameter matrices. A contact matrix, $[C_{ij}]$, gives the number of contacts that persons in group i make with persons in group j per unit of time. The mixing matrix, $[\rho_{ij}]$, gives the fraction of the contacts of persons in group i that are made with persons in j per unit of time. The transmission parameter matrix includes the effects of the probability of transmission per contact, and so, it gives the transmission rate to susceptibles in i resulting from contacts with infectious individuals in j.

In the literature, there are two main lines of development in the attempts to take into account the effects of heterogeneity on disease transmission and its implications for immunization programs. One line is empirical, the other is based on a model of mixing in the population; there may be mixtures.

a. Empirical

The empirical approach is to try to fill in the elements of a contact matrix directly from data. For example, in their study of the effect of immunization on the spread of influenza A, Longini et al. (1978) divided the population into five subgroups, based on age. They used what they called an infectious contact rate matrix to define effective contact rates between an infectious individual in group i and individuals in group j, and estimated the elements of the matrix by comparing the attack rates predicted by their deterministic model with those given by a stochastic model which simulated field data from previous epidemics. In a model of the global spread of influenza, Rvachev and

Longini (1985) used uniform mixing within major cities of the world and a symmetric matrix for the daily movement of individuals from city i to j and from city j to i. They then used statistics on air traffic to fill in their movement matrix.

The difficulties with direct empirical fitting of the elements of the contact or mixing matrix increase rapidly with the number of subgroups, because the information needed soon outstrips the information available from the data. For this reason, we want to build in natural constraints on the entries of the matrix. The idea is to use information about the processes that generate contact patterns to structure the mixing matrix in the hope that knowledge about the basic causes will provide enough constraints so that the n^2 elements of the contact matrix can be determined by no more than about n basic factors which then have to be estimated from data.

b. Models of Mixing

In the literature, one can discern two somewhat different approaches to the development of mixing models. In the first approach, one starts with uniform mixing in subgroups and tries to directly specify non-random mixing between subgroups. The second approach uses proportional mixing as a starting point and tries to introduce restrictions on random mixing.

Approach 1.

In this approach, the model consists of a number of subgroups with uniform mixing within the subgroups, and then a matrix for mixing between groups is specified. In an early attempt to treat heterogeneity in a model of a simple epidemic in a population with m subgroups, Rushton and Mautner (1955) assumed homogeneous mixing within each subgroup with a common within-subgroup transmission parameter α and homogeneous mixing between subgroups with a different but common transmission parameter β for transmission between individuals of different subgroups. In another early paper, Haskey (1957) looked at a stochastic model of transmission for two isolated subgroups for which the two transmission parameters for within-group and the two for between-group transmission all differed. Bartlett (1956) also studied a two subgroup model. Watson (1972) looked at the stochastic and deterministic versions of the SIR model with subgroups, using two values for the transmission parameter. Post et al. (1983) looked at the criteria for endemicity in a stratified SIR model in which the transmission from group j to i is a function of the number of susceptibles in i, the number of infectives in j, and the fraction T_{ij} of the time group i contacts group j. Anderson and May (1985) used essentially the same approach as Rushton and Mautner (1955), a common within-group transmission parameter β and a weaker between-group rate $\epsilon\beta$, $0 \leq \epsilon \leq 1$, in their study of immunization programs in an SIR model with subgroups; two parameters defined all entries in their transmission parameter matrix. In later work, on age dependent changes in the transmission of infectious diseases, Anderson and May (1985) examined the implications of a number of transmission parameter matrices for transmission between age classes. In all of the matrices they examined, they used n values to fill in the entries of an $n \times n$ matrix. Travis and Lenhart (1987) generalized this by using a common within-group transmission rate parameter β and between-group parameters,

$\epsilon_{ij}\beta$, $0 \leq \epsilon_{ij} \leq 1$; this approach still requires n^2 parameters to specify between-group mixing.

In her work on modeling the spread of hepatitis A, Sattenspiel (1987) developed an interesting model for mixing of geographically separated subgroups. As in other work, mixing within the geographically separate subgroups is uniform. The mixing between the subgroups occurs in the following way. A subset of each subgroup travels to social facilities associated with each group, where again homogeneous mixing occurs. The contacts at these social facilities are specified in terms of a migration matrix which gives the fraction of those individuals in each traveling subgroup that go to each social facility. This requires the estimation of $n \times (n-1)$ components. This model has been analyzed in detail by Sattenspiel and Simon (1988) and has been one of the stimuli to the present work.

Approach 2.

The second approach starts with proportional mixing which is a random allocation method for a heterogeneous population. In proportional mixing, the contacts of a group are divided among all groups, including itself, in proportion to the 'contact activity' of each group. Let N_i be the number in group i and c_i be the mean number of contacts per unit time of an individual in group i. Then c_iN_i is the total contact rate of all individuals in group i. The fraction of group i's contacts that are made with group j is given by equation (1):

$$\rho_{ij} = \frac{c_jN_j}{\sum_k c_kN_k}. \tag{1}$$

Note that for given j, ρ_{ij} is the same for all groups. Furthermore, if the contact rate per person is the same for all groups, then ρ_{ij} is proportional to group size N_j. Nold (1980) introduced a model for mixing in which the mixing matrix was a convex combination of random mixing within groups ($\rho_{ij} = \delta_{ij}$), and of proportional mixing. That formulation is equivalent to reserving a fixed fraction, ρ, of each group's contacts for within-group mixing; the rest of the groups' contacts are then subject to proportional mixing. That approach provides a way of specifying a uniform preference for mixing with individuals with similar characteristics and has been used by Hethcote, Yorke and Nold (1982) and Hethcote and Yorke (1984) to model the spread of gonorrhea and also by Hethcote and Van Ark (1987). Our group at the University of Michigan (Jacquez et al. 1988) has generalized this approach to give what we call "preferred mixing." In preferred mixing one can reserve an arbitrary fraction of each group's contacts for within-group contacts and the remaining contacts are subject to proportional mixing. Thus if ρ_i is the fraction reserved for within-group contacts for group i, equations (2) and (3) give the contact fractions for within-group and between-group contacts for preferred mixing:

$$\rho_{ii} = \rho_i + (1-\rho_i)\frac{c_i(1-\rho_i)N_i}{\sum_k c_k(1-\rho_k)N_k}, \tag{2}$$

$$\rho_{ij} = (1-\rho_i)\frac{c_j(1-\rho_j)N_j}{\sum_k c_k(1-\rho_k)N_k}; j \neq i. \tag{3}$$

Preferred mixing has been extended by Hyman and Stanley (1988,1989) and Blythe and Castillo-Chavez (1989) to include some preference beyond the identity group for continuously distributed characteristics.

3. Mixing in Models of AIDS

As might be expected, the first models of HIV transmission were for the most part based on a single group with homogeneous mixing or on multiple groups with proportional mixing (Pickering et al. 1986; Anderson et al. 1986; May and Anderson 1987; May et al. 1988; Hethcote, 1989; Mode et al. 1988). Later models allowed for more complex transmission possibilities.

However, models of sexually transmitted diseases require a symmetry condition for sexual contacts between two-groups. The number of sexual contacts group i has with group j must equal the number group j has with group i.

Knox (1986) modeled HIV transmission in a multigroup population in which the groups were defined by sexual preference. He used a contact matrix which was to be filled in from data. DeGruttola and Mayer (1988) looked at a two group model for heterosexual spread, the two groups being low risk and high risk groups. To introduce a preference for within-group mixing, they calculated the probability of a contact between the members of the two groups in the following way. Let N_A and N_B be the numbers in groups A and B respectively. The probability that a member of A chooses a member from B as a partner is $\phi N_B/(N_A + \phi N_B)$; the probability that the partner is from A is $N_A/(N_A + \phi N_B)$. For $\phi = 0$, A's contacts are all within group; for $\phi = 1$, there is proportional mixing if the number of contacts per person is assumed to be the same for groups A and B. It is not clear that this model satisfies the contact symmetry constraint. Abramson and Rothschild (1988) proposed a multiple group model that has a number of problems. For one, their contact matrix does not meet the symmetry constraint. In addition, the number of contacts per person in i with persons in j is taken to be constant in their model. However, this number must change as the population composition changes, even if the total number of contacts per person in i remains constant.

In our models (Jacquez et al. 1988; Koopman et al. 1988), we divided the population into subgroups by degree of sexual activity and introduced preferred mixing which allowed us to reserve an arbitrary fraction of a group's contacts for within-group contacts. This approach enabled us to examine the implications of a spectrum of models ranging from mixing only within the population subgroups, called restricted mixing, to full proportional mixing. The important finding was that even small amounts of mixing between low and high activity groups markedly increased the rate of spread and the endemic infected fraction in the low activity groups while having only small effects on the high activity groups. Hyman and Stanley (1988) report the same results for a model in which the rate of new partnership formation varies continuously over the population.

A contact factor that plays an important role in HIV transmission is the phenomenon of pair formation. Pair formation markedly decreases the number of contacts involved in general transmission by concentrating the contacts within pairs. Dietz and

Hadeler (1988) and Dietz (1988b) have introduced pair formation into models of transmission that include heterosexuals and homosexuals.

4. Where Are We Now?

Up to now, we have not had a method of specifying mixing that can be used to describe arbitrary patterns of potential contacts in a natural way while still satisfying the inherent constraints on mixing and contact matrices. In the next section, we present a method that describes a wide variety of mixing patterns for discrete subgroups; extension to continuously distributed characteristics should be straightforward. As will be seen, we model selectivity of mixing in heterogeneous populations with a two step process. The first step involves the choice of an activity group in which to make contacts. The second step involves selection of contacts within the activity group.

For AIDS, we have reached an important plateau in the development of models of mixing. In the model studies so far, it is clear that the pattern of mixing plays a major role in determining the time course of spread of the disease and the sizes of the endemic infected groups. Now the challenge is to find and work out the effects of the actual patterns of mixing that play a role in the spread of AIDS.

The problem facing us is the perennial problem of "detail versus simplicity" in the models we design. There is much discussion of the complexity of contact networks in the spread of AIDS and the need to incorporate this complexity in our models. We believe this has been overstated and mistakes the role of modeling. Models that become too complex do not serve their intended function, which is to provide insight. The papers of Anderson et al. (1986) and May and Anderson (1987) show that relatively simple models can provide lots of insight. The essence of modeling is to capture the main processes at work. Not only does that give insight into main effects, it provides the background against which other effects can be evaluated. We do not believe that we need to incorporate much detail on social networks in our models, but that we need at least some information on contact networks to help fill out the mixing matrices. We need to identify the main groups and then construct a mixing matrix which captures the main effects of the social interactions whose complexity has been stressed so much.

5. Specification of Mixing in Heterogeneous Populations

a. Contact Matrices and Mixing (Contact Fraction) Matrices

First let us distinguish between contact and mixing matrices in more detail. A contact matrix gives the *rate* of making contacts between different groups, whereas mixing matrices give the *fractions* of a group's contacts that are with other groups. Contact and mixing matrices are useful for describing many types of processes in heterogeneous populations, not just epidemic spread. For that reason, we keep separate the probability of an interaction, such as disease transmission, that follows a contact. For example, suppose c_i is the number of contacts per person in group i per unit time, X_i and Y_i are the numbers of susceptibles and infectives in i, respectively, ρ_{ij} is the fraction of the contacts of group i that are with group j, and β_{ijr} is the probability of disease transmission given a contact between a susceptible in group i and an infective in group j in stage r of the infection. If the contacts between groups i and j are random with respect to infection status and stage of infection, the rate of transmission from infectives in j that are in stage r to susceptibles in i must be

$$c_i X_i \rho_{ij} \beta_{ijr} \frac{Y_{jr}}{X_j + Y_j}.$$

Let U_i be the recruitment rate into group i and μ be the non-AIDS fractional mortality rate constant. Then for our model for HIV transmission (Jacquez et al. 1988), in which the infecteds pass through m stages before the development of AIDS, the rate of change of the susceptibles in group i is given by equation (4) in which n is the number of groups:

$$\frac{dX_i}{dt} = -c_i X_i \sum_{j=1}^{n} \rho_{ij} \sum_{r=1}^{m} \beta_{ijr} \frac{Y_{jr}}{X_j + Y_j} - \mu X_i + U_i. \tag{4}$$

In this example, the mixing matrix is ρ and the contact matrix is $\mathbf{C}$, given by equation (5), wherein $N_i = X_i + Y_i$:

$$\mathbf{C} = \begin{pmatrix} c_1 N_1 \rho_{11} & c_1 N_1 \rho_{12} & \dots & c_1 N_1 \rho_{1n} \\ c_2 N_2 \rho_{21} & c_2 N_2 \rho_{22} & \dots & c_2 N_2 \rho_{2n} \\ \vdots & \vdots & \ddots & \vdots \\ c_n N_n \rho_{n1} & c_n N_n \rho_{n2} & \dots & c_n N_n \rho_{nn} \end{pmatrix}. \tag{5}$$

The problem has been to find a formulation for ρ that allows one to describe any sort of mixing pattern and meets the constraints on ρ and $\mathbf{C}$, namely $\sum_j \rho_{ij} = 1$ and the symmetry constraint on the contact matrix, $c_i N_i \rho_{ij} = c_j N_j \rho_{ji}$.

b. Introduction to Structured Mixing and Selective Mixing.

We divide the population into subgroups using characteristics relevant to the problem at hand. These subgroups could be called characteristic or structural subgroups, but to avoid the implication that they are immutable, we will use the term population subgroup. In previous work, mixing matrices have been treated as matrices that describe the fractions of the contacts of one population subgroup with another, and they were therefore always $n \times n$ matrices. Thus ρ in the previous section is an $n \times n$ matrix. That view of mixing matrices unnecessarily restricts the mixing processes that they can represent. We think of mixing as occurring in terms of the activities, in this case the contacts, of the population subgroups. The contacts of the population subgroups are partitioned by assigning them to groups, the activity groups, in which mixing occurs. That viewpoint leads to a definition of a new type of mixing matrix that we have named an **activity group matrix**. An activity group matrix specifies the allocations of the contacts of the population subgroups to activity groups. Note that such activity groups do not change the structure of the population; they provide us with a new and malleable structure for describing mixing processes.

A related concept, that of mixing groups, has been used before in stochastic simulations, with random mixing within mixing groups (Elveback et al. 1971, 1976), but as far as we have been able to determine, it has not been used in deterministic modeling in epidemiology. Important differences between the two applications should be kept in mind. Stochastic simulations involve integral units (individuals) whose contacts are allocated to mixing groups in discrete time steps. In deterministic modeling, the total contacts of susceptibles or of infectives are treated as continuous variables in continuous time.

With the use of activity groups, non-random or selective mixing can occur at either or both of two levels. It can occur in the definition of activity groups as well as in the selection of contacts within an activity group. We call the former ***structured mixing*** and the latter ***selective mixing***. This paper is concerned primarily with structured mixing; our companion paper in this volume (Koopman et al. 1989) concentrates on selective mixing.

c. The Background to Structured and Selective Mixing.

The formulation in terms of activity groups and structured and selective mixing was derived to generalize both preferred mixing (Jacquez et al. 1988) and the mixing defined by Sattenspiel (1987). In preferred mixing, one can reserve a fraction of a group's contacts for within-group contacts. However, it is not possible to specify the fraction of a group's contacts with each other group. The other group may not have enough contacts available, so one cannot count on satisfying the symmetry constraint by setting aside arbitrary fractions of a group's contacts for different groups. One solution is to assume that the group with the smaller number of available contacts dominates, i.e., let the smaller of $c_i N_i \rho_{ij}$ and $c_j N_j \rho_{ji}$ determine the ρ_{ij} and ρ_{ji}, as has been done by Hyman and Stanley (1988) for the continuous case. In the mixing used by Sattenspiel (1987), a migration matrix was used to specify the fraction of each group that went to a social facility associated with each group, giving a square mixing matrix; the number of contacts between two groups in a facility was taken as the product of the numbers from the two groups.

The previous work of the Michigan group (Jacquez et al. 1988; Koopman et al. 1988) was limited by two major restrictions. One was that no preferential mixing beyond that specifiable by preferred mixing could be examined. The other was that the number of contacts per person per unit time, c_i, was taken to be constant. Structured mixing goes a long way towards solving the first problem: it allows one to define a much wider range of preferences in mixing. The second limitation is easily overcome in simulations: it is easy to allow c_i to vary with the population available to mix with i. For example, we expect the actual number of contacts to be zero when none are available and to rise monotonically with the number of available contacts to approach some saturation level. That approach is included in our formulation of selective mixing within mixing groups (Koopman et al. 1989).

d. Structured Mixing.

Let the population be divided into n **population subgroups**. The breakdown may be based on a number of different ways of dividing the population. For example, one could partition the population by gender, sexual preference, and drug-use; then one population subgroup would be "non-drug-using homosexual males." In our model of HIV transmission among homosexuals (Jacquez et al. 1988; Koopman et al. 1988), we divided the population into five population subgroups based on the number of new sexual contacts per person per unit time.

Next, partition the contacts of the population into **activity subgroups**. The number M of activity groups may be less than, equal to, or greater than the number n of population subgroups. These activity groups are defined in terms of the mixing processes going on in the population. For example, one can divide the contacts of a population of male homosexuals according to the locations where sexual contacts are sought.

Then, we form the activity group matrix $\mathbf{f} = ((f_{ik}))$, where f_{ik} is the fraction of population subgroup i's contacts allocated to activity group k. This activity group matrix $\mathbf{f}$ is an $n \times M$ matrix. Its elements must satisfy $\sum_k f_{ik} = 1$. The columns of $\mathbf{f}$ give the activity groups; the rows give the allocation of each population subgroup's contacts to the activity groups. The elements of $\mathbf{f}$ need not be constant.

An activity group may contain contributions from any number of population subgroups, and the contacts of a given population subgroup may appear in any number of activity groups. In particular, if an activity group contains a contribution from only one population subgroup, this situation is equivalent to reserving that fraction of the population subgroup's contacts for within-group mixing, as in preferred mixing.

Given such a matrix $\mathbf{f}$, we can form the **contact matrix** $\mathbf{C}(k)$ for the k'th activity group, where the (i,j)'th entry,

$$C(k)_{ij} = C(f_{ik}, f_{jk}, N_i, N_j),$$

denotes the number of contacts per unit time in activity group k that are made between population subgroups i and j. The mixing within activity group k may be by any mechanism that gives a symmetric contact matrix, $\mathbf{C}(k)$. The type of mixing may in fact differ in the different activity groups depending on the mixing processes at work, as long as the contact matrix for each of the activity groups is symmetric. Note that each $\mathbf{C}(k)$ is an $n \times n$ matrix. The overall contact matrix $\mathbf{C}$ is obtained by summing all of the $\mathbf{C}(k)$'s:

$$\mathbf{C} = \sum_k \mathbf{C}(k). \tag{6}$$

The symmetry of the individual $\mathbf{C}(k)$'s ensures the symmetry of $\mathbf{C}$. This process provides a contact matrix for the population subgroups that satisfies the symmetry requirement no matter how complex the underlying mixing.

Examples of mixing mechanisms within activity groups that satisfy the symmetry constraints are proportional mixing and preferred mixing as well as any mixing process of the "chemical reaction" type, in which the contacts of population subgroups in any activity group are symmetric in the products of the number of contacts available from the population subgroups. Another example is given in our companion paper (Koopman et al. 1989) in which the contacts between population subgroups i and j in the kth activity group are given by equation (7):

$$C(k)_{i,j} = \frac{N_i f_{ik} N_j f_{jk} h_i h_j q_{ij} q_{ji} w_{ij}}{\sum_p N_p h_p}. \tag{7}$$

Here h_i is a measure of extroversion (outgoingness) of people in population subgroup i, q_{ij} represents the fraction of group j people acceptable to group i people and w_{ij} is a parameter representing willingness of individuals in group i to have another contact in group j. To ensure the symmetry condition, we must have $w_{ij} = w_{ji}$.

Note that if knowledge of the processes defining the elements of $\mathbf{f}$ does not define all of the f_{ik}, the remaining fractions of the population subgroups must also be mixed by a symmetric mixing. However, the remaining fractions of the population subgroups may be assigned to extra activity groups in many ways, varying from restriction to within-group mixing for each fraction to proportional mixing for all of the leftovers in one additional activity group.

For example, suppose the population is partitioned into groups based on the mean number of contacts per year, $c_1, \ldots, c_n$; these are the population subgroups. Assume that the mixing processes define M activity groups. Of the $c_i N_i$ contacts of population subgroup i, $c_i N_i f_{ik}$ are allocated to activity group k. For this example, suppose the mixing within activity groups is proportional mixing. Let $\rho(k)_{ij}$ be the fraction of group i's contacts with j in activity group k. By proportional mixing, $\rho(k)_{ij}$ is given by equation (8):

$$\rho(k)_{ij} = \frac{c_j N_j f_{jk}}{\sum_p c_p N_p f_{pk}}. \tag{8}$$

Therefore the contact matrix for the k'th activity group is given by (9):

$$\mathbf{C}(k) = \frac{1}{\sum_p c_p N_p f_{pk}} \begin{pmatrix} (c_1 N_1 f_{1k})^2 & \cdots & c_1 c_n N_1 N_n f_{1k} f_{nk} \\ c_1 c_2 N_1 N_2 f_{1k} f_{2k} & \cdots & c_2 c_n N_2 N_n f_{2k} f_{nk} \\ \vdots & \ddots & \vdots \\ c_1 c_n N_1 N_n f_{1k} f_{nk} & \cdots & (c_n N_n f_{nk})^2 \end{pmatrix}. \tag{9}$$

Let $\mathbf{cN}$ be the $(n \times n)$ diagonal matrix of elements $c_i N_i$ and let $\mathbf{f_k}$ be the $(n \times 1)$ column vector of elements f_{ik}. Then $\mathbf{C}(k)$ can also be written as in equation (10):

$$\mathbf{C}(k) = \frac{\mathbf{cN f}_k \mathbf{f}_k^T \mathbf{cN}}{\sum_p c_p N_p f_{pk}}. \tag{10}$$

The (i,j) element of $\mathbf{C}$, given in (6), is then (11):

$$C_{ij} = \sum_{k=1}^{M} \frac{c_i N_i c_j N_j f_{ik} f_{jk}}{\sum_p c_p N_p f_{pk}}. \tag{11}$$

Returning to the AIDS example that gave us equation (4), if there are M activity groups, equation (12) replaces equation (4):

$$\frac{dX_i}{dt} = -c_i X_i \sum_{k=1}^{M} f_{ik} \sum_{j=1}^{n} \rho(k)_{ij} \sum_{r=1}^{m} \beta_{ijr} \frac{Y_{jr}}{X_j + Y_j} - \mu X_i + U_i. \tag{12}$$

As a further illustration, we recast the models of the works that stimulated the development of structured mixing in terms of the population subgroups and activity groups. In our model of preferred mixing (Jacquez et al. 1988) the population was divided into n population subgroups by the average number of contacts per year. In that context, the activity groups are the fractions of each population subgroup reserved for within-group mixing plus one group which contains all of the non-reserved fractions, giving $M = n + 1$. In Sattenspiel's paper (1987), the population subgroups were n geographically separate groups. The activity groups are the fractions of the population subgroups that do not travel plus one activity group for each social facility, giving $M = 2n$.

Structured mixing thus generalizes preferred mixing and the migration matrix approach of Sattenspiel (1987) to allow the specification of arbitrary activity groups.

6. Applications of Structured Mixing

We present in summary form what we see to be potential areas of application. One can use structured mixing to generate near-neighbor types of mixing for age groups, for spatially separate groups or for particular types of mixing between social groups. As an application to mixing between age groups, consider the modeling of sexually transmitted diseases. Sexual contacts tend to be between people close in age, and the number of contacts per person per unit time depends on age. Assume we have a population divided into 5-year age groups and that each group has contacts primarily with itself and the age groups on either side, with smaller contact rates with age groups one-removed. The population subgroups are the age groups; suppose the first is the 10-15 year group. The activity matrix might then look like the following,

$$\mathbf{f} = \begin{pmatrix} f_{11} & f_{12} & f_{13} & 0 & 0 & 0 & 0 & \cdots \\ f_{21} & f_{22} & f_{23} & f_{24} & 0 & 0 & 0 & \cdots \\ f_{31} & f_{32} & f_{33} & f_{34} & f_{35} & 0 & 0 & \cdots \\ 0 & f_{42} & f_{43} & f_{44} & f_{45} & f_{46} & 0 & \cdots \\ 0 & 0 & f_{53} & f_{54} & f_{55} & f_{56} & f_{57} & \cdots \\ \vdots & \vdots & \vdots & \vdots & \vdots & \ddots & \vdots & \vdots \end{pmatrix}. \tag{13}$$

Non-random mixing between spatially separate groups can also be specified in terms of an activity group matrix, with potential applications in epidemiology and ecology. For example, if we think of the spatial organization of a pattern of villages with occasional large cities, the population subgroups are the villages and cities, although each city might contain more than one population subgroup. The activity groups might then be defined in the following way. Each village mixes primarily with itself and the neighboring villages, with a small fraction that mixes with nearby cities. A city subgroup mixes primarily with itself and other subgroups in the same city, with smaller contributions to nearby villages and cities.

Social groups such as clubs, school groups and groups formed in the workplace are obviously activity groups.

7. Applications To AIDS

In the context of AIDS, we think of the choice of a partner as a two phase process. The first is the choice of an activity group in which to interact, the second is in the choice of partner within the activity group. In this paper we have focused on the first of these — structured mixing; our companion paper (Koopman et al. 1989) focuses on the second — selective mixing.

In our work on preferred mixing (Jacquez et al. 1988), the population subgroups were defined in terms of number of contacts per person per year. The activity groups were the reserved fractions of the population subgroups plus a group that picked up the leftover fractions. With preferred mixing we were unable to compare those results with mixing patterns in which the population subgroups mixed primarily with neighboring subgroups. In that context, it seems likely that most mixing is between population subgroups that have similar contact frequencies. Structured mixing allows us to examine the effects of various forms of near-neighbor mixing. In addition, structured mixing enables us to look at mixing between groups defined by preferred type of activity and other characteristics besides preferred contact frequency.

Acknowledgements

This work was supported in part by a Presidential Initiatives Grant from the University of Michigan and by grant RR02176-01A1 from NIH-DRR, DHEW. The work of Jill Joseph and David Ostrow and discussions with them have stimulated us in thinking about mixing and contact patterns. Discussions with E.O. Laumann, Martina Morris and Tony Tam of the University of Chicago have contributed to our thinking, particularly in relation to selective mixing. We thank Ira Longini for pointing out the prior use of mixing groups in stochastic simulations.

REFERENCES

Abramson, P.R. and B. Rothschild. (1988). Sex, drugs and matrices: Mathematical prediction of HIV infection. *J. Sex Res.*, 25, 106-122.

Anderson, R.M. and R.M. May. (1985). Age-related changes in the rate of disease transmission: Implications for the design of vaccination programmes. *J. Hyg. Cam.*, 94, 365-426.

Anderson, R.M., G.F. Medley, R.M. May and A.M. Johnson. (1986). A preliminary study of the transmission dynamics of the human immunodeficiency virus (HIV), the causative agent of AIDS. *IMA J. Math. Appl. Med. Biol.*, 3, 229-263.

Barbour, A.D. (1978). MacDonald's model and the transmission of bilharzia. *Trans. Roy. Soc. Trop. Med. Hyg.*, 72, 6-15.

Bartlett, M.S. (1956). Deterministic and stochastic models for recurrent epidemics. *Proc. 3rd Berkeley Symp. on Math. Stat. and Prob.*, vol. 4, pp 81-109.

Blythe, S.P. and C. Castillo-Chavez. (1989). Like-with-like preference and sexual mixing models. *Math. Biosci.*, (in press).

DeGruttola, V. and K.H. Mayer. (1988). Assessing and modeling heterosexual spread of the human immunodeficiency virus in the United States. *Rev. of Infect. Dis.*, 10, 138-150.

Dietz, K. (1988a). The first epidemic model: A historical note on P.D. Enko. *Austral. J. Stat.*, 30A, 56-65.

Dietz, K. (1988b). On the transmission dynamics of HIV. *Math. Biosci.*, 90, 397-414.

Dietz, K. and K.P. Hadeler. (1988). Epidemiological models for sexually transmitted diseases. *J. Math. Biol.* 26, 1-25.

Dietz, K. and D. Schenzle. (1985). Mathematical models for infectious disease statistics. In *A Celebration of Statistics. The ISI Centenary Volume*, A.C. Atkinson and S.E. Feinberg, (eds.), Springer, New York, Ch. 8, 167-204.

Elveback, L., E. Ackerman, L. Gatewood and J.P. Fox. (1971). Stochastic two-agent epidemic simulation models for a community of families. *Am. J. Epidem.*, 93, 267-280.

Elveback, L.R., J.P. Fox, E. Ackerman, A. Langworthy, M. Boyd and L. Gatewood. (1976). An influenza simulation model for immunization studies. *Am. J. Epidem.*, 103, 152-165.

Fox, J.P., C.E. Hall and L.R. Elveback. (1970). *Epidemiology.* The MacMillan Co., New York.

Haskey, H.W. (1957). Stochastic cross-infection between two otherwise isolated groups. *Biometrika*, 44, 193-204.

Hethcote, H.W. (1989). A model for HIV transmission and AIDS. (in press)

Hethcote, H.W. and J.W. Van Ark. (1987). Epidemiological models for heterogeneous populations: proportionate mixing, parameter estimation and immunization programs. *Math. Biosci.*, 84, 85-118.

Hethcote, H.W., J.A. Yorke and A. Nold. (1982). Gonorrhea modeling: A comparison of control methods. *Math. Biosci.*, 58, 93-109.

Hethcote, H.W. and J.A. Yorke. (1984). *Gonorrhea Transmission Dynamics and Control.* Lecture Notes in Biomath., No. 56, Springer-Verlag, Berlin.

Hyman, J.M. and E.A. Stanley. (1988). Using mathematical models to understand the AIDS epidemic. *Math. Biosci.*, 90, 415-474.

Hyman, J.M. and E.A. Stanley. (1989). The effect of social mixing patterns on the spread of AIDS. *Proc. Math. Appr. to Environmental and Ecological Problems.*, Springer-Verlag, (to appear)

Jacquez, J.A., C.P. Simon, J. Koopman, L. Sattenspiel and T. Perry. (1988). Modeling and analyzing HIV transmission: The effect of contact patterns. *Math. Biosci.*, 92, 119-199.

Kermack, W.O. and A.G. McKendrick. (1927). A contribution to the mathematical theory of epidemics. *Proc. Roy. Soc. London A*, 115, 700-721.

Knox, E.G. (1986). A transmission model for AIDS. *Eur. J. Epidem.*, 2, 165-177.

Koopman, J., C.P. Simon, J. Jacquez, J. Joseph, L. Sattenspiel and T. Park. (1988). Sexual partner selectiveness effects on homosexual HIV transmission dynamics. *J. AIDS*, 1, 486-504.

Koopman, J., C.P. Simon, J.A. Jacquez, T.S. Park. (1989). Selective contact within structured mixing groups; With an application to the analysis of HIV transmission risk from oral and anal sex. This volume.

Longini, I.M.Jr., E. Ackerman and L.R. Elveback. (1978). An optimization model for influenza A epidemics. *Math. Biosci.*, 38, 141-157.

May, R.M. and R.M. Anderson. (1984). Spatial heterogeneity and the design of immunization programs. *Math. Biosci.*, 72, 83-111.

May, R.M. and R.M. Anderson. (1987). Transmission dynamics of HIV infection. *Nature*, 326, 137-142.

May, R.M., R.M. Anderson and A.R. McLean. (1988). Possible demographic consequences of HIV/AIDS epidemics. I. Assuming HIV infection always leads to AIDS. *Math. Biosci.*, 90, 475-505.

Mode, C.J., H.E. Gollwitzer and N. Herrmann. (1988). A methodological study of a stochastic model of an AIDS epidemic. *Math. Biosci.*, 92, 201-229.

Nold, A. (1980). Heterogeneity in disease transmission modeling. *Math. Biosci.*, 52, 227-240.

Pickering, J., J.A. Wiley, N.S. Padian, L.E. Lieb, D.G. Echenberg and J. Walker. (1986). Modeling the incidence of acquired immunodeficiency syndrome (AIDS) in San Francisco, Los Angeles and New York. *Math. Modeling*, 7, 661-688.

Post, W.M., D.L. DeAngelis and C.C. Travis. (1983). Endemic disease in environments with spatially heterogeneous host populations. *Math. Biosci.* 63, 289-302.

Ross, R. (1911). *The Prevention of Malaria*, 2nd ed., John Murray, London.

Rushton, S. and A.J. Mautner. (1955). The deterministic model of a simple epidemic for more than one community. *Biometrika*, 42, 126-132.

Rvachev, L.A. and I.M. Longini,Jr. (1985). A mathematical model for the global spread of influenza. *Math. Biosci.*, 75, 3-22.

Sattenspiel, L. (1987). Population structure and the spread of disease. *Human Biol.*, 59, 411-438.

Sattenspiel, L. and C.P. Simon. (1988). The spread and persistence of infectious diseases in structured populations. *Math. Biosci.*, 90, 341-366.

Serfling, R.E. (1952). Historical review of epidemic theory. *Human Biol.*, 24, 145-166.

Soper, H.E. (1929). The interpretation of periodicity in disease prevalence. *J. Roy. Stat. Soc.*, 92, 34-73.

Taylor, I. and J. Knowelden. (1964). *Principles of Epidemiology.* Little, Brown & Co., Boston.

Travis, C.C. and S.M. Lenhart. (1987). Eradication of infectious diseases in heterogeneous populations. *Math. Biosci.*, 83, 191-198.

Watson, R.K. (1972). On an epidemic in a stratified population. *J. Appl. Prob.*, 9, 659-666.

SELECTIVE CONTACT WITHIN STRUCTURED MIXING WITH AN APPLICATION TO HIV TRANSMISSION RISK FROM ORAL AND ANAL SEX

James S. Koopman
Department of Epidemiology
Univ. of Michigan
Ann Arbor MI 48109

Carl P. Simon
Depts. of Math., Econ. & Pub. Pol.
Univ. of Michigan
Ann Arbor MI 48109

John A. Jacquez
Depts. of Physiol. & Biostatistics
Univ. of Michigan
Ann Arbor MI 48109

Tae Sung Park
Department of Biostatistics
Univ. of Michigan
Ann Arbor MI 48109

Abstract

This paper presents a mathematical model of heterogeneous mixing which is designed to explore the effects of partner selection on the transmission patterns of sexually transmitted diseases. The model generates a symmetric matrix of the rate of sexual contacts between individuals categorized into discrete population subgroups. Sexual pairing results from a process with three separate stages: 1) social contact, 2) acceptance as a potential sex partner, and 3) initiation of sex in response to the needs and standards of each partner. This model can define the contact pattern within any single activity group of the structured mixing model presented by Jacquez et al (1989) in this volume. In such a formulation, the rate of new sexual partnership formation is determined by the number of available partners as well as by sexual needs and moral standards and can vary throughout the course of an epidemic. This approach provides a framework for exploring the potential consequences on infectious disease transmission of different sociological factors while at the same time providing a framework for testing specific sociological theory. We present an example of an epidemic in a male homosexual population where all sexual partnerships are short term. The parameters relating the acceptance of one group by another as potential sexual partners vary by the relative sexual activity rates of individuals and by their relative preference for oral or anal sex. Per sex act transmission probabilities for anal sex were made four times as high as oral sex. Proportional mixing results in a corresponding fourfold difference in risks of oral and anal sex. A moderate degree of selective mixing, however, generates a thirty two fold difference in the risk of oral and anal sex during the stage of the epidemic corresponding to that in which epidemiologic studies have been used to assess the relative risks of oral and anal sex.

1. Introduction

a. Why Models of Heterogeneous Mixing are Necessary

A fundamental problem that has yet to be addressed in epidemiology is what determines the pattern of flow of an infection through different social, geographic, and exposure population subgroups. AIDS has created an urgent need to address this question. This question is quite different from the questions addressed by previous mathematical models of AIDS. Key determinants in previous models have been the natural history of infection and contagiousness and variations in exposure rates. The key determinants of flow patterns, however, are likely to be contact patterns. We present here a flexible and meaningful model of contact patterns where the number of contacts that one population subgroup has with a second corresponds to the number of contacts the second has with the first.

Even when the focus of inquiry is the predicted total size and shape of an epidemic rather than the flow pattern of infection, consideration of contact patterns can be crucial. For HIV transmission, contact patterns are obviously far from random. In recent analyses and simulations of HIV transmission among homosexuals, we have shown that populations with identical distributions of individuals by frequency of sex and sex partners could experience markedly different total epidemics depending on the pattern of contacts between individuals (Jacquez et al. 1988; Koopman et al. 1988). Models with heterogeneity of risk factors but random or proportionate mixing would miss this important determinant of epidemic size and shape.

But there are even more important reasons for analyzing contact patterns. If we are to predict the path that an infection is going to take as it spreads through a population, we must describe and analyze who has infection transmitting contact with whom. Such an analysis should help us focus our intervention efforts on the population subgroups where our efforts are going to have the greatest effect in cutting off new chains of transmission before they branch out into ever multiplying ramifications. Without such an analysis, we might waste our efforts in seeking to stop either unlikely transmissions or unimportant transmissions where blocking one source of infection is like trying to patch up a hole in a dam when the flood waters have broken through elsewhere. Whereas contact heterogeneity may be viewed as an inconvenient complication of models examining the total size and shape of an AIDS epidemic, it is the essential determinant that determines how infection might flow from one population subgroup or one geographic area to another.

b. Models of Heterogeneous Contact and the Estimation of Risk Factor Effects:

Another reason for describing contact patterns relates to the estimation of risk factor effects. It is most difficult to get information on the infection status of sex partners of a study subject at the time the study subject had sex with them. As a result, all studies examining the risk of oral or anal sex present parameters which disregard the probability that one's partners are infected (Moss et al. 1987; Goedert et al. 1984; Goedert et al. 1985; Melbye et al. 1984; Jeffries et al. 1985; Winkelstein et al. 1987; Kingsley et al. 1987; Goedart et al. 1987; Chmiel et al. 1987; Polk et al. 1986; Darrow et al. 1987; Stevens et al. 1986, Nicholson et al. 1985; Lyman et al. 1986; Schechter et al. 1986). We will illustrate one particular importance of heterogeneous contact formulations by showing how psychosocial factors could create patterns of infection in a population which would markedly distort risk assessment which ignores such factors. Most analyses of the risks of oral and anal sex have used standard multivariate techniques. These techniques distort risk assessment in four ways: 1) relationships between risks of different types of sex acts may not reflect the relationships between risks of these sex acts with infected individuals because the partners with whom different sex acts are performed might have different probabilities of infection, 2) standard multivariate analyses assume that outcome in one study subject is independent of outcome in other study subjects even though this is clearly untrue where infection in some individuals increases the risk of transmission to others, 3) relative risks of different sex acts do not provide adequate comparisons between absolute risks of different sex acts because the relative risks compare individuals with a behavior to those without it and the denominators, the risks in those without the behavior, are incomparable, 4) risk estimates in standard analyses fail to distinguish sex acts with single partners from sex acts with multiple partners even though, theoretically, each individual sex act should contribute less to the total risk when all sex acts are with the same partner as compared to the situation where most sex acts are with different partners.

The illustration of the effects of heterogeneous contact patterns in this paper will concentrate wholly on the first type of distortion which derives from not considering the probability that the sexual partners of a study subject might be infected. It is heterogeneous mixing that creates different probabilities of partners being infected. With random mixing everyone would be drawing partners from the same pool and therefore everyone's partners would have the same probability of being infected. We will show that the probability that an anal or oral sex partner is infected can vary markedly. This variability will distort risk assessments for oral and anal sex that do not take the likelihood that a partner will be infected into account.

c. Overcoming the Deficiencies of Previous Models of Heterogeneous Mixing:

The models we used to show the importance of contact patterns on the total epidemic used a formulation called "preferred" mixing to create heterogeneous or non-random mixing patterns (Jacquez et al. 1988; Koopman et al. 1988). However, preferred mixing, like a related formulation suggested by Hethcote and Van Ark (1987), has difficulty creating balanced preferences for groups other than one's own and thus cannot provide the basis for a comprehensive theory of contact patterns. Moreover, the basic parameters of preferred mixing are not derived from any theory of human behavior and would be difficult to estimate from data. Because of these limitations, we have devised two formulations of heterogeneous mixing that operate at two levels and that are more comprehensive and more theoretically meaningful than preferred mixing. These two formulations correspond to the two major forces generating heterogeneous mixing: namely, 1) the social or geographical settings where one meets partners, and 2) the psychosocial factors leading to sexual partnership formation between individuals who meet in different social settings. A companion article (Jacquez et al. 1989) presents a model formulation capturing the first source of heterogeneous mixing, a formulation we call *structured mixing*. The major purpose of this article is to present a model which corresponds to the psychosocial factors leading to sexual partnership formation. We call this a *selective mixing* model.

In presenting this selective mixing model, we are not advocating any sociological theory related to the specific mathematical formulation of the model. Nor do we pretend to present sociologically correct theory. What we do is present a framework for the formulation of symmetric contact matrices which increases our ability to examine the consequences of contact patterns on transmission dynamics. For factors which we show to be epidemiologically important, we would hope that sociologists will proceed to test and alter specific sociological theory. Since both the inputs and the outputs of our structured and selective mixing models should be sociologically observable, such testing might be fairly straight forward. As much as possible, we try to point out alternative formulations that might be explored with sociological science.

2. Selective Mixing Model Formulation:

a. A Structured Mixing Framework within which Selective Mixing Can Act:

Heterogeneous contact formulations are reviewed in an article accompanying this one (Jacquez et al. 1989). That paper presents a formulation in which heterogeneous contact between individuals with different characteristics can be determined by differential involvement of individuals in different activity groups. That formulation, called *structured mixing*, assumes that individuals are categorized into one of a number of distinct *population subgroups* on the basis of some set of characteristics of interest. Those characteristics might be race, age, gender, levels of sexual drive, degrees of acceptance of promiscuous behavior, sexual orientation, sexual act preferences, or any number of other factors. All individuals within a population subgroup are assumed to have comparable risk behaviors and comparable determinants of partner selectiveness. The social contacts made by each member of a population subgroup are apportioned into a number of distinct *activity groups*. All members of a specific population subgroup are assumed to have comparable distributions of their contacts into different activity groups.

Activity groups should be defined in terms of the mixing processes occurring in a population. For example, one criteria could be the locations or social groups where potential sexual partners might be met. Then the contacts made by members of each population subgroup can be apportioned into the different activity groups in different ways. The apportionment might be on the basis of the actual number of sexual partners encountered in different settings in the past. It might be on the basis of social contacts where one felt some sexual attraction. Or it might be on the basis of all types of social contact. The structured mixing formulation then constructs an overall *contact matrix* $\mathbf{C}=((C_{ij}))$ between population subgroups where the elements C_{ij} are the rate of new sexual partnerships per unit time between individuals in population subgroups i and j. It does this by summing across the contact matrices $\mathbf{C}(k)$ of each activity group where $C(k)_{ij}$ is the number of new sexual partnerships per unit time between individuals in population subgroups i and j that occur within the k'th activity group. The differential involvement by members of different population subgroups in different activity groups is then able to generate heterogeneous contact matrices even when there is random contact within each activity group.

Note that the contact matrix, $\mathbf{C}=((C_{ij}))$, of new sexual partnership formation rates, together with a matrices describing the type of frequency of sex acts in partnerships between different subgroups, describes sexual contact patterns.

This structured mixing formulation can use any within-activity-group contact formulation that meets the consistency requirement of sexual contact, namely that any one group have the same number of insertive contacts with a second group as the second has receptive contacts with the first. Since we will not be distinguishing insertive and receptive contacts in this presentation, this requirement implies that each **C**(k) will be a symmetric matrix.

We will present here a within-activity-group contact formulation that takes into account the factors determining selectiveness of contacts within a chosen activity group. The formulation to be presented here will be called *selective mixing* and can be used within the structured mixing formulation presented in the companion paper. For simplicity of notation, an example with only one activity group will be examined.

b. A Theoretical Framework for Selective Mixing:

The framework we present here is intended to achieve a flexible formulation of symmetric within-activity-group contact matrices in a manner corresponding to sociological factors which we see as potentially important determinants of sexually transmitted disease transmission patterns. As a starting point for the formulation of selective mixing, we divide the process of partner formation into three stages once a member of a population subgroup is within an activity group. These are: 1) the initial visual or conversational encounter or "social contact", 2) the recognition that someone encountered in a social context is an acceptable sex partner, and 3) the decision to have sex with that partner.

There are various ways to expand or collapse these stages and to alter the specific formulations we present for each stage. We will point out some of these but will not attempt to be comprehensive.

c. The Social Contact Stage of Selectivity:

Let h_i denote the number of social contacts per person in population subgroup "i" (in activity group "k"). In general, h_i will depend on the "expansiveness" or extroversion of persons in group i and on their relative attractiveness. If N_i is the number of persons from population subgroup i (in activity group k), then $N_i h_i$ is the number of social contacts by persons in group i. To compute the number of social encounters between members of group i and group j, note that $N_j h_j \div (\Sigma_m N_m h_m)$ is the fraction of the total number of social contacts that are initiated by persons in group j. We begin by assuming that social contact is always mutual, that the rate at which social contact is made is not dependent upon the number of people in an activity group, and that mixing is proportional to $N_i h_i$. Under the proportional mixing hypothesis, the total number of social contacts with persons in group j by a typical person in group i is $h_i N_j h_j / (\Sigma_m N_m h_m)$; and the total number of social contacts between all persons in population subgroup i and population subgroup j (in activity group k) is

$$A_{ij} = \frac{N_i N_j h_i h_j}{\Sigma_m N_m h_m} . \qquad [1]$$

Alternative formulations might have created a dependence between the number of social contacts made and the number of individuals encountered in a social setting. Functions with a shape similar to that seen in figure one presented when we talk about the third stage, could have been used. For convenience, we leave the incorporation of any such dependence until the third stage.

d. The Mutual Acceptability Stage of Selectivity:

Not all social contacts will be between individuals who might find each other satisfactory sex partners. If both groups i and j, for example, are strictly heterosexual males, none of the contacts between them would be mutually acceptable for sex. We denote by q_{ij} the fraction of group j individuals encountered that a person in group i finds acceptable for sex. If group i finds only a fraction of group j acceptable as sex partners and vice versa, then, under the assumption of random mixing between structural subgroups i and j (as usual in activity group k), the fraction of social contacts that are *mutually* acceptable for sex is $q_{ij} q_{ji}$. If we denote by B_{ij} the rate of making social contacts between groups i and j which are mutually acceptable for sex, then

$$B_{ij} = \frac{N_i N_j h_i h_j q_{ij} q_{ji}}{\Sigma_m N_m h_m} . \qquad [2]$$

The total rate at which an individual in group i makes mutually acceptable encounters given a particular q_{ij} matrix is

$$B_i = \frac{\Sigma_j B_{ij}}{N_i} = \frac{h_i \Sigma_j (N_j h_j q_{ij} q_{ji})}{\Sigma_m N_m h_m} . \qquad [3]$$

Note that if there is more than one activity group, B_i would have to be summed across all activity groups. Only for the sake of simplicity are we assuming a single activity group.

Instead of separating stages one and two, we could have combined them by making a single parameter equivalent to $h_i q_{ij}$. This parameter is equivalent to the rate at which individuals in population subgroup i make social contact with individuals in population subgroup j that they judge to be potentially acceptable sex partners. When population subgroup characteristics are obvious, such as race, these parameters might be estimated in studies which ask individuals to assess these rates. The decision that someone is an acceptable sexual partner, however, might not be determinable on the basis of superficial social contact. Indeed when individuals engage in any assessment of the HIV status of partners in order to determine their acceptability, there is a clear separation of the social contact stage and the determination of acceptability stage. Since one of the uses to which we intend to put this model in the future is the evaluation of the effects of counseling and testing programs, where indeed acceptability might be a function of test results, we will keep stages one and two separate.

Note also that we have made the q_{ij} independent of the total number of potentially acceptable individuals encountered. In fact the availability of sexual partnerships might affect how choosy one is and therefore alter the relationships of q_{ij} between different population subgroups. If this were the case, increasing numbers of social contacts might increase partner selectiveness along attractiveness scales. Since we do not anticipate evaluating the effects of numbers of social contacts, and since we do not anticipate important fluctuations in the total number of social contacts in the simulations we might undertake, we will disregard for now any effect of the availability of sexual partnerships on one's pattern of selectiveness with regards to population subgroups.

e. The Proportion of Mutually Acceptable Encounters Resulting in Sex:

Not all encounters which are mutually acceptable for sex will result in sexual partnerships. The actual decision about whether to form a sexual partnership will depend, among other things, on the individual's sexual drive, on the constraints which morals or fear of sexually transmitted diseases place on behavior, and on current partnership status. We will consider the first two of these factors here and will delay considering the dependence on current partnership status until section 2j.

Let c_i represent the rate of new partnership formation at which population subgroup i members have a satisfactory balance between their sexual drives and their internalized moral standards when there are no limits on the number of acceptable contacts and no extraordinary pressures by contacts to have sex. Thus c_i may be interpreted as an asymptotic level for members of group i when partners of desired types are readily available. In our previous models (Jacquez et al. 1988; Koopman et al. 1988), c_i represented the actual rate of new sexual partnership formation, a rate which we assumed to be fixed. This fixed characteristic of the actual rate of new sexual partnership formation could lead to some unrealistic situations where high rates of new partnership formation were maintained within quite small populations. The new parameter c_i presented here represents the new sexual partnership formation rate *goals* of individuals in group i rather than their actual new partnership formation rate. The actual rate will be lower when the desired partners are not freely available. It will result in a higher actual rate when group i members are sought after by a large number of individuals who are acceptable sexual partners to group i. We formulate a new parameter, w_{ij}, the proportion of mutually acceptable contacts between members of groups i and j that actually result in sex in a way that corresponds to these influences.

The proportion of mutually acceptable contacts that result in sex, w_{ij}, should increase as c_i or c_j increase. It should also increase as the number of potential partners increases, but only to a point. Once some saturation level of sexual partnership formation has been achieved, the needs of group i or j individuals should drive it no higher. If one of the groups, say "j", has no other source of partners than the other group "i", then the needs of group "j" might drive the actual rate of partnership by group "i" above their ideal level of c_i. We present in [4] one equation among a large number of possible ones that manifests these relationships:

$$w_{ij} = \sqrt{\frac{c_i c_j}{(K_i + \lambda_i B_i)(K_j + \lambda_j B_j)}}\,, \qquad [4]$$

where K_i and λ_i are shape parameters. The value of K_i must be equal to or greater than c_i to insure that w_{ij} will always be a proportion.

To motivate this choice, let us first consider a situation where the B_j for all $j \neq i$ are large. For this special situation, let us denote the actual proportion of mutually acceptable encounters that group i makes which result in sexual partnerships as Ω_i. Now this will not depend upon the desires or needs of any group other than "i". The actual rate of new sexual partnership formation for group "i" members will be $B_i\Omega_i$. When B_i is small, it would seem natural that $B_i\Omega_i$ would be proportional to B_i. When B_i is large, $B_i\Omega_i$ should equal c_i. A simple mathematical realization of such a function is $\Omega_i = \frac{c_i}{K_i + B_i}$, where K_i is a shape parameters with $K_i \geq c_i$. The ratio of $\frac{c_i}{K_i}$ represents the proportion of mutually acceptable encounters that will result in a sexual partnership when B_i is small. In the absence of sociological theory to define Ω_i, we set $K_i = c_i$. One can generalize the above with another parameter, λ_i, as in [4]. The graph of $B_i\Omega_i = \frac{c_i B_i}{K_i + \lambda_i B_i}$ versus B_i is presented in figure 1 and illustrates that this function has the desired properties.

There are alternative ways that w_{ij} might be determined as a function of Ω_i and Ω_j. Equation [4], which is what we have chosen, represents a geometric mean. This has the

Figure 1
Relationships between the rate of social contacts with individuals mutually acceptable for sex B(i), and the rate of new sexual partnership formation given that all B(j) are large and c(i) = 5

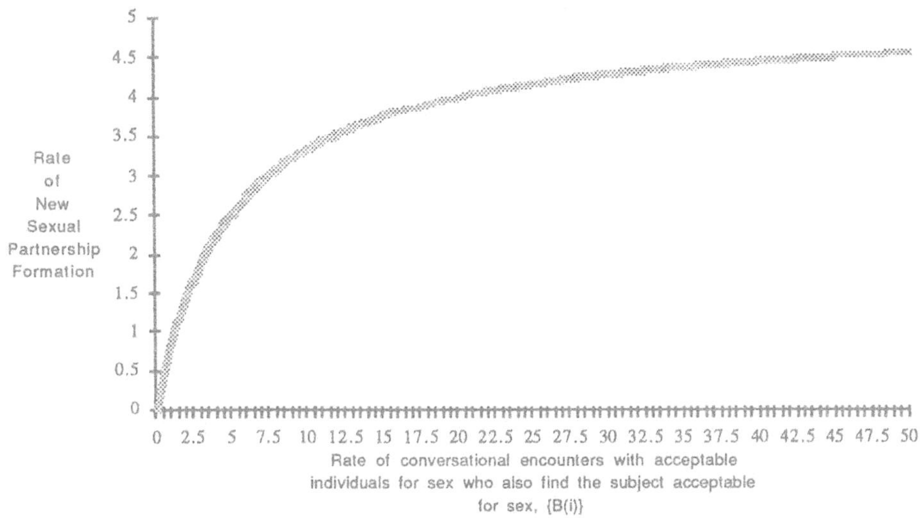

required symmetry properties. It also has the asymptotic property that w_{ij} tends to 0 as either Ω_i or Ω_j tends to 0. The arithmetic mean, however, would appear to be equally acceptable since the number of contacts between two groups will always be a multiplicative function of the total number of partnerships made by a group. This means that w_{ij} would not necessarily have to tend to zero as Ω_i or Ω_j tend to zero. The arithmetic mean moreover makes it easier to calculate a set of c_i parameters to correspond to a set of observed new partnership formation rates. One referee suggested that we treat Ω_i as a probability and define $w_{ij}\frac{\Omega_i\Omega_j}{1-(1-\Omega_i)(1-\Omega_j)}$. With our geometric mean formulation of w_{ij}, the graph of the actual rate of new partnership formation versus B_i is very similar to Figure 1 with the difference that the shape of the curve and the level of the asymptote reached will be dependent upon values of B_j where $j \neq i$.

f. The Formula for Selective Mixing:

Finally, we pull all this together to obtain the formula for C_{ij}, the elements of the contact matrix, which are the number of new sexual partnerships (per unit time) between individuals in population subgroups i and j:

$$C_{ij} = B_{ij}\, w_{ij} = \frac{N_i N_j h_i h_j q_{ij} q_{ji} w_{ij}}{\Sigma_m N_m h_m} . \qquad [5]$$

This C_{ij} has the same meaning as in our companion paper (Jacquez et al. 1989), except that we have been working with only one activity group. For complete correspondence with the notation in (Jacquez et al. 1989), we should designate [5] as $C(k)_{ij}$, where k refers to the activity group. Note that the symmetry requirement is met as $C(k)_{ij} = C(k)_{ji}$.

In our previously published models (Jacquez et al. 1988; Koopman et al. 1988) of HIV transmission in heterogeneous populations, we used ρ_{ij} matrices to summarize the contact patterns in the population, where ρ_{ij} represented the proportion of group i's contacts that were with members of group j. The C_{ij} matrix presented above is related to these ρ_{ij} matrices by

$$\rho_{ij} = \frac{C_{ij}}{\Sigma_m C_{im}} . \qquad [6]$$

g. Selective Mixing without Constraints on Desired Partnership Rates:

In many situations, B_i and B_j could be large enough so that $w_{ij} \approx \sqrt{\frac{c_i c_j}{B_i B_j}}$. In this case, the selective mixing formulation yields the following formula for C_{ij}:

$$C_{ij} = \frac{N_i N_j q_{ij} q_{ji} \sqrt{c_i c_j h_i h_j}}{\sqrt{(\Sigma_k N_k h_k q_{ik} q_{ki})(\Sigma_k N_k h_k q_{jk} q_{kj})}} . \qquad [7]$$

Note that, as long as the B_i's are reasonably large, if we proportionately increase the N_i or c_i values in *all* the population subgroups, the C_{ij} values are proportionately increased. If we proportionately increase all the h_i or q_{ij} values, there is no change in the C_{ij} matrix, again as long as the B_i's are reasonably large.

h. Comparison to Proportionate Mixing:

Selective mixing is more flexible than proportionate mixing as it permits selective forces rather than just random forces to act. Even when there are no selective factors acting in selective mixing, however, there are differences between selective and proportionate mixing. For example, under selective mixing, the actual rate of sexual partnership can change in response to the number of potential partners in the environment. In proportionate mixing, the actual rate of new partnership formation is usually fixed.

For a simple comparison between selective and proportionate mixing, assume that all B_i are large enough so that $w_{ij} \approx \sqrt{\frac{c_i c_j}{B_i B_j}}$. To consider a selective mixing model with no selective factors acting, assume that $q_{ij} = q_{ji} = 1$ so that all social contacts are potential sexual partners and therefore by [3], $B_i = h_i$. Under these assumptions, where no selective factor is acting, the selective mixing formulation [5] becomes:

$$C_{ij} = \frac{N_i N_j \sqrt{c_i h_i c_j h_j}}{\Sigma_m N_m h_m}, \qquad [8]$$

while the proportional mixing formulation is

$$C_{ij} = \frac{N_i N_j c_i c_j}{\Sigma_m c_m N_m}. \qquad [9]$$

The way some third group "g" can affect the rate of pairing between groups "i" and "j" is different under selective mixing even with no selective factor acting and under proportional mixing. Under proportional mixing, if some third group raises its sexual partnership need level, c_g, the number of partnerships between groups "i" and "j" decreases even though the number of direct encounters between groups "i" and "j" and their sexual partnership needs should not be changed by this change in a third group's sexual partnership needs. Under selective mixing, a change in the need level c_g of a third group has no effect on the rate of pairing between groups "i" and "j". If, however, a third group raises its social contact level, the number of social contacts between groups "i" and "j" will decrease under selective mixing. If a third group raised its social contacts in proportion to its sexual partnership needs, there would be no difference between the effects of third groups in selective mixing with no selective factors acting and proportional mixing. Such a proportional increase, however, seems to be improbable when the number of mutually acceptable encounters B_g of the third group is large. Most likely, the new needs would be met within the existing B_g merely by raising the w_{ij}. Remember that a large B_g means that one is on the flat asymptote of Figure 1.

When c_g is large relative to B_g, then there may be motivation for a group to increase its social contact rate because its sexual partnership needs are not being met. We discussed in section 2)c that alternative formulations might be considered to account for this. For now, however, we will not consider situations where c_g is large relative to B_g.

In other ways, both proportional mixing and selective mixing with no selective factor acting behave similarly. In either case, as the number of individuals N_g in a third group "g" increases, the number of partnerships between "i" and "j" groups will decrease. This is logical since the number of social contacts should be decreased because "i" and "j" are smaller proportions of the pool in which social contacts are made.

i. Comparison to a Mass Action Formulation by Gail:

A heterogeneous mixing formulation presented by Gail et al. (1989) provided some of the inspiration for selective mixing. Gail's formulation of heterogeneous mixing makes an analogy to the mixing of gases in an enclosed space. His attractiveness parameter corresponds to our $h_i h_j$ parameter. Gail introduces heterogeneity that deviates from proportionate mixing into his model by assuming that attractiveness parameters are structurally defined for some "ij" pairings. Thus his attractiveness parameters also take on the role of our q_{ij} parameters. For example, all strictly heterosexual male groups "i" have zero attractiveness terms with all other male groups "j". All other attractiveness terms are then calculated to maximize randomness (minimize information) under the constraint of symmetric contact matrices. Gail makes no provision for a w_{ij}-like term; consequently, as the number of individuals in a population is increased, the number of sexual contacts each individual makes is proportionately increased. This is not a realistic situation. If all population subgroups change only minimally in size, this would not be a major source of error in a model of a real sexual contact system. But in the course of an AIDS epidemic, there can be rather considerable changes in the sizes of some population subgroups. Moreover, in Gail's formulation, the role of changes in third group behavior on pairing rates between two other groups is similar to that of proportionate mixing.

By defining the determinants of social contacts and encounters mutually acceptable for sexual partnership separately, we hope to clarify the meaning of the separate terms presented in Gail's formulation and make clear the need for a term which represents the proportion of encounters mutually acceptable for sexual partnership which will actually result in sexual partnership. The introduction of this term further specifies how changes in third groups will affect pairing rates between two other groups.

j. Using Selective Mixing in Long Term Partnership or Paired Mixing Models:

If we are dealing with a situation where no long-term partnerships are made (such as in the homosexual casual and anonymous sex scene), little is lost by assuming that the duration of all partnerships is equal. In the opposite situation of long-term partnerships, we see two approaches. In a first approach, one could adjust the c_i's so that the actual rates of new partnership formation correspond to the inverse of the average duration of partnerships between population subgroups "i" and "j". This is similar to what we have done previously with our preferred mixing formulation (Koopman et al. 1988). In this more realistic model, however, the shape parameters for w_{ij} will affect how the actual rates of new sexual partnership formation relate to the c_i's.

In a second approach, one could use a pairing model in the style of those presented by Dietz (1988) and Dietz and Hadeler (1988). In pairing models, one has the same problems in relating observed pairing rates to c_i's. But the combination of structured and selective mixing would add a great deal of flexibility to the pairing models. In a paired state space model in the style of Dietz, where selective (and perhaps also structured) mixing is acting, the c_i's could be formulated as a function of pairing status (c_{ip}) where a very low value would be assigned to paired individuals and a much higher value to unpaired individuals. This would take care of the dependence of c_i mentioned in the first paragraph of section 2e. Of course, one would want to make some reasonable assumptions about the effect of pairing on c_i in order to reduce the total number of parameters. Similarly, the h_i and q_{ij} values could be made functions of pairing status (h_{ip} and q_{ijp}); and N_{ip} would correspond to the number of individuals in population subgroup i which are in each pairing status. Appropriate sociological theory about the determinants of h_{ip} and q_{ijp} could reduce the total number of model parameters needed. With this pairing formulation, paired individuals could have different levels and different types of infidelity corresponding to h_{ip} and q_{ijp} value patterns.

k. Efficient use of Structured and Selective Mixing Formulations:

There is some redundancy in the f_{ik} parameter of structured mixing (the proportion of population subgroup i's contacts which are made in activity group k) and the h_i, w_{ij}, and q_{ij} parameters of selective mixing. Careful modeling should use this redundancy to minimize the total number of parameters.

In a detailed model of the sexual pairing process, the f_{ik} parameter presented in the companion paper might be the proportion of time group i members spend in activity group k. Then the h_i parameters will be needed to reflect different intensities of social contact in different activity groups, the q_{ij} parameters will be needed to reflect the different average acceptabilities for sexual partnership of individuals going to different activity groups, and the w_{ij} parameters would be needed to reflect the proportion of acceptable contacts that would actually result in sex.

In a simpler model of the sexual pairing process, we might make f_{ik} equal to the proportion of sexual partnerships that are made in different activity groups. Then there would be no need for h_i or w_{ij} type parameters. In this case, q_{ij} parameters could be limited to values of one or zero corresponding to those population subgroups that can have contact (e.g. male bisexuals with female heterosexuals) and those that cannot have contact (e.g. strictly heterosexual male groups with other male groups). To use this type of data to make projections, however, one would have to assume that changes in w_{ij} over the course of the epidemic would not be significant. This is equivalent to assuming that changes in B_i will not have a marked effect on w_{ij}. Certainly when one considers what has happened in the homosexual community, the decreasing c_i of a majority of the homosexual population, together with the closing of bathhouses, has probably decreased the B_i of individuals who did change their c_i. Even in individuals who have had no decrease in their c_i, the decreasing c_j of other groups will decrease the actual contact rate, w_i. Thus it may not always be wise to simplify by disregarding w_{ij} type parameters.

An intermediate approach might be to define the f_{ik} on the basis of the site where acceptable partners are encountered. How one decided to define acceptable partners would have a big influence on the results. One could ask about all the settings and individuals where one actually felt some sexual desire for other individuals in order to define the f_{ik}. One could ask about situations where there was some response in the individual encountered that also indicated some degree of sexual attraction. Or one could ask about situations where any individuals in the broad gender, age, sexual orientation, or race categories which a subject finds acceptable are encountered. In this case there is certainly redundancy between the $q_{ij}q_{ji}$ and the w_{ij} parameters so that the w_{ij} value will depend upon how q_{ij} are defined.

Jacquez et al. (1989) have shown how only a few parameters might be used in the structured mixing formulation to define fairly intricate heterogeneous mixing. Thus one of these simpler strategies might markedly reduce the total number of parameters needed to describe heterogeneous mixing when a selective mixing formulation is needed.

3. Model Simulation in a Male Homosexual Population

a. Oral and Anal Sex Contact Patterns in a Male Homosexual Population:

Within a male homosexual population, different types of population subgroups might be defined so that insertive and/or receptive oral and/or anal sex would be practiced by different population subgroups in different proportions and at different rates depending on the population subgroup membership of their contacts. For the sake of simplicity in our illustration, we make some simplifying assumptions. First we assume that we are dealing only with transient relationships so that each new sexual partnership consists of one sexual encounter. Second, we disregard insertive and receptive distinctions and assume all sexual encounters are mutually insertive and receptive. Third, we assume that all sex can be divided into oral and anal. Fourth, we use only two dimensions to divide our simulation population into population subgroups. One dimension will be determined by c_i and h_i values which we will make perfectly correlated. There will be three categories along this dimension. A second dimension will be determined by the proportion of sexual encounters that members of a population subgroup would prefer to be anal. We label this proportion P_i. Again there will be three categories along this dimension so that in total there will be nine population subgroups. We define the preferred proportion of anal sex, P_i, in population subgroup i as the proportion of sexual encounters that would involve anal sex when members of population subgroup i have sex with other members of their same population subgroup. Since we assume only two types of sex, the preferred proportion of oral sex would be $1-P_i$. When members of one population subgroup have sex with members of another population subgroup having a different preferred proportion of anal sex, we assume that the actual proportion of anal sex will be half way between the preferences of the two groups. The proportion R_i of all sexual encounters of group i members that will be anal is given by

$$R_i = \frac{\sum_{j=1}^{9} C_{ij}(P_i + P_j)/2}{\sum_{j=1}^{9} C_{ij}} \qquad [10]$$

Table 1

Initial simulation conditions consistent with observations in the "Coping and Change Study"

		POPULATION SUBGROUPS								
		Prefer all oral sex			Prefer all anal sex			Prefer 20% anal sex		
		1	2	3	4	5	6	7	8	9
Preferred proportion of anal sex.	P_i	0	0	0	100%	100%	100%	20%	20%	20%
Hundred thousands of individuals	N_i	49	67	82	23	32	38	80	90	64
Ideal sex partner rate per month	c_i	15	4.3	1.4	15	4.3	1.4	15	4.3	1.4
Total social contacts per month	h_i	3000	2700	2400	3000	2700	2400	3000	2700	2400

In Table 1 we present a distribution of individuals into nine groups with different N_i, c_i, and preferred sex type frequencies that approximate the observed frequencies of partners and oral and anal sex practices seen in individuals under study in the Chicago Coping and Change Study (CCS) cohort (Joseph et al. 1987). Note that this is a very rough approximation for several reasons:

1) we have disregarded differences that may exist between insertive and receptive behaviors because we only have information on receptive behaviors;
2) we have disregarded information on the frequency of other types of sex besides oral and anal;
3) we have to make estimates of new partnership formation rates from information on the number of different partners per month.

We have no information in our data pertinent to the h_i or q_{ij} values; so the values of h_i included in Table 1 and q_{ij} in Table 2 are purely hypothetical. The patterns of h_i in Table 1 correspond to a slight increase in social contact rate as desired sexual partnership levels c_i increase.

Table 2

The proportion of the column population subgroups which the row population subgroups find acceptable for sex (q_{ij}).

	POPULATION SUBGROUPS								
	Prefer all oral sex			Prefer all anal sex			Prefer 20% anal sex		
	1	2	3	4	5	6	7	8	9
1	0.78	0.86	0.90	0	0	0	0.39	0.43	0.45
2	0.58	0.70	0.86	0	0	0	0.29	0.35	0.43
3	0.48	0.58	0.78	0	0	0	0.24	0.29	0.39
4	0	0	0	0.78	0.86	0.90	0.195	0.215	0.225
5	0	0	0	0.58	0.70	0.86	0.145	0.175	0.215
6	0	0	0	0.48	0.58	0.78	0.12	0.145	0.195
7	0.39	0.43	0.45	0.195	0.215	0.225	0.78	0.86	0.90
8	0.29	0.35	0.43	0.145	0.175	0.215	0.58	0.70	0.86
9	0.24	0.29	0.39	0.12	0.145	0.195	0.48	0.58	0.78

Table 2 presents the q_{ij} values that we use for this simulation. These values exclude direct contact between the groups that would want all oral and all anal sex. There is considerable overlap, however, with the group that has a mixed preference. To set up the pattern of q_{ij} values in Table 2, we assumed that partners with lower partnership formation rates would be more acceptable to other individuals. We also assumed that groups with a 20% anal sex preference would find members of the pure oral preference group half as acceptable as other individuals with a 20% anal preference; similarly they would find those with a pure anal preference only one fourth as acceptable. For the sake of simplicity, we assume that the acceptances of the pure anal and oral sex groups for the 20% anal sex groups were equal to the symmetric acceptances by the 20% anal sex group. Many other formulations could be equally or more plausible. Since the purpose of this example is merely to illustrate the potential importance of contact patterns and not to assess the actual effects of contact patterns, we proceed to simulate this one contact pattern. Given the values in Table 1 and the values of q_{ij} shown in Table 2, and setting K_i equal to c_i, the resulting $\underline{C}=((C_{ij}))$ matrix is shown in Table 3. Once again, this is a plausible contact matrix, but many other formulations could be equally plausible.

Table 3

The overall rate C_{ij} of new sexual partnership formation in millions of contacts per year between different population subgroups.

	POPULATION SUBGROUPS								
	Prefer all oral sex			Prefer all anal sex			Prefer 20% anal sex		
	1	2	3	4	5	6	7	8	9
1	182.36	112.90	64.64	0	0	0	69.79	35.60	11.95
2	112.90	83.76	56.37	0	0	0	43.21	26.41	10.42
3	64.64	56.37	45.45	0	0	0	24.74	17.77	8.40
4	0	0	0	75.63	51.12	29.23	11.24	5.73	1.92
5	0	0	0	51.12	41.40	27.82	7.59	4.64	1.83
6	0	0	0	29.23	27.82	22.40	4.34	3.12	1.47
7	69.79	43.21	24.74	11.24	7.59	4.34	427.36	218.0	73.15
8	35.60	26.41	17.77	5.73	4.64	3.12	218.0	133.25	52.55
9	11.95	10.42	8.40	1.92	1.83	1.47	73.15	52.55	24.83

b. The Effects of Changing Selective Mixing Patterns Selectively by Population subgroups:

Before we discuss the results of simulations which use the values in Tables 1, 2, and 3, let use expand our intuition for the behavior of selective mixing by examining the sensitivity of contact patterns to changes in basic selective mixing parameters. As we remarked after equation [7], for reasonably large values of B_i, proportional increases in *all* the N_i's and c_i's lead to proportional increases in the C_{ij}'s and proportional increases in all the h_i's and q_{ij}'s lead to little change in the C_{ij}'s. More interesting changes occur as we change the values of one set of population subgroups disproportionately to other population subgroups. The proportionate changes in Table 3 created by decreasing the N_i's or h_i's of the pure anal preference groups i= 4 through 6, to one fourth of their Table 1 values are presented in Tables 4 and 5. These changes are very similar. They show greater than one fourth decreases in rate of contacts in the anal group with itself, slightly less than one fourth decreases in the interactions of the anal group with other groups, and there are compensatory increases in the rate of contacts between groups not involving the anal group. Tables 4 and 5 are similar because both equally reduce the total rate of social contacts made by each group. As seen in Table 6, there are, as a consequence, compensatory increases and decreases in the proportion of acceptable encounters that actually result in sex and in the total rate of encounters made which are acceptable for sex.

Table 4

Proportionate changes from Table 3 in sexual partnership formation created by decreasing the N_i of the groups i=4 through 6 to one fourth of the values in Table 1.

	POPULATION SUBGROUPS								
	Prefer all oral sex			Prefer all anal sex			Prefer 20% anal sex		
	1	2	3	4	5	6	7	8	9
1	1.03	1.02	1.01	--	--	--	1.03	1.02	1.02
2	1.02	1.01	1.01	--	--	--	1.02	1.02	1.01
3	1.01	1.01	1.00	--	--	--	1.02	1.01	1.01
4	--	--	--	0.11	0.13	0.14	0.34	0.34	0.34
5	--	--	--	0.13	0.14	0.15	0.39	0.38	0.38
6	--	--	--	0.14	0.15	0.16	0.41	0.41	0.41
7	1.03	1.02	1.02	0.34	0.39	0.41	1.04	1.03	1.03
8	1.02	1.02	1.01	0.34	0.38	0.41	1.03	1.02	1.02
9	1.02	1.01	1.01	0.34	0.38	0.41	1.03	1.02	1.02

Note that changing the N_i or h_i of the anal preference group creates a rather dramatic actual decrease in anal sex in this group even though there is presumably no change in the psychological determinants of behavior. The behavior change is wholly due to the change in available opportunities for anal sex. It is thus theoretically possible given this formulation that the anal preference group generates more than one secondary case for each primary case at the beginning of the epidemic but less than one secondary case later so that the epidemic dies out. A similar scenario is possible if just the high contact rate anal preference groups decreased their desired frequencies of sexual partnerships.

Table 5

Proportionate changes from Table 3 in sexual partnership formation created by decreasing the h_i of the groups i=4 through 6 to one fourth of the values in Table 1.

	POPULATION SUBGROUPS								
	Prefer all oral sex			Prefer all anal sex			Prefer 20% anal sex		
	1	2	3	4	5	6	7	8	9
1	1.03	1.02	1.01	--	--	--	1.03	1.02	1.02
2	1.02	1.01	1.01	--	--	--	1.02	1.02	1.01
3	1.01	1.01	1.00	--	--	--	1.02	1.01	1.01
4	--	--	--	0.17	0.22	0.28	0.41	0.41	0.41
5	--	--	--	0.22	0.29	0.37	0.55	0.55	0.55
6	--	--	--	0.28	0.37	0.46	0.69	0.68	0.68
7	1.03	1.02	1.02	0.41	0.55	0.69	1.04	1.03	1.03
8	1.02	1.02	1.01	0.41	0.55	0.68	1.03	1.02	1.02
9	1.02	1.01	1.01	0.41	0.55	0.68	1.03	1.02	1.02

The proportionate changes in Table 3 created by decreasing the c_i's of the pure anal preference groups 4 through 6 to one fourth of their Table 1 and 2 values are presented in Table 7 where we see that the groups not interacting with the pure anal preference group are not affected by this change. The effect of reducing the acceptance of the mixed preference group for the pure anal preference group to one fourth of the original values is shown in Table 8. Here we see nearly a one fourth reduction in the rate of contacts between these groups with very small compensatory responses elsewhere.

The effects of all the changes leading to Tables 4, 5 ,7, and 8 on the total rate of encountering sexually acceptable individuals (B_i) and the proportion of these with whom sex results ($w_i = \frac{\Sigma_j w_{ij} B_{ij}}{\Sigma_j B_{ij}}$) and the actual proportion of encounters that are anal, R_i, is summarized in Table 6 below. Here we can see that the situations we have been presenting are in the part of the curve in Figure 1 that relates the actual rate of new partnership formation (which equals w_iB_i) to the total rate, B_i, of sexually acceptable encounters where there is a perceptible effect of a changing B_i. Thus random mixing formulations of the populations we have specified, which either fix c_i or make it proportional to the number of individuals in contact groups, would give considerably different results.

Table 6

Changes in the total number of sexually acceptable individuals encountered and in the proportion of acceptable contacts that result in sex in each group as various parameters relevant to the anal group are changed

		POPULATION SUBGROUPS								
		Prefer all oral sex			Prefer all anal sex			Prefer 20% anal sex		
Change from original		1	2	3	4	5	6	7	8	9
Table 3										
None	w_i	.13	.08	.04	.25	.15	.09	.13	.07	.04
	B_i	741.7	650.1	601.8	309.7	272.2	252.8	868.4	744.2	672.9
	R_i	.025	.024	.023	.957	.958	.960	.195	.195	.195
Table 4										
Reduce # preferring	w_i	.12	.07	.04	.35	.25	.16	.11	.07	.04
pure anal by 1/4	B_i	853.9	748.4	692.9	127.5	111.0	102.0	985.4	844.1	762.8
	R_i	.025	.024	.024	.899	.902	.906	.188	.188	.187
Table 5										
Reduce pure anal	w_i	.12	.07	.04	.54	.47	.36	.11	.07	.04
social contacts by 1/4	B_i	853.9	748.4	692.9	31.9	27.8	25.5	985.4	844.1	762.8
	R_i	.025	.024	.024	.921	.925	.929	.190	.189	.189
Table 7										
Reduce pure anal ideal	w_i	.13	.08	.04	.09	.05	.03	.13	.07	.04
partner rate by 1/4	B_i	741.7	650.1	601.8	309.7	272.2	252.8	868.4	744.2	672.9
	R_i	.025	.024	.023	.928	.930	.932	.190	.190	.190
Table 8										
Reduce mixed	w_i	.13	.08	.04	.27	.17	.10	.13	.07	.04
acceptance of anal	B_i	741.7	650.1	601.8	276.3	243.9	227.3	856.0	733.23	662.62
by 1/4	R_i	.025	.024	.024	.989	.989	.989	.187	.187	.186

Table 7

Proportionate changes from Table 3 in sexual partnership formation created by decreasing the c_i of the groups i=4 through 6 to one fourth of the values in Table 1.

	POPULATION SUBGROUPS								
	Prefer all oral sex			Prefer all anal sex			Prefer 20% anal sex		
	1	2	3	4	5	6	7	8	9
1	1.0	1.0	1.0	--	--	--	1.0	1.0	1.0
2	1.0	1.0	1.0	--	--	--	1.0	1.0	1.0
3	1.0	1.0	1.0	--	--	--	1.0	1.0	1.0
4	--	--	--	0.35	0.31	0.30	0.59	0.59	0.59
5	--	--	--	0.31	0.28	0.27	0.53	0.53	0.53
6	--	--	--	0.30	0.27	0.26	0.51	0.51	0.51
7	1.0	1.0	1.0	0.59	0.53	0.51	1.0	1.0	1.0
8	1.0	1.0	1.0	0.59	0.53	0.51	1.0	1.0	1.0
9	1.0	1.0	1.0	0.59	0.53	0.51	1.0	1.0	1.0

Table 8

Proportionate changes from Table 3 in sexual partnership formation created by decreasing the acceptance of the mixed preference for the pure anal group to one fourth of the values in Table 2

	POPULATION SUBGROUPS								
	Prefer all oral sex			Prefer all anal sex			Prefer 20% anal sex		
	1	2	3	4	5	6	7	8	9
1	1.00	1.00	1.00	--	--	--	1.01	1.01	1.01
2	1.00	1.00	1.00	--	--	--	1.01	1.01	1.01
3	1.00	1.00	1.00	--	--	--	1.01	1.01	1.01
4	--	--	--	1.07	1.08	1.09	0.26	0.26	0.26
5	--	--	--	1.08	1.10	1.10	0.26	0.26	0.26
6	--	--	--	1.09	1.10	1.10	0.26	0.26	0.26
7	1.01	1.01	1.01	0.26	0.26	0.26	1.01	1.01	1.01
8	1.01	1.01	1.01	0.26	0.26	0.26	1.01	1.01	1.01
9	1.01	1.01	1.01	0.26	0.26	0.26	1.01	1.01	1.02

c. Simulating HIV Epidemics with Separate Oral and Anal Transmission Risks

Given our assumptions of c_i, h_i, q_{ij}, and initial N_i values, we use simulation models such as those we have used previously (Jacquez et al. 1988; Koopman et al. 1988) to generate expected distributions of infection and illness at different times during an epidemic for our nine population subgroups. In these models, new individuals entering the population flow into the uninfected populations. Once an uninfected individual makes an effective contact with an infected individual, that is to say a contact in which infection is successfully transmitted, the previously uninfected individual passes through five stages: 1) a stage Y_{i1} where he is infected and possibly infectious but does not have detectable antibodies, 2) a stage Y_{i2} where he has detectable antibodies, but his immune function and T cell levels remain normal, 3) a stage Y_{i3} where the symptoms of AIDS-related complex or T cell deficiencies are evident, 4) an initial AIDS condition Y_{i4} during which he continues sexual activity, and 5) an AIDS stage Y_{i5} with no sexual activity. Finally death ensues. In the uninfected state and at each stage of infection before the last AIDS stage, individuals are assumed to die from non-AIDS causes at the rate μ of 1% per year. The rate U_i at which individuals flow into state X_i is set to give a stable population if there is no HIV infection.

The rate at which individuals flow from one infected stage to another is a constant proportion of the number of individuals in a particular stage. As a result, when stages are chained together, the distribution of times it takes individuals to reach the AIDS state or death is bell shaped but skewed to the right (Jacquez, 1985). Flow rates for the transitions between infected stages have been estimated by Longini et al. (1989). These estimates, their standard errors, and the corresponding mean periods of time spent in each stage are presented in our previous paper (Koopman et al. 1988). The analysis of Longini et al. (1989) did not use determinations as to whether individuals were sexually active to divide AIDS cases into two stages as we have done. Our choice of 8 months as a likely period of sexual activity after the onset of AIDS was arbitrary but consistent with available literature (Fischl et al. 1987).

The rate at which uninfected individuals in activity group i become infected is a function of: a) the number of susceptible individuals in that activity group (X_i), b) the rate at which they form new sexual partnerships with each population subgroup ($\frac{C_{ij}}{N_i}$), c) the proportion of individuals in each population subgroup who are at each stage of infection ($\frac{Y_{js}}{N_j}$), and d) the likelihood of transmission given that a sexual partnership is made with an individual in a particular activity group who is at a given stage of infection (β_{ijs}). Mathematically this rate is expressed as

$$\frac{X_i}{N_i}\sum_{j=1}^{9} C_{ij} \sum_{s=1}^{4} \frac{Y_{js}}{N_j}\beta_{ijs}. \qquad [11]$$

The C_{ij} are defined by the selective mixing formulations of equations 1-6. Initially 1/100,000 of each subgroup i was placed in stage 1 of infection.

The resulting set of differential equations used in the simulations is as follows:

$$\frac{dX_i}{dt} = U_i - \mu X_i - \frac{X_i}{N_i}\sum_{j=1}^{9} C_{ij}\sum_{s=1}^{4} \beta_{ijs}\frac{Y_{js}}{N_j}, \qquad [12]$$

$$\frac{dY_{i1}}{dt} = \frac{X_i}{N_i}\sum_{j=1}^{9} C_{ij}\sum_{s=1}^{4} \beta_{ijs}\frac{Y_{js}}{N_j} - k_1Y_{i1} - \mu Y_{i1}, \qquad [13]$$

$$\frac{dY_{is}}{dt} = k_{s-1}Y_{i,s-1} - k_sY_{is} - \mu Y_{is} \quad ; \quad s = 2,3,4, \qquad [14]$$

$$\frac{dY_{i5}}{dt} = k_4Y_{i4} - k_5Y_{i5}. \qquad [15]$$

A summary of all parameters is presented in Table 9.

When considering only casual and anonymous sex, b_{ijs} is not influenced by the rate of new sexual partnership formation in subgroups i or j since we assume that all relationships are equally transient. The value of b_{ijs} will be influenced, however, by the proportion of the transient partnerships that involve oral or anal sex and the probabilities of transmission given oral (a_{os}) or anal (a_{as}) sex at stage s of infection. The frequency of oral or anal sex in partnerships between i and j individuals is assumed to be half way between the preferred frequencies of each component group as discussed above. Therefore:

$$\beta_{ijs} = \left(\frac{P_i + P_j}{2}\right)\alpha_{as} + \left(1 - \frac{P_i + P_j}{2}\right)\alpha_{os}. \qquad [16]$$

d. Simulation Results:

Because our purpose is to illustrate the selective mixing formulation, we present here only selective results of simulations corresponding to the parameters in Tables 1 and 2. The aspects that are presented were chosen to illustrate the distortion in classical multivariate risk analysis of different sexual acts due to the failure to consider that the partners of each sexual act might have different probabilities of being in the various stages of infection. To examine the distortion, we

Table 9

Summary of terms used in formulating selective mixing and in modeling HIV transmission.

N_i	=	The number of individuals in population subgroup i (within a given activity group).
h_i	=	The number of social contacts per person by an individual group i per unit time.
A_{ij}	=	The average number of social contacts initiated between all individuals in groups i and j per unittime.
q_{ij}	=	The proportion of individuals in group j with whom group i individuals converse that group i individuals would potentially accept as sex partners.
B_{ij}	=	The number of social contacts that are mutually acceptable as potential sexual partners between groups i and j per unit time.
B_i	=	The number of social contacts with potentially acceptable new sex partners for an individual in group i per unit time.
w_{ij}	=	The proportion of social contacts between mutually acceptable sexual partners in groups i and j that actually result in sexual partnership.
Ω_i	=	the actual proportion of mutually acceptable encounters that group i makes which result in sexual partnerships given that every other group has very large B_j.
C_{ij}	=	The rate at which new sexual partnerships are initiated between members of groups i and j.
ρ_{ij}	=	The proportion of new sexual partnerships made by individuals in group i that are with individuals in group j.
c_i	=	The rate of new sexual partnership formation at which group i individuals would satisfy both their sexual desires and their moral standards, when the number of acceptable contacts in sufficiently large.
w_i	=	The proportion of mutually acceptable sexual partners with whom an individual in group i converses which would be taken as sexual partners if the needs and standards of their potential sexual partners were not taken into consideration.
p	=	Subscript p's added to any of the above terms refer to pairing status.
P_i	=	The preferred proportions of anal sex for group i members.

Table 9 Continued

R_i = The actual proportions of anal sex for group i members.

X_i = The number of uninfected individuals in population subgroup i.

Y_{js} = The number of individuals in population subgroup j who are in infection state s.

β_{ijs} = The average probability over the entire course of a partnership that a susceptible from group i will be infected by a partner from group j who was in stage s of infection when the partnership began.

U_i = The rate at which individuals flow into population subgroup i.

μ = The death rate of all individuals not in the last stage of AIDS.

k_s = The rate at which individuals in stage s of infection progress to the next stage.

α_{os} = The probability that oral sex between a susceptible and an infected in stage s of infection will result in HIV transmission.

α_{as} = The probability that anal sex between a susceptible and an infected in stage s of infection will result in HIV transmission.

$\bar{\alpha}_a$ = The average probability of transmission from an anal sex act at one point in time during the epidemic.

$\bar{\alpha}_o$ = The average probability of transmission from an oral sex act at one point in time during the epidemic.

present the average probability of transmission from oral and anal sex at different stages of the epidemic.

The probability of transmission in the average anal sex act we will call $\bar{\alpha}_a$. It can be calculated at a given point in time of the epidemic as the average over all anal sex acts of product of the probability of transmission given anal sex with an infected individual and the probability that the individual is infected. The formula for such an average is:

$$\bar{\alpha}_a = \frac{\sum_{i=1}^{9}\sum_{j=1}^{9} C_{ij}\frac{P_i + P_j}{2}\sum_{s=1}^{4}\alpha_{as}\frac{Y_{js}}{N_j}}{\sum_{i=1}^{9}\sum_{j=1}^{9} C_{ij}\frac{P_i + P_j}{2}}. \qquad [17]$$

Similarly the probability of transmission in the average oral sex, $\bar{\alpha}_o$, act can be calculated as:

$$\bar{\alpha}_o = \frac{\sum_{i=1}^{9}\sum_{j=1}^{9} C_{ij}\left\{1 - \frac{P_i + P_j}{2}\right\}\sum_{s=1}^{4}\alpha_{os}\frac{Y_{js}}{N_j}}{\sum_{i=1}^{9}\sum_{j=1}^{9} C_{ij}\left\{1 - \frac{P_i + P_j}{2}\right\}}. \qquad [18]$$

The ratio of oral and anal sex act transmission probabilities has been fixed in our simulations at 4. Deviations of this ratio from four should reflect the degree of distortion in risk estimates that would be due to not taking into account the proportion of contacts in the different stages of infection. Simulations were performed at the values of parameters in Tables 1 and 2 which gave the C_{ij} matrix in Table 3. The value of α_{os} was set at one fourth the value of α_{as} so that $\alpha_{a1} = 0.04$, $\alpha_{a2} = 0.002$, $\alpha_{a3} = 0.02$, $\alpha_{a4} = 0.04$, $\alpha_{o1} = 0.01$, $\alpha_{o2} = 0.0005$, $\alpha_{o3} = 0.005$, $\alpha_{o4} = 0.01$.

The resulting epidemic curves in the pure oral preference, the pure anal preference, and the mixed preference groups are presented in Figure 2. An equal proportion, 1 in every 100,000, of each of the 9 groups are originally seeded with infection. It takes considerable time to generate an epidemic. The epidemics generated, however, seem consistent with the patterns that have been observed in the MACS cohorts. We can see that selective mixing with the parameters used in this simulation has determined quite separate epidemics in the pure oral preference and the pure anal preference populations.

The average probabilities of transmission in an anal and in an oral sex act at different times during the epidemic and their ratio are presented in Figure 3 along with their ratio. There is considerable deviation in the ratio from four, with a peek difference of 31.5 reached at year 20 after introduction. By the time the actual epidemic of AIDS becomes quite noticeable, however, there is not a marked disparity in the risk of oral or anal sex from the programmed differences in per sex act risks of anal and oral sex. By varying acceptability parameters, it is possible to get considerably greater deviances of the observed risk ratios of anal to oral sex from the programmed differences. Before any conclusions are made regarding relative anal and oral sex risks, more information on contact patterns should be obtained and more thorough exploration of model possibilities should be pursued.

Figure 2
Number of New AIDS Cases Throughout a Simulated Epidemic where the Anal and Oral Preference Groups Mix with the Mixed Preference Group

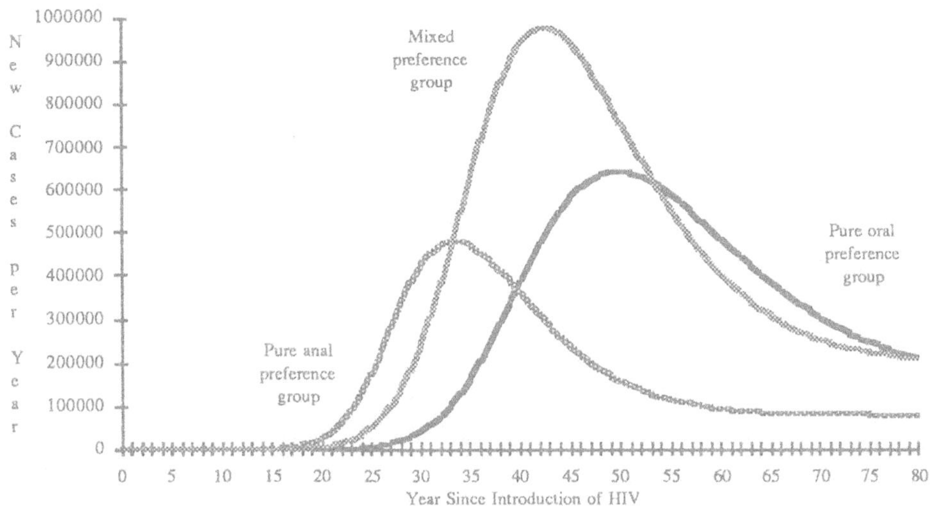

4. Discussion

The crucial influence of sexual partner selectivity patterns on the sum total of AIDS cases at different points in the epidemic has been demonstrated earlier (Jacquez et al. 1988; Koopman et al. 1988). Until now, however, there has been no way to model contact patterns consistent with reasonable causal hypotheses whose parameters are capable of being estimated by collectable data.

This need has motivated our development of the combination of selective and structured mixing. This combined modeling approach proceeds from the assumption that there are two forces creating heterogeneous sexual contact patterns in a population. The first is the choice of social contexts for meeting potential sexual partners. The second is the degree of selectivity exercised in choosing partners among those who are encountered in these social contexts. A consideration of these same two forces has motivated the group of researchers who won the NIH contract to design a National Sexual Behavior Survey (Laumann et al. 1987).

Figure 3
Average Absolute and Relative Risks of Anal and Oral Sex Throughout a Simulated Epidemic

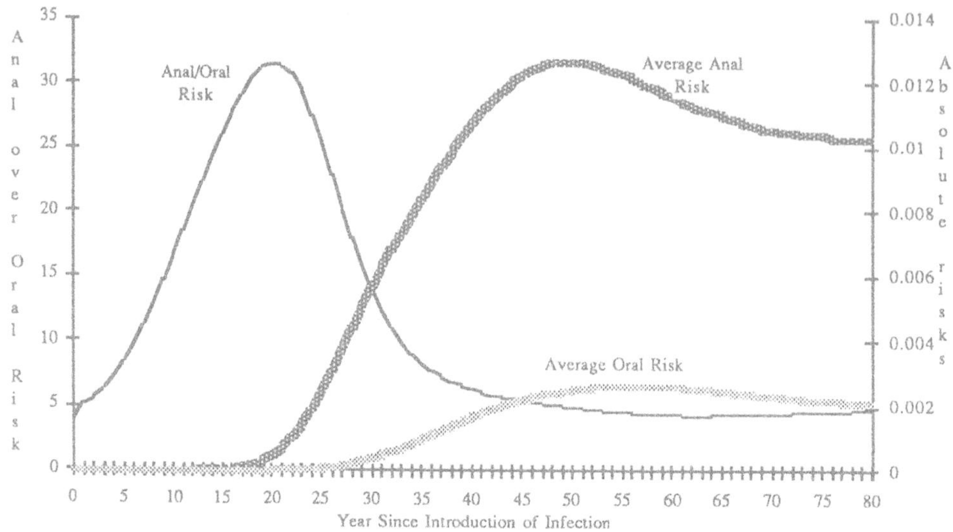

A major advantage of this approach is that the description of contact patterns does not require that study subjects specify all the characteristics of all their sexual contacts. Such a specification is an impossible task for some characteristics, like new sexual partnership formation rate. Instead, the approach presented here describes contact patterns and defines the system of contacts through specification of the social context of encounters that lead to sex and the psychosocial factors acting in partnership selection. Given this type of information, it is possible to use the structured and selective mixing formulations to deduce the likelihood of different types of partners. When information is simultaneously gathered on the characteristics of the sexual partners of study subjects as well as upon the determinants of structured and selective mixing, it should be possible to check the consistency of the structured and selective mixing contact pattern description with the observed contact patterns. In the case of age group and race, it is relatively easy to collect data on the sexual partners of study subjects. For those characteristics, models of structured and selective mixing can be readily checked against easily collectable data. Given this testability characteristic of structured and selective mixing models, there is hope that sociologists might explore appropriate theory so that the h_i and q_{ij} parameters might be specified by models with a smaller number of parameters.

The specification of h_i may, however, not be necessary to employ selective mixing for many purposes. When one has an observed new partnership formation rate for each subgroup in a set of data, then one will have to write a set of simultaneous equations and solve for the ci. Different sets of h_i will lead to different sets of ci. But the specified sets of h_i seem to have little influence on the resulting contact matrix C_{ij}. The value of a formulation with the h_i, which may be approximated by a single average social encounter rate for all subgroups, is seen when one considers what the magnitude of this parameter does to the responsiveness of new partnership formation rates to changes in availability of partnerships. In general, smaller values of h_i will make the system more responsive, while larger values that get one out on the flat part of figure 1, will make the system less responsive.

This paper presented an example of the use of the selective mixing formulation to describe contact patterns by preference for type of sex and new partnership formation rate in a homosexual population having predominantly casual and anonymous sex. That example was not meant to reflect any real pattern of selective mixing since no data is currently available to determine several key parameters of selective mixing. It represents one moderately plausible contact pattern. The example shows that it is quite possible that our perception of the relative safety of oral sex is incorrect due to a failure to take contact patterns into consideration. To show whether indeed our perception is being so distorted and to provide a basis to estimate the transmission probabilities of oral and anal sex, we need a more complete model of heterogeneous mixing involving both structured and selective mixing; we need to include other types of sex besides oral and anal, we need to distinguish insertive and receptive behavior, and we need data on the magnitude of several of the parameters in the model, including those which determine the patterns of contact.

Acknowledgements

The contributions of Jill G. Joseph PhD and David G. Ostrow MD PhD through provision of the Coping and Change Study data and through many stimulating discussions were an important part of this work. Discussions with Martina Morris, Tony Tam and Ed Laumann at the University of Chicago were also an important stimulus for this work. We would also like to thank an anonymous referee for a useful suggestion as to how w_{ij} might be better formulated.

References

Chmiel, J.S., R. Detels, R.A. Kaslow, L. VanRaden, M. Kingsley, R. Brookmeyer. (1987). Factors associated with prevalent Human Immunodeficiency Virus (HIV) infection in the multicenter AIDS cohort study. *Am J Epidemiol* ; 126(4): 568-577.

Darrow, W.W., D.F. Echenberg, H.W. Jaffe HW, P. O'Malley, R.H. Byers, J.P. Getchell, J.W. Curran. (1987). Risk factors for Human Immunodeficiency Virus (HIV) infections in homosexual men. *Am J Public Health*; 77(4): 479-483.

Dietz, K., (1988). On the transmission dynamics of HIV. *Math Biosci*; 90: 397-414

Dietz, K., K.P. Hadeler. (1988). Epidemiological models for sexually transmitted diseases. *J Math Biol* 26:1-25.

Fischl, M.A., G.M. Dickinson, G.B. Scott GB, N. Klimas, M.A. Fletcher, W. Parks. (1987). Evaluation of heterosexual partners, children and household contacts of adults with AIDS. *JAMA* 257: 640-4.

Gail, M.H., D. Preston, S. Piantados. (1989) Disease prevention models of voluntary confidential screening for Human Immunodeficiency Virus (HIV) in isolated low risk and high risk populations and in mixed gay/heterosexual populations. *Statistics in Medicine*; 8:59-81.

Goedert, J.J. (1984). Determinants of retrovirus (HTLV-III) antibody and immunodeficiency conditions in homosexual men. *The Lancet*; (September 29) 711-715.

Goedert, J.J., R.J. Biggar, D.M. Winn. (1985). Decreased helper T lymphocytes in homosexual men: Sexual Practices. *American Journal of Epidemiology*; 121(5): 629-36.

Goedert, J.J., R. J. Biggar, M. Melbye, D.L. Mann, S. Wilson, M.H. Gail, R.J. Grossman, R.A. DiGioia, W.C. Sachez, S.H. Weiss, W.A. Blattner. (1987). Effect of T4 count and cofactors on the incidence of AIDS in homosexual men infected with Human Immunodeficiency Virus. *JAMA*; 257(3): 331-334.

Hethcote, H.W., J.W. Van Ark. (1987). Epidemiological models for heterogeneous populations: proportionate mixing, parameter estimation, and immunization programs. *Math. Biosci.* 84:85-118.

Jacquez, J.A. (1985) *Compartmental analysis in biology and medicine*, Chapter 7, second edition. Ann Arbor: The University of Michigan Press.

Jacquez, J.A., C.P. Simon, J.S. Koopman, L. Sattenspiel, T. Perry. (1988). Modeling and analyzing HIV transmission: the effect of contact patterns. *Mathematical Biosciences*, 92:119-199.

Jacquez, J.A., J. Koopman, C.P. Simon. (1989). *Structured mixing: heterogeneous mixing by the definition of activity groups. A new general method for describing contact patterns with special reference to AIDS*. (This volume).

Jeffries, E., B. Willoughby, W.J. Boyko, M.T. Schecter, B. Wiggs, S. Fay, M. O'Shaughnessy. (1985). The Vancouver Lymphadenopathy-AIDS Study: 2. Seroepidemiology of HTLV-III antibody. *Can Med Assoc J*; 132: 1373-1377.

Joseph, J.G., S.B. Montgomery, C.A. Emmons, D.G. Ostrow. (1987). Magnitude and determinants of behavioral risk reduction: longitudinal analysis of a cohort at risk for AIDS. *Psychology and Health*; 1987: 73-95.

Kingsley, L.A., R. Kaslow, C.R. Rinaldo, K. Detre, N. Odaka, M. VanRaden, R. Detels, B.F. Polk , J. Chmiel, S.F. Kelsey, D. Ostrow, B. Visscher. (1987). Risk factors for seroconversion to Human Immunodeficiency Virus among male homosexuals. *The Lancet* (February 14) 345-348.

Koopman, J.S., C.P. Simon, J.A. Jacquez, T.S. Park. (1988). Sexual partner selectiveness effects on homosexual HIV transmission dynamics. *Journal of the Acquired Immune Deficiency Syndrome*, 1:486-504.

Laumann, E.O., Gagnon JH; Michael, RT (1987). Social and Behavioral Aspects of Health and Fertility-Related Behavior: Technical Proposal submitted in response to National Institute for Child Health and Human Development RFP no. NICHD-DBS-87-13. September 1, 1987. (Available from the Authors).

Longini, I.M., W.S. Clark, R.H. Byers, J.W. Ward, W.W. Darrow, G.F. Lemp, H.A. Hethcote. (1989). Statistical analysis of the stages of HIV infection using a Markov model. *Statistics in Medicine* 8:(In Press)

Lyman, D., M. Ascher, J.A. Levy. (1986). Minimal risk of transmission of AIDS-Associated retrovirus infection by oral-genital contact (letter). *JAMA*; 255(13):1703

Melbye, M., R.J. Biggar, P. Ebbesen, M.G. Sarngadharan, S.H. Weiss, R. Gallo R, W.A. Blattner. (1984). Seroepidemiology of HTLV-III antibody in Danish homosexual men: prevalence, transmission, and disease outcome. *Br Med J* (September 8) 289: 573-575.

Moss, A.R., D. Osmond, P. Bacchetti. (1987). Risk factors for AIDS and HIV seropositivity in homosexual men. *American Journal of Epidemiology*; 125(6): 1035-1046.

Nicholson, J.K.A., J.S. McDougal, H.W. Jaffe, T.J. Spira, M.S. Kennedy, B.M. Jones, W.W. Darrow, M. Morgan, M Hubbard. (1985). Exposure to Human T-Lymphotropic Virus Type III/Lymphadenopathy-Associated Virus and immunologic abnormalities in asymptomatic homosexual men. *Ann Intern Med*; 103: 37-42.

Polk, B.F., R. Fox, R. Brookmeyer, S. Kanchanaraksa, R. Kaslow, B. Visscher, C. Rinaldo, J. Phair, (1986). Predictors of the Acquired Immunodeficiency Syndrome developing in a cohort of seropositive homosexual men. *N Engl J Med*; 316(2): 61-66.

Schechter, M.T., W.J. Boyko, B. Douglas, M. Maynard, B. Willoughby, A. McLeod A,. K.J.P. Craib. (1986). Can HTLV-III be transmitted orally? (letter). *Lancet*; (February 15,1986): 379.

Stevens, C.E., P.E. Taylor, E.A. Zang, J.M. Morrison, E.J. Harley, S.R. Cordoba, C. Bacino, R.C. Ting, A.J. Bodner, M.G. Sarngadharan, R.C. Gallo, P. Rubinstein.

(1986). Human T-cell Lymphotropic Virus infection in a cohort of homosexual men in New York City. *JAMA*; 2556(16): 2167-72.

Winkelstein, W., D.M. Lyman, N. Padian N, R. Grant, M. Samuel, J.A. Wiley, R.E. Anderson, W. Lang, J. Riggs, J. Levy. (1987). Sexual practices and risk of infection by the Human Immunodeficiency Virus; the San Francisco Men's Health Study. *JAMA*; 257(3): 321-25.

V. The Immune System and the HIV

MODELING THE INTERACTION OF THE IMMUNE SYSTEM WITH HIV

Alan S. Perelson

Theoretical Division
Los Alamos National Laboratory
Los Alamos, NM 87545

Santa Fe Institute
1120 Canyon Road
Santa Fe, NM 87501

Abstract

The interactions between the human immune system and HIV are potentially complex. In this paper I review some of these interactions and sketch the beginnings of a general model that can potentially account for many of the immunological consequences of HIV infection. This model involves a large number of ordinary differential equations and many parameters. To make progress, I simplify the general model and develop a four-equation model that involves free HIV and uninfected, latently infected and actively infected CD4$^+$ T cells. Using reasonable guesses for parameter values, I show that this model can account for some of the puzzling features of AIDS: the long latent period, the almost complete absence of free virus particles, the low frequency of infected T4 cells and the slow T cell depletion seen during the course of the disease. Further, the model suggests why the latent period may be significantly shorter in children than in adults.

1. Introduction

The detailed mechanisms of pathogenesis of HIV infection are still unknown. Infection with HIV results in a severe immunosuppression due to selective depletion in CD4$^+$ T cells (T4 cells). A large number of immunological abnormalities accompany HIV infection, and all but a few can be attributed to the decline in T4 cells (Lane and Fauci 1985; Fauci 1988). HIV binds to cells via the CD4 molecule (Dalgleish et al. 1984; Klatzmann et al. 1984). Thus T4 cells, as well as monocytes and macrophages which also express CD4, are targets of HIV infection. While HIV infection is cytopathic in T4 cells, monocytes appear to survive, harboring the virus and possibly playing the role of a reservoir (Gartner et al. 1986; Folks et al. 1987). Persistence of HIV in human monocytes may in part explain the inability of the immune response to clear the body of the virus (Fauci 1988).

A number of puzzles about HIV infection and potential therapies need to be explained. Quantitative models, of the type that I discuss below, may be helpful in this endeavor. For example, immunization normally boosts the population of antigen specific T4 lymphocytes. However, in the case of HIV infection, increasing the T4 population also boosts one of the cell populations that the virus attacks. Further, viral replication is triggered by activation of infected T4 cells. Thus immunization could lead to an increase in the viral population rather than to a reduction. Immunization generally also leads to an increase in serum antibody specific for HIV. When antibody attaches to HIV, it acts as a tag identifying the virus as harmful to non-specific phagocytic cells, such as macrophages and monocytes. These cells, which have receptors for the Fc portion of antibody molecules, bind the antibody coating the virus as a first stage in the phagocytic process. Unfortunately, many cells have Fc receptors. Thus antibody-coated virus can bind to cells which do not express CD4. Once bound to a cell, the antibody-coated virus can fuse to the membrane of the cell and infect it. Thus, coating HIV with antibody can enhance its infectivity of macrophages and monocytes and also allow it to enter cells, which it normally would not infect, by a non CD4-dependent pathway (Takeda, Tuazon and Ennis 1988; Levy 1988). A quantitative model could help determine the precise outcome of immunization under differing circumstances.

Another important puzzle that needs to be quantitatively examined is the long latency period of the disease. Questions about the degree to which the latency results from a balance between death of infected cells that have never produced virus and the infrequent encounter of HIV infected T4 cells with the particular antigen that triggers their viral replication need to be explored. We also need to inquire into the causes of the decline in the T4 lymphocyte population. A number of hypotheses, discussed below, have been proposed, but can they quantitatively account for the observations?

HIV infection can lead to the death of T4 cells, possibly by damaging the cell membrane when large amounts of virus are produced and bud off the cell surface (Fauci 1988), or by introducing large amounts of unintegrated viral DNA (Shaw et al. 1984), or by inducing terminal differentiation of the infected T4 cell, leading to a shortened life-span (Zagury et al. 1986). However, when attempts have been made to quantify the degree of HIV infection, either by the use of fluoresceinated antibodies against viral encoded proteins or by the use of *in situ* hybridization to detect cells with viral mRNA, on the order of 1 in 10^4–10^5 cells in the peripheral blood of HIV infected individuals appear to express the virus at a given time (Fauci 1988; Harper et al. 1986). A larger proportion of cells may be latently infected and not detected by current techniques (Fauci 1988). If the degree of infection is this low, how can one explain the profound depression found in the T4 population of AIDS patients? A likely possibility is that mechanisms other than direct cytopathic effects may be important in T4 depletion (Fauci 1986). For example, HIV may infect a T cell precursor and reduce the rate of production of mature T cells (Fauci 1988; Gluckman, Klatzmann and Montagnier 1986). A quantitative calculation could assess this hypothesis. Alternatively, HIV may infect and deplete a subset of T4 cells that are critical to the propagation of the entire T4 population. In this regard, it is known that AIDS patients have a decreased capacity to secrete lymphokines, especially IL-2, upon T cell stimulation, and have reduced levels of IL-2 receptors on activated T cells (Prince, Kermani-Arab and Fahey 1984). Quantitatively models of the effects of IL-2 have been developed (De Boer and Hogeweg 1987; Kevrekidis, Zecha and Perelson 1988), and such models need to be applied to AIDS.

Autoimmune mechanisms have also been proposed as a means by which non-HIV infected T4 cells could be depleted during HIV infection. For example, envelope protein (gp120), either shed by virus (Gelderblom et al. 1987) or released from HIV-producing lymphocytes, may bind to CD4 molecules on uninfected T4 cells thereby triggering immune clearance of these cells (Klatzmann and Montagnier 1986) or their elimination by antibody-dependent cytotoxicity (ADCC) (Lylerly et al. 1987). Antilymphocyte antibodies have been found in AIDS patients (Kiprov et al. 1984). Stricker et al. (1987) have found an autoantibody that reacts with a previously unknown antigen on $CD4^+$ cells. The antibody suppresses proliferation of T4 cells *in vitro* and induces cytotoxicity in the presence of complement. Ziegler and Stities (1986) have suggested that, because CD4 interacts with both the HIV envelope glycoprotein gp120 and the class II MHC molecule on antigen presenting cells, gp120 may mimic the configuration of a portion of the class II MHC molecule. Thus antibodies and CTLs generated in an immune response to HIV could cross-react with class II MHC. Further, anti-idiotypic antibodies raised during a response to HIV could recognize any $CD4^+$ cells, thus causing destruction of uninfected T4 cells. The degree to which any of these autoimmune mechanisms play a role should be assessed via quantitative models.

2. Model

A number of features of the life history of HIV are important in developing dynamical models of its action. First, when HIV infects a cell it integrates a DNA copy of its RNA genome into the DNA of the infected cell. The viral DNA, called the "provirus," will be duplicated with the cell's DNA every time the cell divides. Thus a cell, once infected, remains infected for life. Further, the provirus can remain latent, giving no sign of its presence for months or years (Ho et al. 1987), or it can be stimulated and lead to the production of new virus particles. New viruses are produced by the usual means of protein synthesis. The viral DNA is transcribed into RNA, some of which is translated into proteins. The proteins and RNA are assembled into new virions that bud from the surface of the infected cell. The budding can take place very rapidly, leading to the lysis of the host cell (this seems to be the case in T4 cell infection), or it can take place slowly and spare the host cell (this seems to occur in macrophage and monocyte infection). The activation of T cells into a proliferative state, say by the T cell recognizing antigen, is required for converting a latent HIV infection into active viral replication.

In order to model these events, I shall consider cells that are uninfected, cells that are latently infected, i.e., that contain the virus but are not producing it, and cells that are actively infected, i.e., that are producing virus. First, I will sketch a rather general model that has the potential of accounting for many of the immunological consequences of HIV infection. However, because of its generality, this model has many unknown parameters. Further, because many phenomena of relevance to HIV have not yet attracted the attention of theorists, tested submodels do not yet exist for all of the phenomena contained in this general model. Thus, some terms will contain functions of yet unknown form. This is meant to pose a challenge to both theorists and experimentalists. After this general model is introduced, a more modest model with few parameters and no unknown functions is presented. Both models are formulated in terms of ordinary differential equations and thus spatial dependence is ignored. For interactions occurring in the blood stream, this is a reasonable approximation. However, to correctly account for interactions in the tissues, more complex models involving partial differential equations may be needed. Also, because the models are deterministic, they do not correctly account for the very early stages of the infection. As one will see, the solutions to the model equations will predict that the number of infected T cells increases continuously from zero and does not jump discontinuously from zero to one to two, etc. Stochastic models, such as the one presented by Merrill (1989), can be used to overcome this deficiency.

2a. A General Model

Because antigen stimulation of T4 cells seems to be required to stimulate HIV replication within latently infected cells, it is important to decompose the T4 population into antigen specific subpopulations. Thus, let T denote the total concentration of uninfected T4 cells and let T_k denote the concentration of uninfected T4 cells specific for antigen k. Thus $T = \sum T_k$. Let a_k be the concentration of antigen k. HIV itself is one type of antigen. Here I will not single out the T cells that are HIV specific, but in many models, it would be of interest to do so. Any subpopulation of

T4 cells can be infected by HIV irrespective of its antigen specificity. I distinguish latently infected cells from their noninfected counterparts by adding a superscript: *. Actively infected cells will be denoted by a superscript: **. Thus, T_k^* and T_k^{**} denote the concentrations of T4 cells specific for antigen k that are latently infected and actively infected, respectively. Similarly, m and m^* denote the uninfected and the actively infected monocyte/macrophage populations, respectively (for simplicity I will generally speak only about monocytes with the understanding that macrophages may be part of this population). *In vivo*, I expect the T4 cell, monocyte and HIV population dynamics to be governed by equations such as the following:

T cell equations:

$$\begin{aligned}\frac{dT_k}{dt} =& s(v) - \mu_T T_k + rT_k\left(1 - \frac{T_k}{T_{max}}\right)e^{-\eta T_{tot}} f_s(a_k, \ldots) - k_1 v T_k \\ & - k_s T_k(T^{**} + m^*) - k_s' T_k S - \mu_{ai} T_k g_{ai}(gp120, \ldots) \ , \end{aligned} \tag{1}$$

$$\frac{dT_k^*}{dt} = -\mu_T T_k^* + k_1 v T_k - k_2 f_s(a_k) T_k^* - k_s T_k^*(T^{**} + m^*) - k_s' T_k^* S \ , \tag{2}$$

$$\begin{aligned}\frac{dT_k^{**}}{dt} =& k_2 f_s(a_k) T_k^* - \mu_b T_k^{**} - k_s T_k^{**}(T_{tot} + m_{tot}) - k_s'' T_k^{**} S \\ & - \mu_{is} T_k^{**} g_{is}(CTL, \ldots) - k_{phag}' m T_k^{**} g_{opson}(A_v) \ , \end{aligned} \tag{3}$$

where the total T4 population, T_{tot}, is composed of

$$T = \sum_k T_k \ , \quad T^* = \sum_k T_k^* \ , \quad T^{**} = \sum_k T_k^{**} \ , \tag{4a}$$

and

$$T_{tot} = T + T^* + T^{**} \ . \tag{4b}$$

Syncytium equation:

$$\frac{dS}{dt} = k_s T^{**}(T_{tot} + m_{tot}) + k_s m^*(T + T^* + m_{tot}) - \mu_s S \ . \tag{5}$$

Virus equation:

$$\frac{dv}{dt} = N\mu_b \sum_k T_k^{**} + k_{vm} m^* + N_s \mu_s S - k_1 v T_{tot} - k_m v m_{tot} - \mu_v v - k_n v h(A_v) \ . \tag{6}$$

Monocyte/macrophage equations:

$$\frac{dm}{dt} = s_m - \mu_m m - k_m v m - k_s m(T^{**} + m^*) - k'_s m S$$
$$- k_{phag} m v h(A_v) - k'_{phag} m T^{**} g_{opson}(A_v) \quad , \tag{7}$$

$$\frac{dm^*}{dt} = k_m v m - k_s m^*(T_{tot} + m_{tot}) - k'_s m^* S$$
$$+ k_{phag} m v h(A_v) + k'_{phag} m T^{**} g_{opson}(A_v) \quad , \tag{8}$$

where

$$m_{tot} = m + m^* \quad . \tag{9}$$

Antigen equation:

$$\frac{da_k}{dt} = s_a(t) + r_a a_k \left(1 - \frac{a_k}{a_{max}}\right) - \mu_a a_k - \mu_{ir} a_k g_{ir}(T_k, \ldots) \quad . \tag{10}$$

In Eq. (1), $s(v)$ is a source term and represents the rate of generation of new (presumably uninfected) T4 cells from precursors in the bone marrow and thymus. HIV can infect precursor cells and may have the effect of decreasing the supply of new cells (cf. Edelman and Zolla-Pazner 1989). Thus $s(v)$ may be a constant or a decreasing function of v. T cells have a finite life-span and die with rate μ_T per cell. In Eq. (2), latently infected T cells are also assumed to have precisely the same natural lifespan ($\sim 1/\mu_T$), although other factors can augment the natural death rate.

If a T_k cell encounters antigen k it may be stimulated to grow. Modeling T cell stimulation is a complex matter. Here I have assumed that a fraction, f_s, of T cells are stimulated to grow, where f_s is a function of the antigen concentration and other factors such as lymphokines and antigen presentation by macrophages. These other factors are not delineated in this preliminary sketch, hence f_s is written as a function of a_k and other unspecified variables. Once T4 cells are stimulated, I assume that their growth is governed by a logistic growth rate law, with the maximal specific growth rate denoted r. Note that the logistic law is based on the fact that T cells (or any normal cells) will stop growing as their population level approaches a threshold, here denoted T_{max}. This logistic term prevents T cells of specificity k from growing too large. Other growth control mechanisms may prevent the total T cell population from enlarging too greatly. As in the work of Segel and Perelson (1988), this effect is accounted for by the term $e^{-\eta T_{tot}}$.

The other terms in Eqs. (1) and (2) deal with the effects of HIV. The term $k_1 v T_k$ models the possibility that free virus v infects a T4 cell. A simple mass-action type term has been used, with the rate of infection denoted k_1. Once a T cell has been infected, it becomes a T^* cell; thus this term is subtracted from Eq. (1) and added to Eq. (2).

Cells expressing the viral antigen gp120 on their surface, i.e., actively infected cells, can fuse with uninfected or latently infected T4 cells to form multinucleated giant cells called syncytia (Lifson et al. 1986a,b; Sidroski et al. 1986). The term $-k_s T_k(T^{**} + m^*)$ in Eq. (1) denotes the loss of uninfected T4 cells due to syncytia formation with any actively infected T cell or monocyte. For simplicity, here and elsewhere in the model, I have assumed that actively infected T cells and infected macrophages have equal ability to form syncytia. This need not be the case, and an extra parameter could be added to distinguish between the two case. It is not clear from the literature whether mixed T cell - monocyte syncytia form. However, I see no reason that they cannot form and thus have included them in the model. In Eq. (2), the term $-k_s T_k^*(T^{**} + m^*)$ denotes the loss of latently infected T4 cells through syncytia formation. Syncytia also express viral antigens and can fuse with $CD4^+$ cells. Because syncytia are larger than single cells, we assume they fuse with a rate constant k_s' different from k_s. The concentration of syncytia is denoted S. The term $-k_s' T_k S$ in Eq.(1) and $-k_s' T_k^* S$ in Eq. (2) account for the loss of uninfected and latently infected cells by fusion with syncytia. It is not clear whether actively infected cells also fuse with syncytia, but I have included the term $-k_s'' T_k^{**} S$ in Eq. (3) to encompass this possibility. Analogous terms appear in Eqs. (7) and (8) for syncytia fusion with monocytes. Equation (5) describes the population dynamics of syncytia. I assume that the fusion of a pre-existing syncytium with a cell does not change the number of syncytia. Syncytia are not viable and usually die within 24–36h (Lifson et. al 1986b). This is accounted for by the term $-\mu_s S$, where μ_s is the death rate of syncytia.

The last term in Eq. (1), $-\mu_{ai} T_k g_{ai}(gp120, ...)$, models the loss of uninfected T4 cells through autoimmune mechanisms. The function g_{ai} determines which immune system influences are important in the autoimmune response. For example, if gp120 shed by virus binds to CD4 molecules on uninfected cells as suggested by Klatzmann and Montagnier (1986), then g_{ai} will depend on the rate of shedding, the fate of the shed gp120 molecules, and the availability of binding sites on T4 cells for gp120. To explicitly construct g_{ai}, one would also need to specify and model the immune system effector functions that would remove a cell with gp120 bound: e.g., antibody and complement, antibody-dependent cellular cytotoxicity (ADCC) or cytotoxic T lymphocytes (CTL). Similarly, the term in Eq. (3), $-\mu_{is} T_k^{**} g_{is}(CTL, ...)$, accounts for the loss of actively infected cells due to an immune system attack. The function g_{is} will depend on the ability of the immune system to recognize viral proteins on the surface of actively infected cells and kill these cells by antibody and complement and mechanisms of cell mediated immunity involving CTL, ADCC, natural killer cells, or other immune system effector functions.

Equation (6) models the free virus population. I assume that when an actively infected T4 cell with specificity k becomes stimulated through exposure to antigen k, replication of the virus is initiated and N viruses are produced before the host cell dies. Because actively infected T4 cells of any specificity may produce virus, a sum over all antigens k is included. Virus is also produced by syncytia at rate $N_s\mu_s$ (Lifson et al. 1986) or infected monocytes at rate k_{vm}. Free virus is lost by binding to monocytes or T4 cells of any antigen specificity. Because virus may bind to cells without successfully infecting them, I have chosen rate constants for binding k'_m and k'_1 greater than the corresponding rate constants for infection, i.e., $k'_1 \geq k_1$, $k'_m \geq k_m$. The next term, $-\mu_v v$, accounts for any viral death and/or clearance from the body. Another means of loss of virus is by antibody neutralization. This can be modeled by the term $-k_n v h(A_v)$, where A_v is the concentration of viral specific antibody; k_n is the rate of virus neutralization. The function $h(A_v)$ determines the amount of antibody bound to HIV; I have already developed rather realistic models for such binding processes (Brendel and Perelson 1987a,b) and these models can be used for $h(A_v)$. The production of HIV specific antibody would also need to be modeled. This task is discussed below. Antibody directed against gp120 can block syncytium formation. The terms corresponding to this effect have not yet been included in the model.

Equations (7) and (8) for the uninfected and infected macrophage/monocyte populations are similar to Eqs. (1) and (2). Uninfected cells are produced at a rate s_m and die at a rate μ_m. Free virus particles can infect $CD4^+$ monocytes at rate $k_m v m$. Note that k_m need not equal k_1; the virus may have different tropisms for macrophages and T cells (Gartner et al. 1986). Syncytia can form between monocytes and infected $CD4^+$ cells. Thus I include the term $-k_s m(T^{**} + m^*)$. I assume that monocytes can also become infected by engulfing free virus at a rate that would depend upon the amount of antibody bound to the virus; in Eqs. (7) and (8) the term $k_{phag} m v h(A_v)$ accounts for the effect of phagocytosis. It is also possible that monocytes phagocytose a virally infected cell, especially if it is opsonized. The rate of this process is modeled by $k'_{phag} m T^{**} g_{opson}(A_v)$. A corresponding term is substracted in Eq. (3) to account for the loss of actively infected cells by phagocytosis. The function $g_{opson}(A_v)$ models the binding of antibody to viral proteins expressed on actively infected cells and the efficiency of opsonization, which depends upon the level of antibody coating. Virus might also spread from T4 cell to monocyte or vice versa during antigen presentation. Such transfer terms have not been included in this formulation.

Equation (10) describes the changes in the concentration of antigen. I assume that antigen can be supplied to the system at rate $s_a(t)$, that it grows according to a logistic law with rate r_a, and that it dies (or is non-specifically eliminated from the body) at rate μ_a. An immune response can also lead to the elimination of the antigen at rate $\mu_{ir} a_k g_{ir}$. The intensity of the immune response will depend on the population level of T4 helpers specific for the antigen through the function g_{ir}. Including a time-dependent source term is important because antigen could be given in single doses, as in vaccination, released continuously, as in the case of shed gp120, or introduced into the system at random times, as might occur for environmental antigens. If the antigen is non-growing, as in the case of a vaccine or gp120, $r_a = 0$. A particularly simple case is to assume that $r_a = 0$, that $s_a(t) =$ constant, and to ignore the immune response. The antigen concentration will then reach a steady level. If the antigen is HIV then Eq. (6) can be used.

One can also construct equations for the changes in B_k and A_k, the population levels of B cells and antibody of specificity k (cf. Perelson, Goldstein and Rocklin 1980). To model the humoral response properly, one needs to take into account the role of T4 cells as helper/inducers and both lymphocytes and monocytes as secreters of lymphokines and monokines, respectively. I have recently developed a model for IL-2 secretion by T4 cells and the role of IL-2 in T cell proliferation (Kevrekidis, Zecha and Perelson 1988). This model could be incorporated into the proposed model to develop a more detailed picture of the role of T4 cells in the immune response. In the autoimmune theory of Ziegler and Stities (1986) or Hoffmann (1988) anti-idiotypic interactions need to be studied. Idiotypic network models that incorporate antigen specificity are under development (cf. Farmer, Packard and Perelson 1986; Perelson 1988; 1989; Segel and Perelson 1988; 1989) and could be included in a global model of HIV–immune system interactions. It seems clear that a realistic models of HIV infection must take into account the central role of T4 cells, the lymphokines that they secrete, both the humoral and cell mediated immune responses, as well as network interactions. To develop such a model is an enormous undertaking, since it in essence requires modeling the entire immune system. This is a task that will require the efforts of many people over many years.

As in any complex model, the means of proceeding is to initially study simple cases in order to build experiençe about the model's behavior. In the next section I propose and analyze a set of simple models in which the T cell population as a whole is analyzed rather than the antigen specific subpopulations. One goal of these models is see if the long latent period and slow T cell decline can be accomplished with few actively infected cells and a low concentration of free virus particles.

2b. Simple Models

Let T denote the concentration of uninfected T4 cells and let T^* and T^{**} denote the concentrations of latently infected and actively infected T4 cells. The concentration of free infectious virus particles is v. Antigen is not explicitly included in the model. I assume that the dynamics of the various T4 cell populations is governed by the following equations:

$$\frac{dT}{dt} = s - \mu_T T + rT(1 - \frac{T + T^*}{T_{max}}) - k_1 v T, \tag{11}$$

$$\frac{dT^*}{dt} = k_1 v T - \mu_T T^* - k_2 T^*, \tag{12}$$

$$\frac{dT^{**}}{dt} = k_2 T^* - \mu_b T^{**}, \tag{13}$$

$$\frac{dv}{dt} = N \mu_b T^{**} - k_1 v T - \mu_v v \ . \tag{14}$$

The T^{**} term has been omitted from the logistic term in Eq. (11) since it is expected to be negligible when compared with $T + T^*$. For simplicity, I have chosen s to be constant and assume all virus is infectious, i.e., $k_1' = k_1$. Even though antigen is not explicitly included in the model, I assume that there is antigen present and it is responsible for some background level of T cell stimulation. Thus the the fraction of cells stimulated, $f_s(a)$, has been incorporated into the constants r and k_2. Syncytium formation, which is ignored here, will be put back in a later model developed below.

Although this model is very simple and leaves out all of the details of the immune response, it can be used to illustrate one important point. If one chooses parameter values that correspond to infrequent antigen exposure, the model can predict the long lag times seen in AIDS. Further, if one allows s to be a function of v, then T4 cell depletion is predicted, and even differences in the average time to AIDS in children and adults can be explained. I illustrate these points by numerically solving these equations for reasonably realistic parameter values (see Fig. 1). Before discussing the numerical solutions, there are a number of features of this system worth noting.

First, in the absence of virus, the T cell population has the steady state value

$$T_0 = \frac{T_{max}}{2}\left[1 - \frac{\mu_T}{r} + \sqrt{(1 - \frac{\mu_T}{r})^2 + \frac{4s}{rT_{max}}}\,\right] . \tag{15}$$

Thus reasonable initial conditions for this system of equations are $T(0) = T_0$, $T^*(0) = 0$, $T^{**}(0) = 0$, and $v(0) = v_0$.

Second, because actively infected cells are produced slowly by activation of latently infected cells and then live only a brief time before death by excess viral replication, I expect one can make a quasi-steady state assumption, i.e., after a fast transient:

$$T^{**} = \frac{k_2 T^*}{\mu_b} . \tag{16}$$

Thus if $k_2/\mu_b << 1$, then only a small fraction of T4 cells will be actively infected. In Fig. 1 $k_2/\mu_b = 10^{-4}$ and $T^{**}/T^* \simeq 10^{-4}$ as predicted by Eq. (16).

Third, if the infection is slow, over a rather long time scale one would expect T to be relatively constant and T^* to be in quasi-steady. During the period of validity of these assumptions

$$T^* = \frac{k_1 v T}{\mu_T + k_2} . \tag{17}$$

For the parameters in Fig. 1 with $N = 700$, Eq. (17) reduces to $T^* \simeq 3\times10^2 v$ and T is approximately constant, until day 2000. At this time, $v \simeq 10^4$ and $T^* \simeq 3 \times 10^6$ as predicted.

The system of equations, (11) - (14) with the quasi-steady state assumptions (16) and (17), and T assumed constant, reduces to a single linear equation

$$\frac{dv}{dt} = \left[\left(\frac{N k_2}{\mu_T + k_2} - 1\right) k_1 T - \mu_v\right] v . \tag{18}$$

Thus, virus will grow only if the term in parenthesis is positive, i.e. if

$$N > \frac{\mu_T}{k_2} + 1 . \tag{19}$$

For the parameters of Fig. 1, this condition becomes $N > 601$. Solution of the full nonlinear system shows that the critical value of N is somewhat larger than 650. Thus Eq. (19) only provides an approximate guideline. However, it does point out that the number of virus particles produced by an actively infected cell is a crucial parameter in determining the course of HIV infection. If N is less than a critical value, approximately given by Eq. (19), then virus population ultimately decreases to zero. From Eq. (19), one sees that this is due to fewer viruses being produced by actively infected cells per time unit than are eliminated by the death of latently infected cells. Measuring N is crucial to understanding the dynamics of HIV infection. I know of no precise measurements in the literature, although Layne et al. (1989) estimate $N > 300$ from data on the minimum concentration of soluble CD4 needed to block HIV infectivity in an *in vitro* assay.

Lastly, observe that if $T =$ constant, then Eqs. (12)-(14) becomes a linear system characterized by three eigenvalues. The two quasi-steady state assumptions made above would then correspond to having two relatively large negative eigenvalues.

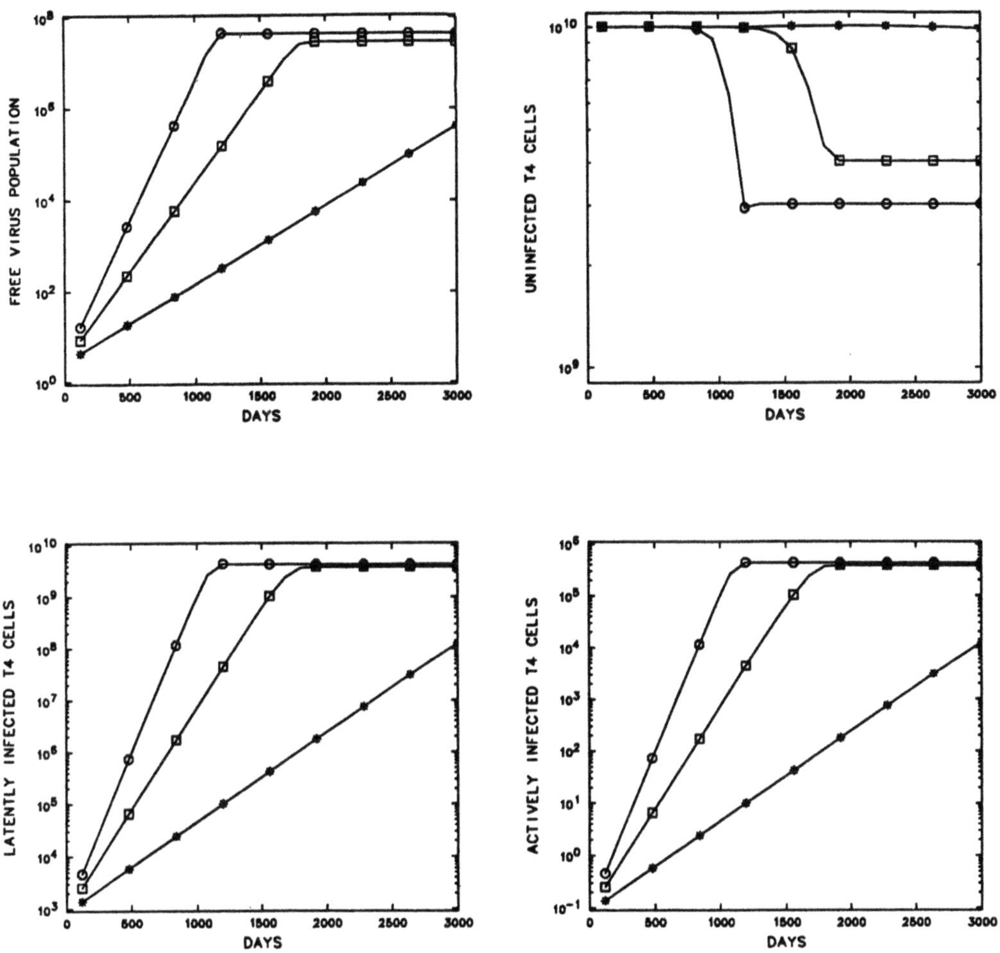

Fig. 1. Solution of Eqs. (11)-(14) with $s = 1.5 \times 10^7$, $\mu_T = 0.003$, $r = 4.5 \times 10^{-3}$, $T_{max} = 1.5 \times 10^{10}$, $k_1 = 10^{-10}$, $k_2 = 5 \times 10^{-6}$, $\mu_b = 0.05$, $\mu_v = 0.1$, $v_0 = 10^3$, $T_0 = 10^{10}$, and $N = 700$ (*), 750 (□), 800 (○). The first time point is at 40 days, so that a fast initial decline in the initial free virus population due to binding uninfected cells is not shown. If $N = 600$ (not shown), the virus population decays to less than one virus particle in about 135 days, and the uninfected T cell population remains approximately constant at 10^{10}.

Equation (19) should be the condition for the third eigenvalue to be positive. When this occurs, the dynamics will be dominated by the process of viral growth, and one should see a slow increase in virus without many cells being latently or actively infected. Eventually, the virus population will build up to a point where the assumption that $T =$ constant is no longer valid, and the uninfected population will decline while the infected population will increase. This event would then correspond to the end of the latent period and beginning of active disease, e.g., ARC or AIDS. Whether this scenario is a correct reflection of the solutions to Eqs. (11) - (14) or not will depend upon the parameter values. A detailed analysis of the validity of the two quasi-steady state assumptions and the dynamics of the resulting model involving only v and T will be presented elsewhere.

The choice of appropriate parameter values is a difficult issue. The number of T4 cells in the peripheral blood of man is approximately 10^{10}. For a blood volume of 10 liters, this then corresponds to a T4 cell concentration of $1000/mm^3$, the level normally found in peripheral blood (cf. Lane and Fauci 1985). Thus I choose as the initial condition, $T_0 = T(0) = 10^{10}$. This number could increase by 50% to 100% or so during infection. Thus T_{max} is between 1.5×10^{10} and 2.0×10^{10}.

I assume that activated T cells divide every 12 to 18 h. Therefore the growth rate of an activated cell is $0.1 - 0.05h^{-1}$. This growth rate needs to be multiplied by the fraction of T4 cells that are dividing. This is probably on the order of a few percent. To this is added a death rate, so that r represents the net increase in the population when cell death is taken into account. In the simulations reported here, I let $r = 4.5 \times 10^{-3}h^{-1}$, which is 50 % larger than the death rate used (see below). Smaller growth and death rates would also be reasonable.

The lifetime of unactivated T cells is variable. Recent work of Gray (1989) indicates that memory T cells may live 2 to 6 weeks (336 - 1000 h) in the absence of antigen stimulated replication. Thus I take $\mu_T = 0.003 - 0.001h^{-1}$.

The supply of new T cells from precursor populations must be less than the number required to maintain the T cell population constant. Thus $s \leq \mu_T T_0$. With $T_0 = 10^{10}$, and μ_T as above, $s \leq 3 \times 10^8$ to $10^8 h^{-1}$. I have taken $s = 1.5 \times 10^7 h^{-1}$. With r as given above, half of the T cell replenishment is by proliferation in the periphery and half from the supply term. The parameters r, s, and μ_T have been chosen so that, in the absence of virus, the population of T4 cells is maintained at its initial value $T_0 = 10^{10}$. Other choices of these parameters, of course, can also maintain this steady state population level.

Estimating the rate k_1 at which virus infects T cells is difficult. Because k_1 is a bimolecular rate constant, it has the dimensions of one over cell concentration per unit time. A useful scaling is therefore to consider $k_1 T_0$ which has the units of one over time. Here I have chosen $k_1 T_0 = 1h^{-1}$. This is roughly the same magnitude that is estimated by assuming that free virus particles are transported in a diffusion limited process to the surface of uninfected T4 cells. Convective transport may also play some role, thus raising the rate. However, once a virus particle encounters a cell, it need not infect it. Thus, only a fraction of the encounters will be successful. As an initial guess, I have taken these factors to cancel.

Latently infected cells behave the same as normal T cells and thus have the same death rate. However, I assume that when they see antigen, rather than dividing, they become actively infected. The time for death of an actively infected cell is probably less than a day. Thus $\mu_b = 0.1 - 0.05h^{-1}$. The number of viruses released N is not known precisely; estimates vary between 100 and 1000.

The rate of conversion of a latently infected cell to an actively infected cell by interaction with antigen is k_2. Only T cells which recognize and respond to the antigen activate HIV replication. Thus k_2 is the rate of T cell activation (e.g., $0.05h^{-1}$) times the fraction of cells activated. I assume that at the low level of antigen present in the environment, activation of latently infected cells will be rare. Say only a few percent of antigen specific cells might become activated. Further, I assume that only a few percent of T cells will be specific for antigen present at any given time. Thus I have chosen $k_2 = 5 \times 10^{-6}h^{-1}$. Clearly, during times of infection by other disease causing agents, this situation could change. Models by Cooper (1986), Intrator, Deocampo and Cooper (1988), McLean (1988) and Reibnegger et al. (1987) all consider this situation.

Figure 1 shows that with the number of viruses released on T cell death $N = 700$, the course of the infection is over 9 years. No T cell depletion is evident, and although free virus is growing exponentially, there are still less than 10^{-4} free virus particles per T cell. Also at the end of 9 years, only 1% of T cells are latently infected and 1 in 10^6 are actively infected. However, if N is increased to 800, T4 cell depletion occurs in 3 years, and the number of latently infected cells grows to more than 10% of the population.

In this model, the total T cell population (infected plus uninfected) never decreases to 10% of its initial value. One can obtain such depletion, but only if the virus population grows to be comparable to the T cell population. To kill T cells with few viruses, I have added to the model syncytia formation and infection of T cell precursor cells. The latter I model by making the T cell source term s be a function of the viral load v. For example, assuming $s = s(v) = se^{-\gamma v}$ with γ small, say $\gamma = 10^{-5}$, no effect is seen until v is approximately 10^4 to 10^5, then the source decreases and T cell depletion occurs. In Fig. 2, I show the effects of changing γ from zero (i.e., Fig. 1) to $\gamma = 10^{-5}$. T cell depletion now is more gradual, occurs earlier, and is somewhat more profound particularly with regard to latently infected T cells.

The average time to AIDS in children is approximately 2 years, whereas it is significantly longer in adults. Medley et al. (1987) and Anderson and May (1988) suggest that it may be eight years, whereas other workers estimate somewhat longer,

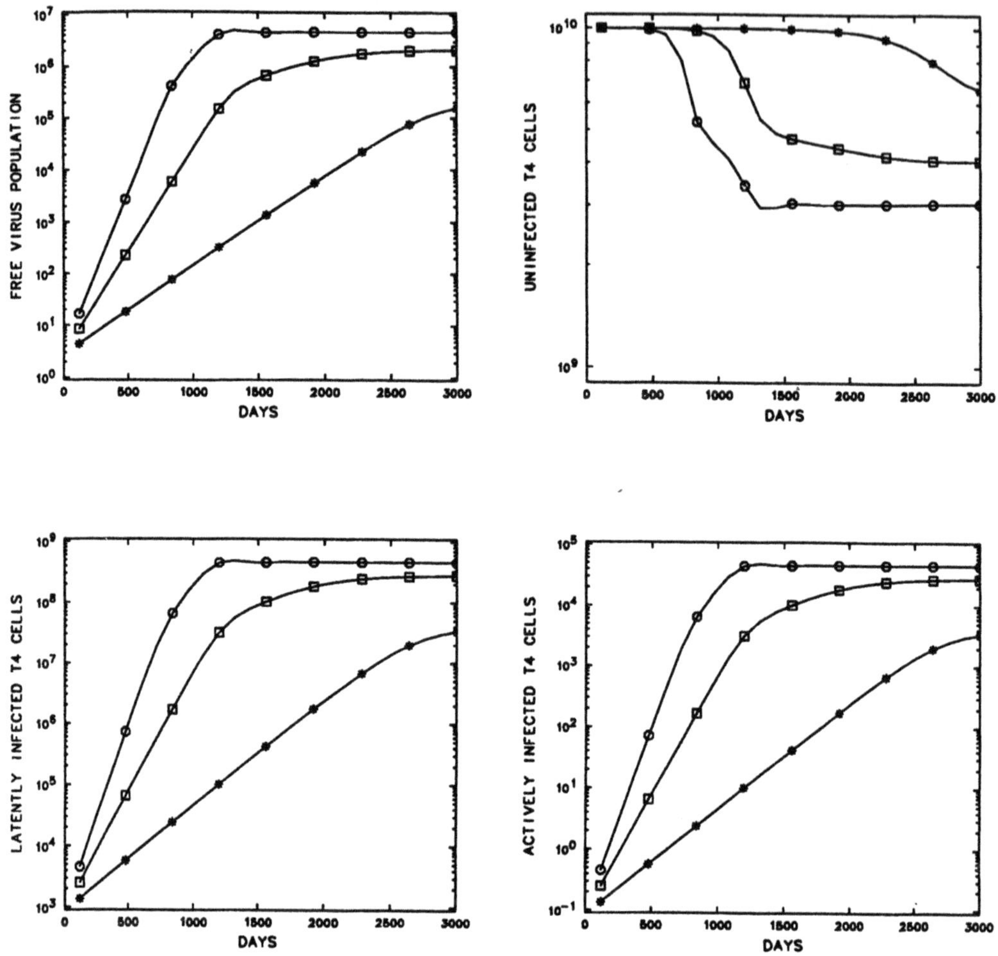

Fig. 2. Parameters same as Fig. 1 except $s = s(v) = se^{-\gamma v}$ and $\gamma = 10^{-5}$. $N = 700$ (*), 750 (□), 800 (○).

9.8 years (Bacchetti and Moss 1989) or shorter, 5.3 years (Costagliola et al. 1989) incubation times. While these estimates are continually being revised as new data becomes available, it seems clear that the incubation period is substantially longer in adults than in children. What can cause this difference? In adults, the thymus slowly atrophies, and thus T cells must maintain their population size mainly by proliferation in the periphery. In children, the thymus is still growing, and I assume it is being used to generate new T cells. Thus bone marrow or thymic infection, which reduces s, should have a greater effect on children than on adults and may contribute to the difference in latent periods. In Fig. 3, I show the results of assuming that 90% of T4 cells are supplied by the bone marrow, 10% from growth, and $\gamma = 10^{-5}$. Examining the $N = 800$ curve one sees that there is major T cell depletion by day 700. The oscillations that are seen are of an amplitude that might not be noticed in a patient. Making γ smaller (e.g. $\gamma = 10^{-4}$) will result in increased and earlier depletion for $N = 700$.

A very interesting feature of Fig. 3 is that it seems to fit many of the puzzling quantitative features of HIV infection. For all values of N the number of latently infected cells is at most 10^7, i.e., 1/1000th of the normal T cell population level. This is in accord with recent (unpublished) polymerase chain reaction measurements. Further, the number of actively infected cells is less than 10^3 and thus below the estimates of 1 in 10^4 or 10^5 cells expressing viral RNA. The total T4 cell population decays to about 30% of normal. Lastly, the number of free virus particles is also low, 10^5 in 10 liters or 0.01 virus particles per μl.

Another means of T cell depletion is syncytium formation. The general structure of a model of syncytia formation was discussed in Section 2a. Adding syncytium formation to the simple model given above yields the following:

$$\frac{dT}{dt} = se^{-\gamma v} - \mu_T T + rT(1 - \frac{T + T^*}{T_{max}}) - k_1 vT - k_s TT^{**} - k_s' TS, \tag{20}$$

$$\frac{dT^*}{dt} = k_1 vT - \mu_T T^* - k_2 T^* - k_s T^* T^{**} - k_s' T^* S, \tag{21}$$

$$\frac{dT^{**}}{dt} = k_2 T^* - \mu_b T^{**} - k_s (T + T^*) T^{**}, \tag{22}$$

$$\frac{dv}{dt} = N \mu_b T^{**} + N_s \mu_s S - k_1 vT - \mu_v v, \tag{23}$$

$$\frac{dS}{dt} = k_s (T + T^*) T^{**} - \mu_s S, \tag{24}$$

where μ_s is the death rate of syncytia, N_s is the number of virus particles released by a syncytium during its life, and k_s and k_s' are the rate constants describing syncytium formation and the addition of a cell to an existing syncytium. In this simple model, I have assumed $k_s'' = 0$, i.e., that actively infected cells do not fuse to syncytia. Since syncytia are thought to live only for one or two days, $\mu_s = .04 - .02h^{-1}$ (Lifson et al.

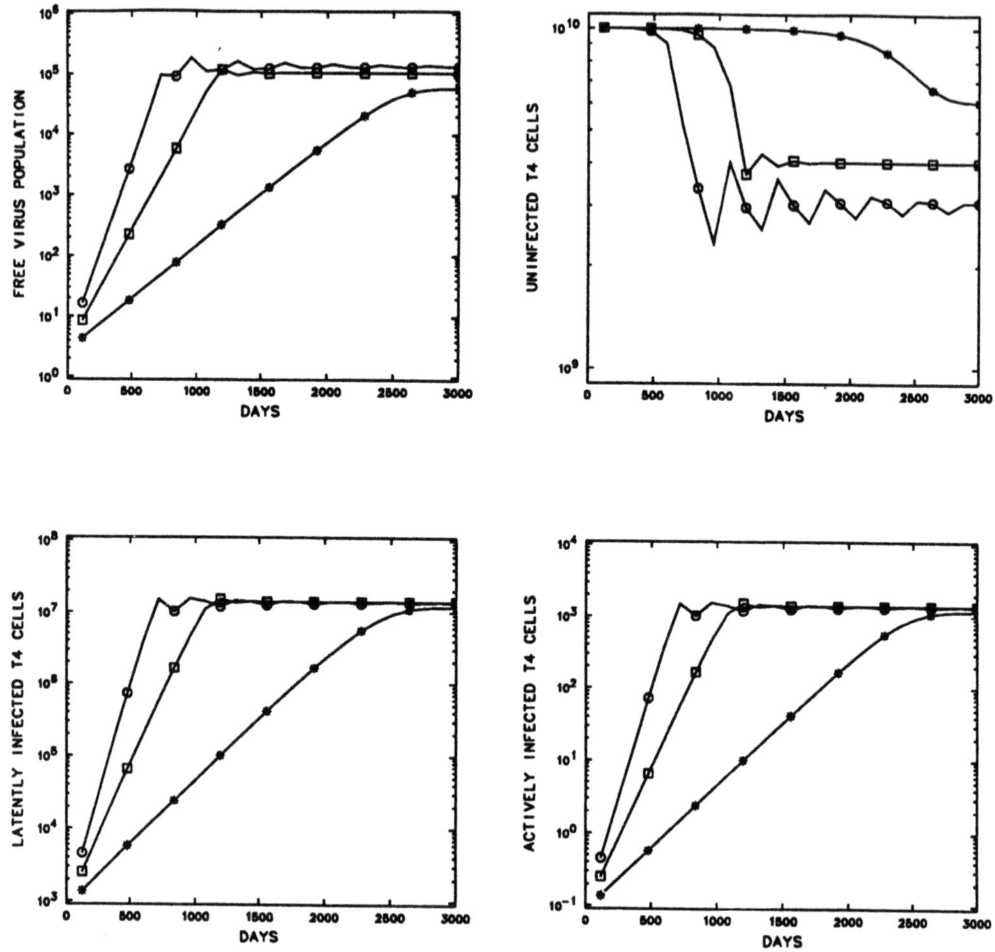

Fig. 3. Parameters same as Fig. 2 except now 90% of uninfected T cells are contributed by the source, i.e., $s = 2.7 \times 10^7$ and $r = 9 \times 10^{-4}$. $N = 700$ (*), 750 (□), 800 (○).

1986b). The number of virus particles produced by a syncytium is not known, but it seems reasonable to assume that $N_s > N$.

Preliminary simulations (not shown) indicate that syncytium formation can reduce the T cell population. However, as one might expect, the behavior of the system is sensitive to the choice of N_s and μ_s. Because actively infected T cells are converted to syncytia, the relationship between the number of viral particles produced by an actively infected T cell during its lifetime and the number of virus particles produced by the syncytium it forms is important in determining the long-term behavior of the system. If the syncytium produces fewer virus particles than the T cell, the infection can be dissipated through syncytium formation.

Macrophage and monocytes may serve as reservoirs for the virus. A simple way of incorporating these effects is to add a source term to equation (23).

A more complete exploration of this simple model is underway and will be reported in a future publication.

Acknowledgements

This work was completed under the auspices of the U.S. Department of Energy. It was supported in part by grant # R89LANL003 from the University of California Universitywide Task Force on AIDS. Conversations with Charles DeLisi contributed to the formulation of the models presented here. Also a workshop on the interaction of HIV with the immune system, sponsored by the Santa Fe Institute, generated ideas that were helpful in the modeling process. George Nelson assisted with the computer simulations and provided helpful discussions.

REFERENCES

Anderson, R.M. and R.M. May. (1988). Epidemiological parameters of HIV transmission. *Nature*, 333, 514-518.

Bacchetti, P. and A.R. Moss. (1989). Incubation period of AIDS in San Francisco. *Nature*, 338, 251-253.

Brendel, V. and A.S. Perelson. (1987a). A note on stochastic models for bacterial adhesion. *J. Theoret. Biol. 126, 247-249.*

Brendel, V. and A.S. Perelson. (1987b). Kinetics of adsorption processes. *SIAM J. Appl. Math.*, 47, 1306-1319.

Cooper, L.N. (1986). Theory of an immune system retrovirus. *Proc. Natl. Acad. Sci. USA*, 83, 9159-9163.

Costagliola, D., J.-Y. Mary, N. Brouard, A. Laporte, and A.-J. Valleron. (1989). Incubation time for AIDS from French transfusion-associated cases. *Nature*, 338, 768-769.

Dalgleish, A.G., P.C.L. Beverley, P.R. Clapham, D.H. Crawford, M.F. Greaves, and R.A. Weiss. (1984). *Nature*, 312, 763-767.

De Boer R.J. and P. Hogeweg. (1987). Immunological discrimination between self and non-self by precursor depletion and memory accumulation. *J. Theoret. Biol.*, 124, 343-369.

Edelman, A.S. and S. Zolla-Pazner. (1989). AIDS: a syndrome of immune dysregulation, dysfunction and deficiency. *FASEB J.*, 3, 22-30.

Farmer, J.D., N.H. Packard, and A.S. Perelson. (1986). The immune system, adaptation, and machine learning. *Physica*, 22D, 187-204.

Fauci, A.S. (1986). Current issues in developing a strategy for dealing with the acquired immunodeficiency syndrome. *Proc. Natl Acad. Sci USA*, 83, 9278-9283.

Fauci, A.S. (1988). The human immunodeficiency virus: infectivity and mechanisms of pathogenesis. *Science*, 239, 617-622.

Folks, T.M., J. Justement, A. Kinter, C.A. Dinarello, and A.S. Fauci. (1987). Cytokine-induced expression of HIV-1 in a chronically infected promonocyte cell line. *Science*, 238, 800-802.

Gartner, S., P. Markovits, D.M. Markovitz, M.H. Kaplan, R.C. Gallo, and M. Popovic. (1986). The role of mononuclear phagocytes in HTLV-III/LAV infection. *Science*, 233, 215-219.

Gelderblom, H.R., E.H.S. Hausmann, M. Ozel, G. Pauli, and M.A. Koch. (1987). Fine structure of human immunodeficiency virus (HIV) and immunolocalization of structural proteins. *Virology*, 156, 171-176.

Gluckman, J.C., D. Klatzmann, and L. Montagnier. (1986). Lymphadenopathy associated virus infection and acquired immunodeficiency syndrome. *Ann. Rev. Immunol.*, 4, 97-117.

Gray, D. (1989). T cell and B cell memory are short-lived in the absence of antigen. *J. Cell. Biochem.*, Suppl. 13A, C010.

Harper, M.E., L.M. Marselle, R.C. Gallo, and F. Wong-Stall. (1986). *Proc. Natl. Acad. Sci USA*, 83, 772-776.

Ho, D.D., R.J. Pomerantz, and J.C. Kaplan. (1987). Pathogenesis of infection with human immunodeficiency virus. *N. Engl. J. Med.*, 317, 278.

Hoffmann, G. (1988). On I-J, a network centre pole and AIDS. In *The Semiotics of Cellular Communication in the Immune System*, E. Sercarz, F. Celada, N. A. Mitchison and T. Tada (eds.), pp. 257-271. Springer-Verlag, New York.

Intrator, N., G.P. Deocampo, and L.N. Cooper. (1988). Analysis of immune system retrovirus equations. In *Theoretical Immunology, Part Two*, A. S. Perelson (ed.), pp. 85-100. Addison-Wesley, Redwood City, CA.

Kevrekidis, I.G., A.D. Zecha, and A.S. Perelson. (1988). Modeling dynamical aspects of the immune response. I. T cell proliferation and the effect of IL-2. In *Theoretical Immunology, Part One*, A. S. Perelson (ed.), pp. 167-197. Addison-Wesley, Redwood City, CA.

Kiprov, D.D., D.F. Busch, D.M. Simpson, P.R. Monrad, G. P. Tardelli, J.H. Gullett, R. Lippert, and H. Mielke. (1984). Antilymphocyte serum factors in patients with acquired immunodeficiency syndrome. In *Acquired Immune Deficiency Syndrome*, M. Gottlieb and J. Groopman (eds.), pp. 299-308. Alan Liss, New York.

Klatzmann, D., E. Champagne, S. Chamaret, J. Gruest, D. Guetard, T. Hercend, J.C. Gluckman, L. and Montagnier. (1984). T-lymphocyte T4 molecule behaves as the receptor for human retrovirus LAV. *Nature*, 312, 767-768.

Klatzmann, D. and L. Montagnier. (1986). Approaches to AIDS therapy. *Nature*, 319, 10-11.

Lane, H.C. and A.S. Fauci. (1985). Immunologic abnormalities in the acquired immunodeficiency syndrome. *Ann. Rev. Immunol.*, 3, 477-500.

Layne, S.P., J.L. Spouge, and M. Dembo. (1989). Quantifying the infectivity of HIV. *Proc. Natl. Acad. Sci. USA*, 86, 4644-4648.

Levy, J.A. (1988). Mysteries of HIV: challenges for therapy and prevention. *Nature*, 333, 519-522.

Lifson, J.D., G.R. Reyes, M.S. McGrath, B.S. Stein, and E.G. Engleman. (1986a). AIDS retrovirus induced cytopathology: Giant cell formation and involvement of CD4 antigen. *Science*, 232, 1123-1127.

Lifson, J.D., M.B. Feinberg, G.R. Reyes, L. Rabin, B. Banapour, S. Chakrabarti, B. Moss, F. Wong-Staal, K.S. Steimer, and E.G. Engleman, E. G. (1986b). Induction of CD4-dependent cell fusion by the HTLV-III envelope glycoprotein. *Nature*, 323, 725-728.

Lyerly, H.K., T.J. Matthews, A.J. Langlois, D.P. Bolognesi, and K.J. Weinhold. (1987). Human T-cell lymphotropic virus III_B glycoprotein (gp120) bound to CD4 determinants on normal lymphocytes and expressed by infected cells serves as a target for immune attack. *Proc. Natl. Acad. Sci. USA*, 84, 4601-4605.

McLean, A. (1988). HIV infection from an ecological viewpoint. In *Theoretical Immunology, Part Two*, A. S. Perelson (ed.), pp. 77-84. Addison-Wesley, Redwood City, CA.

Medley, G.F., F.M. Anderson, D.R. Cox, and L. Billard. (1987). Incubation period of AIDS in patients infected via blood transfusion. *Nature*, 328, 719-721.

Merrill, S. (1989). Modeling the interaction of HIV with cells of the immune response. This volume.

Perelson, A.S. (1988). Toward a realistic model of the immune system. In *Theoretical Immunology, Part Two*, A. S. Perelson (ed.), pp. 377-401. Addison-Wesley, Redwood City, CA.

Perelson, A.S. (1989). Immune network theory. *Immunol. Rev.*. In press.

Perelson, A.S., B. Goldstein, and S. Rocklin. (1980). Optimal strategies in immunology. III. The IgM-IgG switch. *J. Math. Biol.*, 10, 209-256.

Prince, H.E., V. Kermani-Arab and J.L. Fahey. (1984). Depressed interleukin 2 receptor expression in acquired immune deficiency and lymphadenopathy syndromes. *J. Immunol.* 133, 1313-1317.

Reibnegger, G., D. Fuchs, A. Hausen, E.R. Werner, M.P. Dierich, and H. Wachter. (1987). Theoretical implications of cellular immune reactions against helper lymphocytes infected by an immune system retrovirus. *Proc. Natl. Acad. Sci. USA*, 84, 7270-7274.

Segel, L.A. and A.S. Perelson. (1988). Computations in shape space. A new approach to immune network theory. In *Theoretical Immunology, Part Two*, A. S. Perelson (ed.), pp. 321-343. Addison-Wesley, Redwood City, CA.

Segel, L.A. and A.S. Perelson. (1989). Shape Space Analysis of Immune Networks. In *Cell to Cell Signalling: From Experiments to Theoretical Models*, A. Goldbeter (ed.), pp. 273-283. Academic Press, New York.

Shaw, G.M., B.H. Hahn, S.K. Arya, J.E. Groopman, R.C. Gallo, and F. Wong-Staal. (1984). Molecular characterization of human T-cell leukemia (lymphotropic) virus type III in the acquired immune deficiency syndrome. *Science*, 226, 1165-1171.

Sidroski, J., W.C. Goh, C. Rosen, K. Campbell, and W.A. Haseltine. (1986). Role of the HTLV-III/LAV envelope in syncytium formation and cytopathicity. *Nature*, 322, 470-474.

Stricker, R B., T.M. McHugh, D.J. Moody, W.J. Morrow, D.P. Stities, M.A. Shuman, and J.A. Levy. (1987). An AIDS-related cytotoxic autoantibody reacts with a specific antigen on stimulated $CD4^+$ T cells. *Nature*, 327, 710-713.

Takeda, A. C.U. Tuazon, and F.A. Ennis. (1988). Antibody-enhanced infection by HIV-1 via Fc receptor-mediated entry. *Science*, 242, 580-583.

Zagury, D., J. Bernard, R. Leonard, R. Cheynier, M. Feldman, P.S. Sarin, and R.C. Gallo. (1986). Long-term cultures of HTLV-III-infected T cells: A model of cytopathology of T-cell depletion in AIDS. *Science*, 231, 850-853.

Ziegler, J. L. and D.P. Stities. (1986). Hypothesis: AIDS is an autoimmune disease directed at the immune system and triggered by a lymphotropic retrovirus. *Clin. Immunol. Immunopathol.*, 41, 305-313.

MODELING THE INTERACTION OF HIV WITH CELLS OF THE IMMUNE SYSTEM

Stephen J. Merrill
Department of Mathematics, Statistics and Computer Science
Marquette University
Milwaukee, WI 53233

Abstract

Several mathematical models describing the interaction of HIV with T4 lymphocytes and macrophages are presented. The primary problems addressed involve the decline of immunocompetence as mirrored by the T4 cell number, the role of macrophages in the disease process, the interaction in early stages of AIDS, and the fraction of infected circulating T4 cells.

1. Introduction

The interaction of a pathogenic agent with the immune response usually generates both the elimination of the agent and a variety of disease symptoms, some caused by the pathogen, some by the immune response itself, and some caused by the interaction of the two. Effective treatment of an illness requires an understanding of the cause of each symptom, what that indicates about the stage of interaction between the pathogen and the defenses, and how that interaction may be modulated by outside agents and medication. In AIDS, the goal is the same. However, the pathogenic agent, HIV, is sufficiently novel and complex that such an understanding is not at all easy to achieve. Moreover, as the primary target cells of HIV are all central figures in the immune response itself, the problem is further knotted.

In this paper, we will describe some preliminary efforts to model the interaction of HIV with two cells of the immune response, the T4 helper-inducer lymphocyte and cells of the monocyte/macrophage lineage (here called collectively "macrophages"). The

T4 cell, the linchpin of the immune response, is the primary host of HIV. This cell, through contact and chemical messengers, initiates and controls most aspects of the immune response. The macrophage is a "sticky" and phagocytic cell which captures and processes antigen, and serves to produce necessary chemical signals in immune responses.

The interaction of HIV with each of these cells has quite a different natural history. The replication phase in the T4 cell is triggered by stimulation of the cell by an antigen recognized by that T4 cell. Until that stimulation, the viral genes are latent. In the macrophage, HIV probably enters primarily through phagocytosis and through the CD4 marker (the site used on the T4 cell). Apparently HIV does not kill the macrophage, but remains latent or slowly replicating, releasing particles in a more or less continuous fashion with a rate depending on the level of maturation of the cell (Orenstein et al. 1988). Due to the nature of the macrophage involvement, it is generally thought that the infected macrophages may act as a reservoir for the virus, both shielding the virus from the immune response and acting as a source of infectious particles (Popovic and Gartner 1987).

Until now, a primary difficulty in understanding the disease process in AIDS has been the lack of a good animal model for AIDS. Hopefully, mathematical models, used primarily to suggest research directions and investigate potential strategies, will help to fill that gap. The following models attempt to deal with the extraordinary complexity of the interaction between HIV and the immune system. They are speculative and theoretical but represent a beginning in the iterative modeling process.

Generally, the models have a "stochastic" as opposed to a "deterministic" setting. This was done for two primary reasons. First, one of the goals is to obtain distributional information, specifically the latency distribution and the variation in the progression of AIDS from individual to individual. Stochastic models are the necessary format for that work. Secondly, these models either are or will soon be made nonlinear (or density dependent). With these processes, depending on the nonlinearities, approximation of the expected value of the process by a solution of an associated ordinary differential equation may not be straightforward. In Kurtz (1981), for instance, it is shown that a differential equation will approximate a jump Markov process but only after assuming a very restrictive form for the variation of the jump probabilities in terms of the state. In other results (e.g. Wofsey 1980), very careful scaling is required and different approximations result from different scalings. The difficulty is also illustrated in the second model below, (3), where the variance is seen to affect the equation for the expected value, E(t). An obvious approximating differential equation will result if, through a change of scale, the associated variance goes to zero (in the appropriate manner along with other technical requirements to insure convergence in some sense).

2. Early Stages: Exposure and Acute Infection

After exposure to HIV, only 10-20% of those individuals infected have acute symptoms of infection (Bull. WHO 1987). Those that do usually present a condition like mononucleosis, which lasts about two weeks and then disappears. In most cases then, HIV causes no symptoms initially, but slowly makes itself known six weeks to a year after exposure, detected eventually by seroconversion (presence of antibody to HIV) (Redfield and Burke 1988). HIV infection usually announces itself clinically through lymphadenopathy, chronically swollen lymph nodes, due to large numbers of stimulated B-lymphocytes (cells responsible for antibody production). Up to the point of seroconversion, the interaction between HIV, T4 cells and macrophages dictates the time course of the disease.

Let $I(t)$ be the number of HIV-infected T4 lymphocytes at time t. We will first examine $I(t)$ under the assumption that there is no macrophage source,and then investigate the same process with the addition of an external source of viral particles. This will enable us to probe the potential of the role of the macrophage population as a reservoir for the virus.

Given an infected T4 cell, at some random time (exponentially distributed with parameter α), the cell will die (when it is stimulated by an antigen), releasing a large number of viral particles. Each of these particles independently tries to infect a new T4 cell. If we assume that the probability of any one virion infecting a T4 cell is small, the number of newly infected T4 cells which results from the death of the cell will follow a Poisson distribution. We take the mean to be some number λ. Assuming that the mean time to a T4 death is much larger than the infective half-life of HIV, we view this process without the free virus stage, that is, one cell dies and gives rise to a number of new daughter cells according to some distribution. As such, it becomes a continuous time branching process. In order to specify such a process, one must specify the infinitesimal probabilities of the process

$$I(t) = \{ \text{ number of infected T4 cells at time } t, \text{ given } I(0) = 1\}.$$

These are of the form (Karlin and Taylor 1975)

$$\delta_{1k} + a_k h + o(h), k = 0, 1, 2, \cdots ,$$

where

$$\delta_{1k} = \begin{cases} 1 & \text{if } k = 1 \\ 0 & \text{otherwise.} \end{cases}$$

These quantities represent the probability that an infected T4 will die giving rise to k daughters during the time interval $(t, t+h)$. (The Dirac delta function, used here to conveniently express the first term, is 1 if both arguments are the same and 0 otherwise.) It is assumed that

$$a_1 \leq 0, a_k \geq 0 \text{ for } k = 0, 2, 3, \cdots,$$

and

$$\sum_{k=0}^{\infty} a_k = 0.$$

In the particular situation being described, there are two (assumed independent) processes involved, one being cell death and the release of the viral particles, and the other being the new infection of T4 cells. As the time to death and release is exponentially distributed with parameter α, the infinitesimal probability of a death and no newly infected T4 cells (assuming the Poisson distribution for the number of newly infected cells) is determined by a_0, where

$$a_0 = \alpha e^{-\lambda}.$$

Similarly, for $k \geq 2$,

$$a_k = \alpha e^{-\lambda} \frac{\lambda^k}{k!}.$$

For $k = 1$, to insure that the sum of the a_k's is zero,

$$a_1 = \alpha(-1 + \lambda e^{-\lambda}) < 0.$$

Much is known about such processes, and several properties can be seen through the generating function of the infinitesimal probabilities (Karlin and Taylor 1975). Using the Poisson form for the a_k's,

$$u(s) = \sum_{k=0}^{\infty} a_k s^k = ae^{-\lambda} e^{\lambda s} - \alpha s. \tag{1}$$

In particular, if the expected (or mean) value of I(t) is $m(t)$,

$$m(t) = \exp(u'(1)t) = \exp(\alpha(\lambda - 1)t).$$

Also, the extinction probability, q (the probability of *not* remaining infected once exposed), is the smallest root of $u(s) = 0$. Here

$$s = e^{\lambda(s-1)}.$$

Note that this is independent of α and depends only on the mean number of newly infected cells, λ. If $u'(1) = \alpha(\lambda - 1) \leq 0$, $q = 1$; otherwise q is a decreasing function of λ (see Figure 1). Unfortunately, no estimate of λ exists to our knowledge.

With infected macrophages adding infectious virions to the blood, and as a result, causing additional T4 cells to be moved to the infected population, one could either model the altered number of infected T4 cells as two separate processes which interact

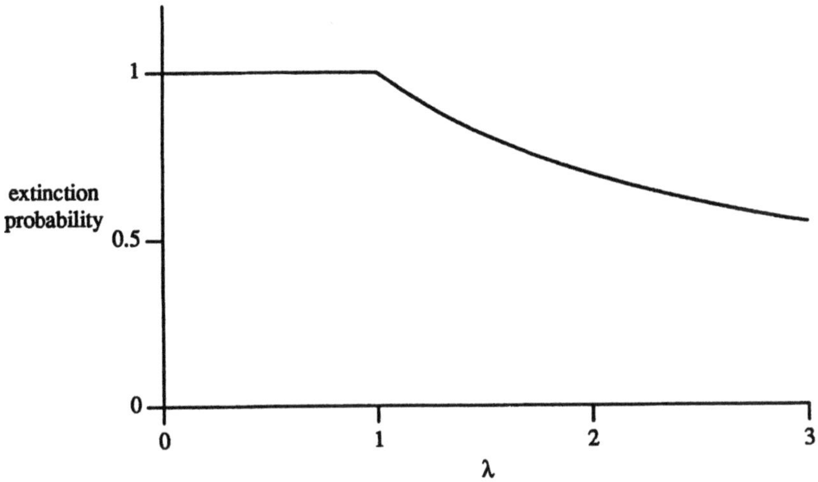

Figure 1. Extinction probability as a function of the mean number of newly infected T4 cells per HIV-killed infected T4 cell.

or, as below, add to the $I(t)$ process through an immigration term. In other words, viral particles released from the macrophages infect T4 cells in a manner which is independent of the process previously described. (By this approach, the additional macrophages infected during the life of the model are ignored.)

Let

$$\delta_{0k} + b_k h + o(h), k = 0, 1, 2, \cdots$$

denote the probability that k T4 cells are added to the infected population during time t to $t + h$ due to the infected macrophage source. Here the general form assumes

$$b_0 \leq 0 \text{ and } b_k \geq 0 \text{ for all other } k,$$

with

$$\sum_{k=0}^{\infty} b_k = 0.$$

Given the "smoother" nature of the HIV lifecycle in the macrophage, we will assume that this immigration acts as a pure birth process so that

$$b_1 = \beta, b_0 = -\beta \text{ and all other } b_k\text{'s are zero.}$$

Then

$$v(s) = \sum_{k=0}^{\infty} b_k s^k = -\beta + \beta s$$

is the infinitesimal generating function for the immigration process.

By writing this process as two interacting continuous time branching processes, one can show (Karlin and Taylor 1975) that if

$$P_k(t) = P\{I(t) = k|L(0) = 0\},$$

and if $\phi(t;s) = \sum_{k=0}^{\infty} P_k(t)s^k$ is $I(t)$'s generating function, then ϕ satisfies

$$\begin{aligned}\frac{\partial\phi}{\partial t} &= u(s)\frac{\partial\phi}{\partial s} + v(s)\phi \\ &= (\alpha e^{\lambda(s-1)} - \alpha s)\frac{\partial\phi}{\partial s} + (-\beta + \beta s)\phi\end{aligned} \tag{2}$$

with initial condition $\phi(0;s) = 1$ and that $E(I(t)) = \frac{\partial\phi}{\partial s}|_{s=1}$. Using techniques outlined in Karlin and Taylor (1975), one can also show that $E(I(t)) \approx \frac{\beta}{\alpha(\lambda-1)}(e^{\alpha(\lambda-1)t} - 1)$ (this may actually hold with equality). If $\lambda > 1$, exponential growth results while when $\lambda < 1, E(I(t)) \to \frac{\beta}{\alpha(1-\lambda)}$.

Before the antibody response is made, it seems likely that $\lambda > 1$ (more than one newly infected cell for each T4 death) as the number of virions released is large (probably on the order of 100,000 from an infected T4 cell). After the primary antibody response (or through therapies using soluble CD4 or other drugs to interfere with the infection process), it may be possible to drive $\lambda < 1$. With the macrophage source however, it appears that a long term (asymptomatic) phase would result and not a cure.

3. Stage 2: Chronic Lymphadenopathy

The previous model predicts that when $\lambda > 1$, an outbreak (and viremia) occurs. This would result in a full-scale immune response against the envelope proteins of HIV (those directly exposed to the response). Important here is the finding that although a large quantity of antibody is produced against HIV at this stage, the fraction of that antibody that is neutralizing (capable of making the virus noninfective) is very low. Moreover, there seems to be little relationship between the antibody "quality" in asymptomatic seropositive individuals and those with AIDS (Bull. WHO 1987). This may be due to "enhancing" effects of antibody produced against HIV, now labeled ADE. As a result, one main aspect of the immune defense against viruses is generally ineffective against HIV. That, when coupled with the cellular mechanisms' relative inability to identify and destroy latently infected cells, results in an immune response that is eventually unable to control the infection. Several models have been proposed to describe this stage: Cooper (1986), Intrator et al. (1988), McLean (1988), Merrill (1988), Reibnegger et al. (1987), and Reibnegger et al. (1989). Most virtually ignore the inhibition of growth by an active immune response, because of the above argument.

In keeping with the mathematical tone of the previous discussion, the model developed in Merrill (1988), based on stochastic considerations, will be presented. The model contains four main quantities which are changing in time:

a) infected macrophages, denoted $M_i(t)$,
b) free infective viral particles, $V(t)$,
c) infected T4 lymphocytes, $I(t)$, and
d) the total cell population $L(t)$.

Assuming $V(t)$ is piecewise continuous, let

$$M_i'(t) = \gamma_1 V(t)(Mac - M_i(t)) - \gamma_2 M_i(t).$$

Here Mac is the (constant) total number of macrophages and γ_1, γ_2 are positive rate constants.

It will be assumed that the half life of infectivity $(\frac{1}{\beta})$ of HIV particles is relatively short, so that at any time, $\frac{dV}{dt} \approx 0$. This means that

$$V(t) = \frac{\alpha}{\beta} I(t) + \frac{\delta}{\beta} M_i(t),$$

except for small transitional times. Here α is the rate at which the infected T4 cells are stimulated (and begin the HIV replication producing N viral partices) and $N\delta$ is the rate at which infected macrophages produce viral particles.

$I(t)$ is a stochastic quantity (non-homogeneous birth-and-death process) satisfying

$$\begin{aligned} &Pr\{I(t+\Delta t) - I(t) = 1 | I(t) = j\} = k_1 v(t)(L(t) - j)\Delta t + o(\Delta t), \\ &Pr\{I(t+\Delta t) - I(t) = -1 | I(t) = j\} = \alpha j \Delta t + o(\Delta t), \text{ and} \\ &Pr\{I(t+\Delta t) - I(t) = 0 | I(t) = j\} = 1 - [k_1 V(t)(L(t) - j) + \alpha j]\Delta t + o(\Delta t). \end{aligned}$$

In Merrill (1988) it was shown that if $E(t) = E(I(t))$ and $Var(t)$ are the expected value and the variance of the process, respectively, then

$$\begin{aligned} E'(t) = &\left(-\alpha + k_1 \frac{\alpha}{\beta} L(t) - k_1 \frac{\delta}{\beta} M_i(t)\right) E(t) \\ &- k_1 \frac{\alpha}{\beta} \left(Var(t) + (E(t))^2\right) + k_1 \frac{\delta}{\beta} M_i(t) L(t). \end{aligned} \tag{3}$$

As similar equations for the variance would involve even higher moments, an appeal to an independent determination of the relationship between $E(t)$ and $Var(t)$ was made.

Consider $R(t)$ viral particles distributed among $L(t)$ cells, each particle choosing independently. Then under conditions when the chance of a random T4 being infected is rare (which seems to almost always be the case), the probability $p(k)$ of a particular

T4 being infected by k particles should follow a Poisson distribution with parameter $\lambda = \lambda(t)$. In particular $P(0) = e^{-\lambda(t)}$ is the probability of picking a non-infected cell at time t. By a binomial argument,

$$E(t) = L(t)\left(1 - e^{-\lambda(t)}\right) \tag{4}$$

and

$$Var(t) = L(t)\left(1 - e^{-\lambda(t)}\right)e^{-\lambda(t)}. \tag{5}$$

We now examine the expected number of T4 lymphocytes at time t, $\hat{L}(t)$, governed by

$$\hat{L}(t) = S_2 - (\varepsilon\hat{L} + \alpha E(t)). \tag{6}$$

Here S_2 is the source, ε the natural removal rate, and excess death depends on the stimulation of infected cells. Using (3), (4), (5), and (6), the following system results:

$$\begin{aligned}
M_i' &= \gamma_1\left(\frac{\alpha}{\beta}\hat{L}\left(1 - e^{-\lambda(t)}\right) + \frac{\delta}{\beta}M_i\right)\left(\frac{S_1}{\gamma_2} - M - i\right) - \gamma_2 M_i,\\
\hat{L}' &= S_2 - \left(\varepsilon\hat{L} + \alpha\hat{L}\left(1 - e^{-\lambda(t)}\right)\right),\\
\lambda' &= \left(1 - e^{-\lambda(t)}\right)\left(-S_2 + \hat{L}\left\{-\varepsilon - \left(\alpha e^{-\lambda(t)} + k_1\frac{\delta}{\beta}M_i + k_1\frac{\alpha}{\beta}e^{-\lambda(t)}\right)\right\}\right.,\\
&\quad \left. + \hat{L}^2\left\{k_1\frac{\alpha}{\beta} + \left(1 - e^{-\lambda(t)}\right)\right\}\right) + k_1\frac{\delta}{\beta}M_i\hat{L}, \text{ and}\\
M_i(0) &= M_0 \geq 0, \hat{L}(0) = L_0 \geq 0, \lambda(0) \geq 0.
\end{aligned} \tag{7}$$

In Merrill (1988), a reduced system involving no macrophage source was examined. Here we present a partial description of the solutions of (7).

Making a change of variable,

$$\theta = 1 - e^{-\lambda(t)} \text{ (θ is the infected fraction)},$$

all solutions of (7) stay within a compact set,

$$D = \left\{\left(M_i, \hat{L}, \theta\right) \middle| 0 \leq \theta \leq 1, \frac{S_2}{\varepsilon + \alpha} \leq \hat{L} \leq \frac{S_2}{\varepsilon}, 0 \leq M_i \leq \frac{S_1}{\gamma_2}\right\}.$$

We also note that $\theta = 1$ is an invariant face, and that there is a unique stable equilibria which is actually globally attracting on that face. The following is true.

THEOREM 1. *If $S_2 > (\alpha + \varepsilon)(\alpha + 2\beta/k_1)$, then the $\theta = 1$ equilibrium point attracts everything in the set D.*

PROOF: Let

$$f(\hat{L},\theta) = -S_2 + \hat{L}\left\{-\varepsilon - \left(\alpha e^{-\lambda(t)} + k_1\frac{\delta}{\beta}M_i + k_1\frac{\alpha}{\beta}e^{-\lambda(t)}\right)\right\}$$
$$+ \hat{L}^2\left\{k_1\frac{\alpha}{\beta} + \left(1 - e^{-\lambda(t)}\right)\right\}.$$

Under the hypothesis, it will be shown below that in D, $f(\hat{L},\theta) > 0$. Thus

$$\theta' = (1-\theta)\left\{\theta f(\hat{L},\theta) + (1-\theta)k_1\frac{\delta}{\beta}M_i(t)\hat{L}(t)\right\}$$

is positive inside D. As a result, $\theta(t)$ is monotone increasing, bounded above, and

$$\lim_{t\to\infty}\theta(t) = 1.$$

Now if $f(\hat{L},\theta) > 0$, $\theta' \geq 0$. And $f(\hat{L},\theta) = 0$ when

$$\theta = \frac{S_2 - \hat{L}\left(\varepsilon - \left(\alpha + k_1\frac{\alpha}{\beta}\right)\right) - \hat{L}^2\frac{k_1\alpha}{\beta}}{\hat{L}\left(\alpha + k_1\frac{\alpha}{\beta}\right) + \hat{L}^2}.$$

The graph of this relationship is given in Figure 2.

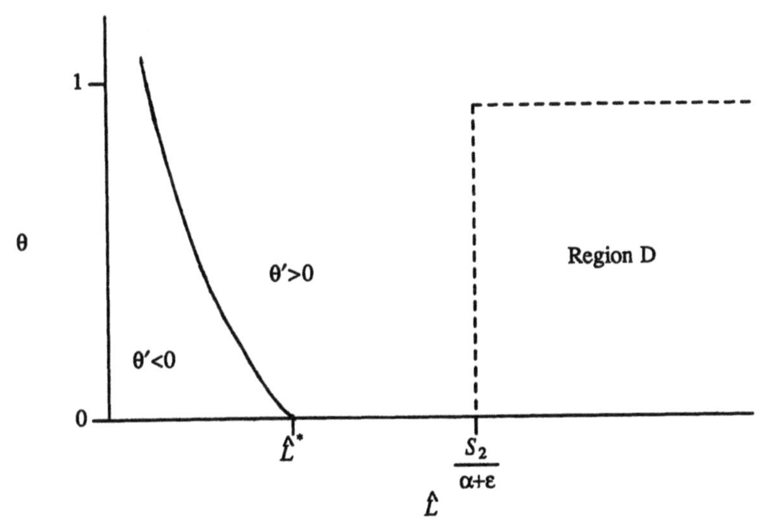

Figure 2. $f(\hat{L},\theta) > 0$ (and thus $\theta' > 0$) when $\hat{L}(t) \geq \frac{S_2}{\alpha+\varepsilon} > \hat{L}^*$. $\hat{L}^*$ is the positive value of $\hat{L}$ where $f(\hat{L},0) = 0$.

To the right of this graph, $\theta' > 0$. As $\hat{L} \geq \frac{S_2}{(\varepsilon+\alpha)}$, if $0 < \hat{L}^* < \frac{S_2}{(\varepsilon+\alpha)}, \theta' > 0$ within D. The complete argument is given in the appendix. From Theorem 1, under some conditions, the infected fraction is monotonically increasing and $\hat{L}(t)$ approaches a number dependent on α and the natural homeostatic parameters. This represents the progressive nature observed in this disease. Much work remains to be done in order to understand this complex system under other conditions; however, preliminary study has shown that this monotonicity cannot always be expected. This raises the possibility of a chronic nonprogressive form for AIDS, which would be seen in the model as a "persistent" solution.

As the number of T4 lymphocytes decreases, there is a corresponding increase in the severity of the immune dysfunctions characterizing AIDS. In fact, the T4 cell count is a natural marker of disease progression (Bull. WHO 1987). This model displays the role of α in this process, α being the stimulation rate by all antigens. eommonly seen antigens are thought to be "cofactors" or even "helpers" modulating the rate of disease progression (Quinn et al. 1987).

4. T4 Lymphocyte Age Distribution

One of the paradoxes uncovered in AIDS research is the very low frequency of infected T4 cells found in peripheral blood. Initial estimates placed the number on the order of 1 out of 10,000 circulating T4 cells. If correct, the primary mechanism responsible for the loss of T4 cells in vitro, the cytopathic nature of HIV, would be hard to propose as the mechanism in vivo. Recent findings now suggest that the fraction of infected cells is increasing with disease progression and may eventually be more on the order of 1 per 100. The following model was constructed to determine the age distribution of all T4 cells if infected cells were preferentially killed. By examining this distribution, the infected cell numbers as a fraction of total population could be compared with that which was observed, thereby providing indirect evidence for or against specific as opposed to nonspecific T4 killing mechanisms. If specific killing of infected cells is the primary mechanism for T4 population reduction in AIDS, then as the process evolves, relatively more young (uninfected) T4 cells are seen, as the disease has preferentially killed the older (and more likely to be infected) ones.

Let $L(a,t)$ be the T4 lymphocyte density of age a at time t. Then using the standard (MacKendrick) aging model,

$$\frac{\partial L}{\partial a} + \frac{\partial L}{\partial t} = -(\text{ age specific death rate}).$$

There are two loss terms: first the natural death, and second, the HIV-dependent death. To derive the second term, we first need to calculate the probability that a lymphocyte at age a is infected. Assuming an exponential (random) time to infection, the probability of infection by age a is $1 - e^{-\mu a}$ where $1/\mu$ is the mean time to infection for a T4 cell. Thus the full age specific death rate is

$$\varepsilon L + \alpha(1 - e^{-\mu a})L,$$

and the full model to be examined is

$$\frac{\partial L}{\partial a} + \frac{\partial L}{\partial t} = -\varepsilon L - \alpha(1 - e^{-\mu a})L \tag{8}$$

with

$$L(a, 0) = \psi(a)$$

and

$$L(0, t) = S_2,$$

the initial and boundary conditions, respectively. Here again, parameters have meanings essentially identical to those in the previous section. The initial condition $\psi(a)$ represents the age distribution before the effects of the disease process, while the boundary condition reflects the source from the bone marrow of new T4 cells (all at the youngest age).

The solution of (8) is

$$L(a, t) = \phi(a - t)e^{-(\varepsilon+\alpha)t - \frac{\alpha}{\mu}e^{-\mu a}},$$

where

$$\phi(\xi) = \begin{cases} \psi(\xi)e^{-\frac{\alpha}{\mu}e^{-\mu a}} & \text{if } \xi > 0 \\ S_2 e^{-(\varepsilon+\alpha)\xi} & \text{if } \xi < 0. \end{cases}$$

Of specific interest is the fraction of lymphocytes found to be infected with HIV at any time. To that end, consider first $t > a$. Then

$$L(a, t) = \tilde{L}_\alpha(a) = S_2 e^{-(\varepsilon+\alpha)a - \frac{\alpha}{\mu}e^{-\mu a}} \tag{9}$$

is seen to be the stationary solution approached for any initial condition ψ.

The stationary solution without the HIV-dependent killing is obtained by setting $\alpha = 0$,

$$\tilde{L}_o(a) = S_2 e^{-\varepsilon a},$$

an exponential age distribution.

Assuming, as before, that the probability of infection by HIV if the cell has attained age a is $1 - e^{-\mu a}$, the number of infected cells under stationary conditions is

$$\int_0^\infty (1 - e^{\mu a})\, \tilde{L}(a)da.$$

As the total number of lymphocytes is

$$\int_0^\infty \tilde{L}(a)da,$$

the fraction infected, I, is

$$I = \frac{\int_0^\infty (1 - e^{-\mu a})\, S_2 e^{-(\varepsilon+\alpha)a} da}{\int_0^\infty \left(S_2 e^{-(\varepsilon+\alpha)a - \frac{\alpha}{\mu} e^{-\mu a}}\right) da}.$$

Making a change of variable

$$u = e^{-\mu a},$$

and using integration by parts,

$$I = \frac{\frac{\mu}{\alpha} e^{-\frac{\alpha}{\mu}}}{\int_0^1 u^{(\frac{\varepsilon+\alpha}{\mu}-1)} e^{-\frac{\alpha}{\mu}u} du} - \frac{\varepsilon}{\alpha}. \tag{10}$$

When $\alpha = 0$ (if infection did not increase the death rate),

$$I = \frac{\mu}{\mu + \varepsilon}.$$

In the expression for I given in (10), note that only two parameters are involved:

$$\gamma = \frac{\alpha}{\mu} \text{ and } \eta = \frac{\varepsilon}{\mu}.$$

In terms of those parameters,

$$I = \frac{\frac{1}{\gamma} e^{-\gamma}}{\int_0^1 u^{(\gamma+\eta-1)} e^{-\gamma u} du} - \frac{\eta}{\gamma}. \tag{11}$$

$I = I(\eta, \gamma)$ is a decreasing function of both variables. As α increases, the infected fraction decreases. Although the analysis is not complete, it appears that I can be made arbitrarily small by choosing the parameters appropriately. For most choices of the parameters, fractions typically on the order of 10were observed. If specific killing is the primary mechanism, the model suggests that infected cell frequencies of a few percent with a predominance of young cells should be obseved.

5. Summary

Several models have been presented, most still in the stages of construction and analysis. All, however, display features of HIV and AIDS which suggest that even models as simple as these may have value in attaining an "understanding" of AIDS.

Many more areas remain to be studied. For example, a further description of the time to reach each stage and the variability would be of use both to health planners and to physicians managing AIDS cases. Also of great use would be a derivation of the infectivity of an individual at various stages and the construction of a modeling platform to evaluate various treatment options.

6. Appendix

The algebraic argument necessary to justify claims made in the proof of Theorem 1 follows. If $S_2 > (\alpha+\varepsilon)\left(\alpha + \frac{2\beta}{k_1}\right)$,

$$\frac{k_1}{\beta} S_2 - 2(\alpha+\varepsilon) > (\alpha+\varepsilon)\frac{k_1\alpha}{\beta}$$

and

$$\frac{k_1\alpha}{\beta} S_2 + (\alpha+\varepsilon)(\varepsilon-\alpha) - (\alpha+\varepsilon)\frac{k_1\alpha^2}{\beta} > (\alpha+\varepsilon)^2.$$

thus

$$1 < \frac{k_1\alpha}{\beta}\frac{S_2}{(\alpha+\varepsilon)^2} + \frac{1}{\alpha+\varepsilon}\left(\varepsilon - \alpha\left(1 + \frac{k_1\alpha}{\beta}\right)\right)$$

and

$$4S_2\frac{k_1\alpha}{\beta} < \left(\frac{2k_1\alpha}{\beta}\frac{S_2}{\alpha+\varepsilon}\right)^2 + \frac{4k_1S_2\alpha}{\beta(\alpha+\varepsilon)}\left(\varepsilon - \alpha\left(1 + \frac{k_1\alpha}{\beta}\right)\right).$$

This implies

$$\sqrt{\left(\varepsilon - \alpha\left(1 + \frac{k_1}{\beta}\right)\right)^2 + 4S_2\frac{k_1\alpha}{\beta}} < 2\frac{k_1\alpha}{\beta}\frac{S_2}{\alpha+\varepsilon} + \left(\varepsilon - \alpha\left(1 + \frac{k_1\alpha}{\beta}\right)\right)$$

and

$$\hat{L}^* = \frac{-\left(\varepsilon - \left(\alpha + \frac{k_1\alpha}{\beta}\right)\right) + \sqrt{\left(\varepsilon - \left(\alpha + \frac{k_1\alpha}{\beta}\right)\right)^2 + 4S_2\frac{k_1\alpha}{\beta}}}{2\frac{k_1\alpha}{\beta}} < \frac{S_2}{\alpha+\varepsilon}.$$

REFERENCES

Bulletin of the World Health Organization. (1987). 65, 453-463.

Cooper, L.N. (1986). Theory of an immune system retrovirus. *Proc. Natl. Acad. Sci. USA*, 83, 9159-9163.

Intrator, N., G.P. Deocampo and L.N. Cooper. (1988). Analysis of immune system retrovirus equations. In *Theoretical Immunology, part two*, A. S. Perelson (ed.). pp.85-100. Addison-Wesley, New York.

Karlin, S. and H.M. Taylor. (1975). *A First Course in Stochastic Processes*, 2nd ed. Academic Press, New York.

Kurtz, T.G. (1981). *Approximation of Population Processes.* Society for Industrial and Applied Mathematics, Philadelphia.

McLean, Angela. (1988). HIV infection from an ecological viewpoint. In *Theoretical Immunology, part two.* A. S. Perelson (ed.). pp.77-84. Addison-Wesley, New York.

Merrill, Stephen J.(1988). AIDS: Background and the dynamics of the decline of immunocompetence. In *Theoretical Immunology, part two*, A. S. Perelson (ed.). pp. 59-75. Addison-Wesley, New York.

Orenstein, J.M., M.S. Melter, T. Phipps and H.F. Gendelman. (1988). Cytoplasmic assembly and accumulation of Human Immunodeficiency Virus types 1 and 2 in recombinant human colony-stimulating factor-1-treated human monocytes: an ultrastructural study. *J. Virol.*, 62, 2578-2586.

Popovic, M. and S. Gartner. (1987). Isolation of HIV-1 from monocytes but not lymphocytes. *Lancet*, ii, 916.

Quinn, T.C., P. Piot, J.B. McCormick, F.M. Feinsod, H. Taelman, B. Kapita, W. Stevens and A.S. Fauci. (1987). Serologic and immunologic studies in patients with AIDS in North America and Africa: the potential role of infectious agents as cofactors in human immunodeficiency virus infection. *Jour. Am. Med. Assoc.*, 257, 2617-2621.

Redfield, R.R. and D.S. Burke. (1988). HIV infection: the clinical picture. *Sci. American*, 259, 90-98.

Reibnegger, G., D. Fuchs, A. Hausen, E.R. Werner, M.P. Dierich and H. Wachter. (1987). Theoretical implications of cellular immune reactions against helper lymphocytes infected by an immune system retrovirus. *Proc. Natl. Acad. Sci. USA*, 84, 7270-7274.

Reibnegger, G., D. Fuchs, A. Hausen, E.R. Werner, G. Werner-Felmayer, M.P. Dierich and H. Wachter.(1989). Stability analysis of simple models for immune cells interacting with normal pathogens and immune system retroviruses. *Proc. Natl. Acad. Sci. USA*, to appear.

Wofsey, C. (Lipow).(1980). Behavior of limiting diffusions for density-dependent branching processes. In *Biological Growth and Spread*, W. Jäger, H. Rost, P. Tautu (eds.), pp.36-49. Springer-Verlag, Berlin.

WHEN HIV MEETS THE IMMUNE SYSTEM: NETWORK THEORY, ALLOIMMUNITY, AUTOIMMUNITY, AND AIDS

Geoffrey W. Hoffmann and Michael D. Grant
Departments of Microbiology and Physics
University of British Columbia
Vancouver, B.C., V6T 1W5
Canada

Abstract

It is suggested that the following facts are relevant to AIDS pathogenesis. Firstly, there is complementarity of the AIDS virus envelope glycoprotein gp120 to a molecule on helper T cells called the CD4 protein, and there is also complementarity of CD4 to certain molecules that are important in the immune system, namely class II MHC. In this respect, gp120 is similar to class II MHC, and the anti-viral immune response may include a component that is directed against class II MHC or V regions resembling class II MHC. Secondly, immunization with foreign lymphocytes can lead to the production of antibodies with V regions that resemble MHC proteins. Since infection with HIV often occurs coincidentally with exposure to allogeneic lymphocytes, infected individuals are likely to make such MHC mimicking antibodies. These facts lead to the idea that AIDS is an autoimmune disease that can be triggered by a combination of HIV and allogeneic cells. These two stimuli would produce mutually complementary "MHC-image" and anti-(MHC image) immune responses that could synergize with each other and destabilize the system. We discuss some recent experimental results on autoantibodies found in AIDS patients and in persons at risk for AIDS that support these ideas.

The theory suggests that vaccines consisting of gpl20 or some related substances may cause AIDS in people belonging to high risk groups. It also leads to new experimentally testable predictions and ideas for preventing the disease. For example, we may be able to prevent AIDS using injections of the viral envelope glycoprotein (gp120 or gp160) together with anti-gp120 or anti-gp160.

Further progress may come from a more detailed understanding of the immune system network. A mathematical model of the symmetrical network theory is reviewed briefly.

1. Introduction

How does AIDS kill? There is general agreement that AIDS is caused by HIV (human immunodeficiency virus), but exactly how HIV manages to wreck the patient's immune system is unclear. One view is that HIV kills the crucial helper T cells directly. This concept is supported by the fact that HIV binds to a molecule on the surface of helper T cells, and the count of helper cells decreases progressively during the course of the disease. But there are difficulties with this theory. HIV infects only about one in a thousand of the helper T cells (Harper et al. 1986; Kingman 1988). The immune system has a lot of regenerative ability, so the catastrophic effects of a virus that effects only a small fraction of the cells is an enigma. Furthermore, the severity of the symptoms does not correlate with the amount of virus present. In contrast to other viral diseases, the production of anti-HIV antibodies does not seem to afford protection against AIDS, even when the antibodies inactivate HIV in laboratory tests. On the contrary, people infected with HIV become ill *after* they make anti-HIV antibodies!

An alternative possibility to direct killing by the virus has been discussed by several investigators. The most important function of HIV could be to act as a foreign substance that induces an immune response (Hsia et al. 1984; Ziegler and Stites 1986; Shearer 1986a; Andrieu et al. 1986; Martinez et al. 1988; Hoffmann 1988). The idea is that the virus triggers the production of antibodies that attack the immune system itself. AIDS would then be an autoimmune disease.

We have formulated a detailed autoimmunity theory of AIDS in the context of a network theory of the the regulation of the immune system (Hoffmann 1988; Hoffmann et al. 1988). The theory makes a number of experimentally testable predictions. We will begin by reviewing the model and some recent experimental data that supports it. We will then briefly discuss the type of mathematical modeling that we feel will be necessary for further quantitative development of the theory.

We apologize for the fact that this contribution does not contain very much mathematics; in fact, we have not attempted to mathematically model the dynamics of HIV infection, which is the theme of this volume. We are, however, attempting to formulate a theory of AIDS pathogenesis, so we feel that our paper is not completely out of place. Our goal is the same as those who are mathematically modeling AIDS, namely to understand the disease. We are using this opportunity to draw attention to an autoimmunity theory of AIDS pathogenesis and some of its implications. If the ideas appeal to readers, they may want to participate in translating the ideas into equations. We believe that understanding AIDS will involve understanding the immune system network, and understanding the immune system network will involve mathematical modeling. In our modeling work, we have been focussing so far on the normal immune system network, in the hope of first gaining an adequate understanding of the healthy immune system. At the end of this paper, we briefly outline an immune system network model.

2. Jerne's Network Hypothesis

In the early 1970's, a revolution in our thinking about the immune system was instigated by a paper entitled "Towards a network theory of the immune system" (Jerne 1974). Jerne reasoned that if animals have repertoires of receptors, such that they can make antibodies against practically anything, they should also be able to make antibodies with V (variable) regions against the V regions of other antibodies. This has since been shown to be true. Jerne pointed out that this could lead to a network of interactions between the cells of the immune system, in which each of the antibodies and lymphocytes specifically stimulate and/or suppress a small fraction of all the other lymphocytes in the system. He postulated that this set of interactions existed, and also that it played a central role in the regulation of the immune system. Jerne's ideas provided a new paradigm for cellular immunology, and the conceptual revolution he started is still in progress. The network way of thinking about the immune system is being assimilated by many immunologists, but there is no unanimity in these matters, and many details of the theory remain to be worked out.

An immune response to an antigen involves firstly the proliferation of a set of lymphocytes specific for that antigen. This first set can stimulate a response by a second set of lymphocytes that are specific for the receptors of the first set. The second set can both back-stimulate the first set and stimulate a response by a third set. Must such responses to responses go on forever? The answer is no; the number of specific interactions is high enough, such that any perturbation is expected to fairly quickly encompass the entire network. The immune response is nevertheless specific; each antigen stimulates a different, characteristic change in the network as a whole.

Network theory leads to a shift in focus in our attempts to understand cellular immunology. In addition to studying events at the level of molecules interacting with receptors at the cell surface, we need to be concerned with events at the level of interacting populations, and we need a description in terms of cellular population dynamics. We therefore formulate and study differential equations that model interactions between populations of cells. In such models, we endeavor to find a correlation between the properties of a simulated network of lymphocytes and the experimentally observed stimulus-response behaviors of the system. Key properties we look for in such models include stability and memory. The immune system can exhibit a very large number of stable steady states (or sets of "memories"), so we look for mathematical models that exhibit many stable states, that are based on known facts about lymphocytes and antibodies, and that are capable of simulating switching between different stable states in response to stimulation by antigen. In fact, the system must have an astronomical number of alternative stable steady states to allow for the myriad of different combinations of immunity that are possible.

3. The Symmetrical Network Theory

A model that has had some success in the above respects is the "symmetrical network theory" (Hoffmann 1980; 1982; Gunther and Hoffmann 1982; Hoffmann et al. 1988). The first postulate of the symmetrical network theory is that interactions between the components of the system are symmetrical to a first approximation. Thus if A and B are two cells of the same type but of different specificities, and if A stimulates, inhibits or kills B via V region interactions, then the converse is also true; B can potentially stimulate, inhibit or kill A. For stimulatory interactions, this assumption is based on the the cross-linking (aggregation) of receptors as the mechanism for the specific stimulation of lymphocytes; if A can cross-link the receptors of B, then B can cross-link the receptors of A. This symmetry can be broken by interactions between V regions and other cell surface molecules such as MHC (major histocompatibility complex) proteins. We have found that it is useful to begin model-building with an idealized system that includes only the symmetric interactions. Extensive experimental evidence supports the concept of symmetrical network interactions (reviewed in Hoffmann 1980).

The symmetrical network theory involves the three major kinds of immune system cells, B cells, T cells and macrophages ("A cells"). B cells are responsible for making antibodies and T cells regulate B cells. There is evidence that T cells regulate via protein molecules called "specific factors." These factors are believed to have a molecular weight of about 70,000, so they are only about half as big as an IgG molecule. On this basis, they are assumed in the theory to be monovalent and hence unable to cross-link receptors, but able instead to block receptors. They are ascribed an important inhibitory role. Specific T cell factors are to immunology what quarks are to fundamental particle physics; we would like to have more direct experimental data about them, but if we assume they exist and have certain properties, we can make a nice theory. There is plenty of evidence showing that the factors exist, but their detailed molecular characterization is proving to be difficult.

The symmetrical network theory provides a framework for understanding many immunoregulatory phenomena in the immune system that cannot be discussed in detail here. The phenomena encompassed include specific suppression, the differences between helper and suppressor T cells, the role of variations in network connectivity, the antigen dose dependence of immune responses, the relation of CD4 and CD8 to class II and class I MHC molecules, the functional phenotype of cells bearing these markers, and more.

4. Complementarities, MHC and HIV

The most fundamental concept in molecular and cellular immunology is complementarity. We are concerned with proteins that fit each other like neighboring pieces of a loosely fitting jigsaw puzzle. One molecule is a rough template for the other and vice versa. In order to determine how the system functions, we need to determine which molecules have complementarity for which other molecules, and we need to characterize the regulatory consequences of the complementarities.

Some important complementarities of the healthy immune system involve the major histocompatibility complex (MHC) cell surface proteins. Different people have different MHC antigens, and these differences are responsible for the strong immune responses we make against organ transplants. The MHC cell surface proteins are self-antigens that exert a strong effect on the repertoire of the T lymphocyte V regions. Each individual's T cells undergo selection to have some complementarity to his or her own MHC antigens. The set of receptors on your T cells constitute a biased repertoire, selected to have some complementarity to your MHC antigens. In particular, your helper T cells have complementarity to a set of your MHC molecules called "class II MHC." For brevity we will often write "class II" when we mean "class II MHC molecules".

Figure 1 shows a sequence in which each cell has specific receptors or antigens on its surface that are complementary to the specific receptors or antigens of the next cell. An important complementarity for the AIDS problem is that of the HIV envelope protein, called gp120, to a molecule on the helper T cell surface called CD4. CD4 in turn has complementarity to class II MHC. These complementarities led Ziegler and Stites (1986) to suggest that the parts of gp120 and class II that are complementary to CD4 could be similar to each other. The relevant part of gp120 would then be an "image" of the corresponding part of class II. Ziegler and Stites therefore suggested that the immune response against the virus could include a response against class II. This model is supported by the finding that a mouse monoclonal antibody against gp120 reacts also with human class II antigens (Beretta et al. 1987). On the other hand, there is little evidence that potent antibodies can be made against self MHC antigens, or in other words, that tolerance to self MHC can be severely broken. If antibodies against class II were important, we would expect to see depletion of the cell types that express significant levels of class II antigen, namely B cells and macrophages, rather than T cells. This is not observed, so anti-class II immunity is presumably not so important.

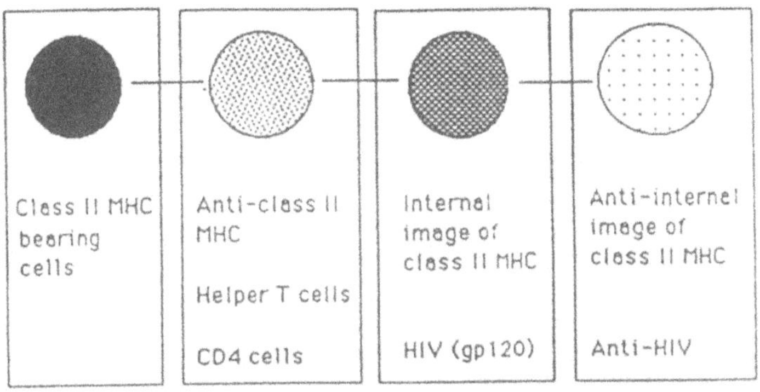

Fig. 1. Relationships between some key components of the immune system and the envelope protein of the AIDS virus (HIV). The cells in this chain have receptors (or antigens) with three-dimensional complementarity to the receptors (or antigens) of their neighbours. The first and third members of this chain have dark shading and the second and fourth members have light shading to suggest similarities in shape in each case.

5. Internal Images

We have considered a slightly more complex model than that of Ziegler and Stites. The V regions of an individual's helper T cells are very diverse, but they all have a weak complementarity to his or her own ("self") class II. This is apparently due to a clonal selection process which ensures that only helper T cells with some anti-class II complementarity survive to become part of the helper T cell repertoire. In a network view of the immune system, it may be expected that the selection of anti-class II helper T cells should be accompanied by the selection of T cells that recognize the V regions of the helper cells. The T cells of this next "generation" have receptors that are complementary to shapes that are complementary to self class II molecules, so they could resemble to some extent the self class II molecules. T cells with receptors that most accurately mimic class II would be most strongly selected, since they interact with the largest number of weakly anti-class II helper T cell clones. In network theory the receptors of these second generation cells are called the *internal image* of the class II antigens. ("Internal" means within the V-region network.) Because of the constraint to recognize as many anti-class II clones as possible, we might expect less diversity at the image-of-self-class-II level than at the anti-self-class-II level (Fig. 2). Mutual stimulation and selection involving the anti-self class II and class II internal image clones could lead to a network topology analogous to an old-fashioned circus tent. Class II image cells correspond to the centre-pole of the tent, and the anti-self-class-II cells (helper cells) correspond to the canvas. The centre-pole

Fig. 2. Clonal selection among T cells interacting with self class II MHC antigens and with each other may lead to this "network focussing" topology. The diverse helper T cells interact with a less diverse set of cells, whose V regions are internal images of self class II MHC.

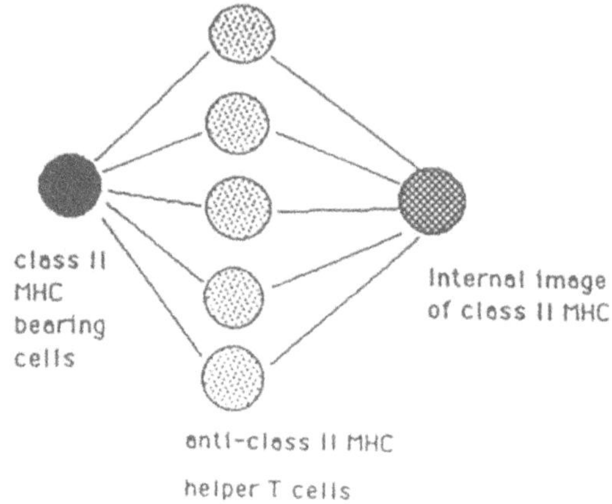

holds up the canvas, and the canvas holds the centre-pole upright. In the same way, positive selection leads to the anti-self-class-II helper T cells stabilizing the class-II-internal-image cells and *vice versa.*

The internal image of class II cannot be exactly identical to class II, since different genes are used. So while people do not seem able to make harmful amounts of antibodies against their own MHC molecules, it may be easier to develop immunity (humoral or cellular) against the slightly different internal image of class II. From the set of complementarities described above, immunity against the envelope of the AIDS virus could also be directed against the internal image of class II, and that is the way we see the immune response to the virus being disruptive. If the class II internal image clones have the role of a stabilizing centre-pole in the network, an attack on these clones could play an important part in destabilizing the system.

An additional complication is that people who contract AIDS typically receive lymphocytes in the blood or ejaculates they receive from their contact person. Shearer (1986b) was the first to emphasize the possible importance of foreign lymphocytes in the etiology of AIDS. He found strong similarities in the pathology observed in AIDS patients and in patients that suffer from graft versus host disease, in which lymphocytes from a graft attack the body of an immunosuppressed patient. Network considerations provide more definite ideas about how the response to lymphocytes could play a role. It has been shown that foreign lymphocytes injected into an animal routinely evoke two immune responses: the first against the foreign MHC antigens on the cell surface (the "anti-foreign" response), and the second against the receptors on the injected cells that recognize the host MHC (Hoffmann, Cooper-Willis and Chow 1986). These receptors are anti-host MHC, so the host's response to the receptors is anti-anti-self MHC. This is a template of a template, so it consists of antibodies with V regions that are internal images-of-self-MHC.

6. Synergy of Two Immune Responses

We are now concerned with two immune responses that can occur in AIDS patients, as shown in Fig. 3. They are both related to self MHC, but are not directed against the MHC itself. The first is the part of the response to gp120 that may be directed also against the V regions that are an internal image of self class II MHC. The second response involves lymphocytes with V regions that are themselves internal images of MHC. We would then have both an *internal image* immune response and an *anti-internal image* immune response, symmetrically directed against each other. It seems probable that there is a synergy between these two responses, with the result that the entire immune system is destabilized at a fundamental level. The two responses are directed against the core of the T-cell network (the internal image of self MHC, or centre pole), and the helper T cells (the canvas that stabilizes the centre-pole). This would explain the collapse of the immune system in AIDS patients even in the absence of much virus.

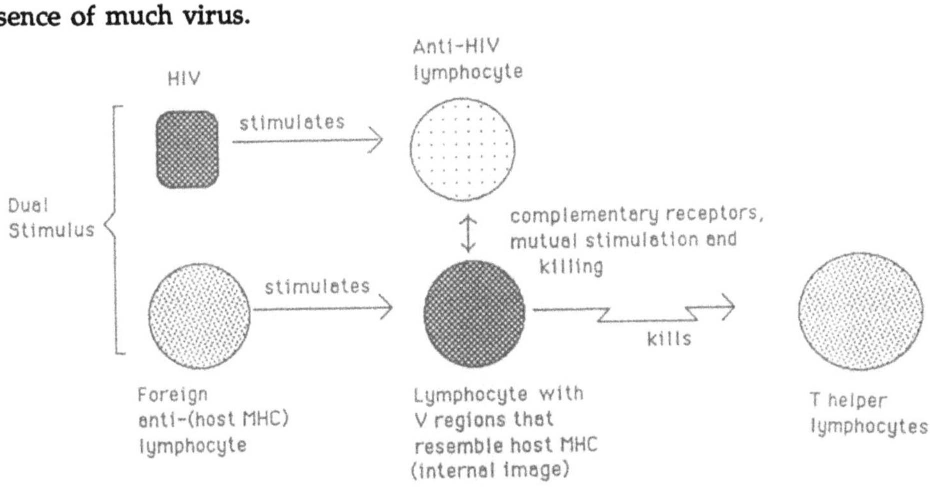

Fig. 3. The set of interactions shown in Fig. 1 leads to this autoimmunity model for the way in which HIV and foreign lymphocytes cause AIDS. Two immune responses are postulated to occur; the first is a response to HIV, the second is a response to the receptors of foreign lymphocytes that recognize host MHC antigens. These two responses are directed against each other, meaning that each perceives the other as an antigen. Synergy between the two responses is postulated to destabilize the system.

This model of pathogenesis leads to several predictions that can be tested. For example, it predicts that internal-image-of-self-MHC antibodies and/or anti-internal-image-of-self-MHC antibodies or corresponding cellular immunities are present in AIDS patients. The theory also suggests new ways of developing animal models for AIDS. Monkeys infected with HIV alone do not get sick. We might be able to find a way to induce AIDS in monkeys by using HIV plus foreign lymphocytes. Another possibility is to immunize animals with a combination of selected anti-CD4 antibodies (which would act as antigens with determinants similar to HIV envelope determinants) and foreign lymphocytes.

7. Autoantibodies

Many autoantibodies have been reported in AIDS (reviewed by Zon and Groopman 1988). Stricker et al. (1987) found antibodies that react with an antigen on T helper cells in 95% of AIDS patients. We have been studying some autoantibodies that occur both in AIDS and in people at risk for AIDS, namely anti-collagen antibodies (Grant, Weaver, Tsoukas and Hoffmann 1989). We found that sera from all 16 members of a group of homosexual AIDS patients in Vancouver contain anti-collagen antibodies. Reactivity against collagen was found also in HIV^+ homosexuals (66%, n=33) and HIV^- homosexuals (32%, n=38). (The anti-collagen antibodies are not just a manifestation of polyclonal B cell activation, since they are present at a much higher level than would be the case if that were so.) Anti-collagen antibodies are found also in graft versus host disease and *systemic lupus erythematosus* (a prototypical autoimmune disease). Graft versus host disease is a form of allogeneic immune response, so the fact that these antibodies are made in those circumstances suggests that the antibodies correlate with alloimmunity. This would be consistent with AIDS being an autoimmune disease that is provoked by a combination of allogeneic cells and HIV.

Systemic lupus erythematosus (SLE), the autoimmune disease mentioned above, has been studied extensively in man and in animal models. Similarities between SLE and AIDS have been noted by Kopelman and Zolla-Pazner (1988). The above theory includes the ideas that AIDS is an autoimmune disease, and that the autoimmunity involves the production of MHC-mimicking antibodies. We have obtained data linking MHC-mimicking antibodies to autoimmunity in a mouse model of SLE (Kion and Hoffmann, 1989). The mouse makes the MHC-mimicking antibodies before it makes the pathological antibodies normally associated with the disease. In view of this timing, it seems possible that such MHC-mimicking antibodies are involved in the development of the disease. It is interesting that this mouse also happens to make anti-collagen antibodies (Tarkowski, et al., 1986).

8. Vaccinate or Tolerize? Implications for Disease Prevention Strategies

Researchers interested in autoimmunity ideas about AIDS are concerned about certain vaccines that are expected to induce the production of antibodies similar to the antibodies induced by the virus. Such substances are predicted to help cause, rather than prevent, the disease. One large vaccine company, Smith-Kline Beckman, is reported to have postponed human vaccine trials on the basis of such concerns. The vaccines in question are firstly the HIV envelope glycoproteins gp160 and gp120, and secondly anti-CD4 antibodies. Glycoprotein gp120 is a fragment of gp160; both gp120 and gp160 include the site that HIV uses to attach to CD4. Anti-CD4 antibodies are being considered as vaccines because part of their V region surface resembles the part of gp120 that binds to CD4.

According to the above model, it is primarily people in high-risk groups that need to be concerned about possible detrimental effects of the vaccines. The theory says the disease is most likely to occur when people receive both allogeneic cells and HIV (or something with a shape resembling HIV, such as the V region of anti-CD4 antibodies). People who do not belong to a high-risk group are relatively unlikely to receive allogeneic cells, so they may have less to worry about. These concerns would not apply to subunit vaccines, consisting of parts of gp120 and gp160 that do not interact with CD4. Autoimmunity concerns also do not apply to p17, a vaccine being tested in England. p17 is a protein of HIV that is not involved in the attachment of the virus to CD4.

The autoimmunity theory of AIDS suggests strategies for combatting the disease that are contrary to most of those currently being explored. The theory suggests we need to dampen the immune response to the envelope protein of HIV rather than immunize to enhance this response. We need to induce tolerance rather than immunity to gp120 and gp160. It may not be very difficult to find ways to suppress this presumptively dangerous part of the anti-HIV response. Specific antibodies can sometimes be used to selectively suppress particular components of an immune response. One possibility would be to use injections of antibodies against the particular V regions that do the damage. Another, simpler possibility is to inject people intravenously with anti-gp120 or anti-gp160 antibodies at about the time of exposure to HIV. It has been known for many years that specific IgG antibodies administered together with a foreign antigen can result in 99% or more suppression of the primary immune response (Uhr and Baumann 1961; Uhr and Möller 1969; Fitch 1974). A "morning after" injection of anti-gp120 may thus be a possibility. Injections of antigen together with antibodies can induce specific immunological tolerance in the sense that a secondary challenge evokes only a weak response (Safford and Tokuda 1971). An injection of antibodies against the relevant part of recombinant gp120 or gp160 together with an injection of recombinant gp120 or gp160 may therefore induce a decreased level of responsiveness to the envelope glycoprotein. This procedure would not preclude the possibility of inducing immunity to other parts of the virus. It is noteworthy that specific antisera have been shown to suppress autoimmunity even in a model system in which an immunogenic form of the antigen is used (Vulpe 1959; Paterson and Harwin 1963; Nakao and Roboz-Einstein 1965; Hughes 1974).

The phenomenon of antibody mediated suppression of the immune response was discovered and investigated most extensively during the 1960's, before the discovery of T cells. Surprisingly, no work seems to have been done on the relationship between antibody mediated suppression and T cell tolerance. Such studies may show that IgG inhibition can be fairly simply understood in the context of the symmetrical network model. An antigen and the its specific antibodies are expected to stimulate antigen specific T cells and anti-idiotypic T cells respectively. Subsequent mutual stimulation between these two populations drives the system towards the symmetrical "suppressed state" of the theory, in which there are elevated levels of both populations. [The reader may wonder how the phenomenon of "IgM enhancement" can then be understood in the context of the model. If specific IgM antibodies are given together with the antigen, they can cause an enhanced immune response (Henry and Jerne 1967). This difference may be related to IgM's greater lytic ability. A single molecule of IgM can kill a cell, while at least two IgG molecules next to each other are necessary to cause lysis of the cell (Borsos and Rapp 1965). Small amounts of IgM may thus kill antiidiotypic T cells more than stimulate them, while the reverse could be true for small amounts of IgG. The IgM antibodies could then drive the system towards the "immune state" of the symmetrical network model.]

Some caution may be necessary with the dual stimulus approach, because the pair of stimuli gp120 and anti-gp120 (for example) are still directed against each other, just as the anti-anti-self response (to allogeneic cells) is directed against the anti-gp120 response. The hope is that a sufficiently small, tolerogenic stimulus will influence mainly the T cell compartment in such a way that specific unresponsiveness to gp120 is induced, and the production of antibodies against the "centre-pole" is inhibited. This can be tested with simian immunodeficiency virus (SIV). SIV causes an AIDS-like disease in the macaque monkey. It is a good model for AIDS in the context of the above model since the envelope protein of SIV binds to CD4, and SIV thus shares the property that is assumed to be the key pathogenic property of HIV.

Since anti-collagen antibodies were found in the serum of all 17 of 17 homosexual AIDS patients studied, one might wonder whether suppression of the production of these antibodies could effect the network in a way that contributes towards suppressing the development of the disease. This would be of interest for HIV positive, anti-collagen negative individuals. We could consider applying a putatively tolerogenic stimulus, perhaps consisting of small amounts of denatured collagen or anti-collagen antibodies (or both, but we again need to be beware of an excessive amount of synergy).

In a recent study by Imagawa et al. (1989), HIV was detected in 31 of 133 seronegative homosexuals who engaged in high risk activity. Of these 31 individuals only four (13 percent) seroconverted within the 28 to 36 month period of the study. Many of the remaining 87 percent that did not seroconvert may be have reached a state of specific immunological tolerance with respect to gp120. Clinicians may be able to promote and/or consolidate the desired tolerant state in such individuals with tolerogenic stimuli such as those mentioned above.

9. Modeling the Immune System Network

We have not modelled the dynamics of the interactions between HIV and the immune system. We are currently still concerned with developing models of the healthy immune system. I will now briefly sketch a mathematical model that has been developed for simulating the interactions of the symmetrical network theory (in the absence of HIV or any other antigen). Since this is not a model of HIV dynamics, the sketch given here is skeletal; fuller descriptions of the model are given in Gunther and Hoffmann (1982) and Hoffmann et al. (1988). Our approach has been to keep the mathematics as simple as possible, and still capture the essence of the network regulatory interactions. Following the example of Richter (1975), we have used only a single variable for cells of each specificity. The simplest system that we have studied that models immunological network interactions is the system

$$\frac{dx_i}{dt} = S_i - x_i \sum_{j=1}^{N} K_{ij} x_j. \qquad (1)$$

Here x_i is the size of the ith population (clone), S_i is a nonspecific rate of influx of the cells of specificity i into the system, and K_{ij} is a symmetric matrix of interaction strengths between clones i and j ($K_{ij} = K_{ji}$), in a system consisting of N clones. This model has the following unusual property. A small, sparsely connected system may be unstable, and as the size (value of N) and/or connectance (fraction of nonzero elements in K_{ij}) increases, the probability of stability increases (Hoffmann 1982; Spouge 1986). The system then has a single attractor. This sytem has been used as a model for the interactions between clones that have not been perturbed by an antigen and are therefore considered to be in a virgin state. The interaction term models the killing of cells by each other, either with antibodies or by a cellular killing mechanism.

The above simple model includes only terms for the constant production of cells and for a killing process that depends linearly on the concentration of "enemies" for each clone. One of the most important properties of the immune system is that it exhibits memory, with a very large number of stable steady states. We add three things to the above model to reflect this, and at the same time, we incorporate more data on the components of the system. Firstly, there are several kinds of killing that occur in the system, some that lead to terms linear in the concentration of "enemies", $\Sigma_j K_{ij} x_j$, and some that have a stronger concentration dependence, which we model with a quadratic term. Secondly, cell death does not depend solely on killing; it seems safe to assume that some lymphocytes die a natural death, and this helps to stabilize the system. Thirdly, we include the specific T cell factors mentioned in Section 3. In our model they have an inhibitory role; they block receptors. Specifically, the factors inhibit both stimulation and killing. (They are also ascribed a second role in switching between stable states, but we won't go into that here). With the above complications we have the following model:

$$\frac{dx_i}{dt} = S_i - k_2 x_i Y_i e_{2i} - k_3 x_i Y_i^2 e_{3i} - k_4 x_i \qquad (2)$$

with $Y_i = \sum_{j=1}^{N} K_{ij} x_j$.

The k_2 and k_3 terms model killing that is linear and quadratic in the concentration of complementary clones, and the k_4 term models natural death. The e_{2i} and e_{3i} factors model inhibition by specific T cell factors and are functions of the x_i and K_{ij}. They go to zero when the concentration of specific factors that inhibit killing of the ith clone reaches a certain level. We assume that the concentration of these factors depends on the concentration of i and i-like clones and on the the concentration of cells that stimulate these clones. We previously used

$$e_{qi} = \begin{cases} 1 & \text{if } x_i Y_i < C_q \\ 0 & \text{if } x_i Y_i > C_q \end{cases} \qquad q = 2,3; \quad i=1,N \qquad (3)$$

for e_{2i} and e_{3i}. As discussed in Hoffmann et al. 1988, equations (3) do not quite reflect the postulates of the model, and an improved formulation is being developed that involves similarity coefficients (Hoffmann, Lyons and

Mathewson, in preparation). We do not know exactly how many stable steady states the system (2) has, but we have reasons to believe that the number is at least of the order of 2^N. The same is true of the improved model.

The dynamics of this N-dimensional system can be portrayed on a 2-dimensional phase plane. We plot x_i against Y_i for each clone i. Solutions of the equation $dx_i/dt = 0$ are lines in this (x_i, Y_i) phase plane and are loci of equilibrium. Different clones can be in qualitatively different stable steady states, called the virgin, immune and suppressed stable states, all of which emerge from this model. These states correspond to separate loci of equilibrium in the phase plane, all of which satisfy $dx_i/dt = 0$. When the trajectories for all clones have converged onto these loci, the system as a whole is at a stable steady state.

We have ideas about how a third cell type, the macrophage, may play a role in switching between stable states, but have so far not attemped to mathematically model the switching, because it involves a rather large number of adjustable parameters.

Recent work by others on network modeling may be found in Perelson (1988). We feel that the scope of the symmetrical network model is clearly greater than that of any of the other models that have been formulated, and that future work is likely to be most productive if it builds on this base, instead of attempting to start from scratch with a new model.

10. Outlook

There are two fundamentally different ways of looking at AIDS. The Standard Model depicts AIDS as a problem in virology. In that picture, the immune system is the passive target and victim of the virus. The other view, presented here, is that the immune system is actively involved in AIDS pathogenesis. If this is the case, attempts to model AIDS without including the active role of the immune system will miss the essence of the problem. (The compromise position that pathogenesis is due to a combination of autoimmune mechanisms and direct virus mediated mechanisms is more complicated and therefore less appealing. It will probably be difficult to exclude this possibility definitively; the best argument against it might be that it violates the principle of Occam's razor.)

A major feature of the network model of pathogenesis is the role ascribed to alloimmunity, with concommitant anti-anti-self immunity. An experimental approach that could clarify the extent to which alloimmunity is important in AIDS is discussed in a recent paper about a method for measuring the level of similarity between sera (Hoffmann and Tufaro 1989).

More progress in understanding the pathogenesis of AIDS in detail can be expected to follow from a greater understanding of the immune system network.

For example, we would like to have a mathematical model of the T cell repertoire that could provide support for the postulated centre-pole topology, or for some other, yet to be formulated topology. We would like to know whether such topologies can be emergent properties of the system that can be seen in dynamical simulations to follow automatically from postulates about the building blocks. This could lead to a more complete understanding of how the great diversity and complexity of the immune system is reconciled with the stability implicit in the system's memory capabilities. When we are confident that we have the right network topology, we will be in a better position to model the interactions between HIV and the immune system.

The fact that the model leads to new ideas about preventing AIDS is exciting. A demonstration that injections of gp120 plus anti-gp120 can induce a suppressed state and protect against AIDS would, of course, not be a proof that the above model is correct in detail. But it would be very strong evidence that AIDS is an autoimmune disease, and would be the attainment of an important goal.

11. Postscript

A currently popular viewpoint in cellular immunology, which a reviewer of this paper suggested we discuss, is that T cells recognise only peptides that are presented on an accessory cell in the cleft of an MHC molecule (Davis and Bjorkman 1988). We are skeptical of this notion when it is expressed in such absolute terms, for reasons that we will discuss briefly in this section. We will try to explain how the experiments that have been interpreted in terms of this "antigen fragment" viewpoint might be better understood in terms of simple selectionist ideas.

The experiments supporting the antigen-fragment-in-the-MHC-cleft concept all involve secondary responses, and they involve three kinds of selective processes. This makes their interpretation more difficult than is sometimes realized. The three selection processes are: (1) a "survival of the fittest" process for T cells in the thymus prior to the involvement of the antigen, (2) a "survival of the fittest" process for T cells during the primary immune response, and (3) a "survival of the fittest" process for antigen fragments during both the primary and the secondary immune responses. The fragments that are broken down most slowly will be stimulatory for the longest time, and fragments that happen to fit into a cleft of the MHC molecules will be protected from degradation, and will presumably be able to stimulate a subset of the T cells that have previously been selected to recognise that particular MHC molecule. The apparent specificity repertoire of T cells, as seen in secondary responses, is a reflection of all three of these selection processes, and it may be a mistake to extrapolate from that apparent repertoire to the T cell repertoire in general. This view is supported by the fact that T cells can in fact be stimulated by reagents that do not include MHC molecules, such as conconavalin A and monoclonal antibodies against T cell receptors (Meuer et al. 1983; Staerz et al. 1985). The key physical property of such reagents is that they are able to cross-link the receptors of the T cell. Additional support for this view comes from work with T cell clones that respond to antigen plus MHC that will respond to antigen alone (without MHC) at higher doses of antigen (Walden et al. 1986; Thomas and Solvay 1986), or that bind antigen directly to their receptors (Siliciano et al. 1986).

Little direct evidence concerning the range of T cell specificities that participate in primary immune responses is available. In these circumstances, we feel it makes sense to be guided by the most basic clonal selection ideas. In a simple clonal selection picture, we would expect *a priori* that T cells should exist that are capable of responding to a wide range of antigens. The T cell repertoire is biased towards recognising MHC and MHC related antigens (by selection in the thymus), but when we take into account the notion of multispecificity that follows automatically from the cross-linking of receptors as the mechanism of specific stimulation of lymphocytes (reviewed in Hoffmann 1980), such biasing does not preclude the possibility of T cells being able to respond to a wider range of stimuli, at least in the early stages of a primary response. The extremely restricted range of specificities typically seen in secondary responses may be partly the result of selection during the primary response, rather than a strict intrinsic restriction in the peripheral T cell repertoire.

ACKNOWLEDGEMENT

This work is supported by grants from the National Health Research and Development Program of Health and Welfare Canada.

REFERENCES

Andrieu, J.M., P. Even, and A. Venet. (1986). AIDS and related syndromes as a viral-induced autoimmune disease of the immune system: an anti-MHC II disorder. Therapeutic implications. *AIDS Research* **2**, 163-174.

Beretta, A., F. Grassi, M. Pelagi, A. Clivio, C. Parravicini, G. Giovinazzo, F. Andronico, L. Lopalco, P. Verani, S. Butto, F. Titti, G. Battista Rossi, E. Ginelli, and A.G. Siccardi. (1987). HIV *env* glycoprotein shares a cross-reacting epitope with a surface protein present on activated human monocytes and involved in antigen presentation. *Eur. J. Immunol.* **17**, 1793-1798.

Borsos, T. and H.J. Rapp. (1965). Complement fixation on cell surfaces by 19S and 7S antibodies. *Science* **150**, 505-506.

Davis, M.M. and P.J. Bjorkman. (1988). T cell antigen receptor genes and T cell recognition. *Nature* **334**, 395-402.

Fitch, F.W. (1975). Selective suppression of immune responses. Regulation of antibody formation and cell-mediated immunity by antibody. *Prog. Allergy* **19**, 195-244.

Grant, M.D., M.S. Weaver, C. Tsoukas, and G.W. Hoffmann. (1989). Distribution of antibodies against denatured collagen in AIDS risk groups and homosexuals AIDS patients suggests a link between autoimmunity and the immunopathogenesis of AIDS. Submitted to *J. Immunol.*.

Harper, M.E., L.M. Marselle, R.C. Gallo, and F. Wongstaal. (1986). Detection of lymphocytes expressing human lymphotropic-T virus type III in lymph nodes and peripheral blood from infected individuals by in situ hybridization. *Proc. Nat. Acad. Sci. (USA)* **83**, 772-776.

Henry, C. and Jerne, N.K. (1968). Competition of 19S and 7S antigen receptors on the regulation of the primary immune response. *J. exp. Med.* **128**, 133-152.

Hoffmann, G.W. (1980). On network theory and H-2 restriction. *Contemp. Topics in Immunobiol.* **11**, 185-226.

Hoffmann, G.W. (1982). The application of stability criteria to the evaluation of network regulation models. In *Regulation of Immune Response Dynamics*, C. DeLisi and J. Hiernaux (eds.), pp. 137-162, CRC Press, Boca Raton, Florida.

Hoffmann, G.W., A. Cooper-Willis, and M. Chow (1986). A new symmetry: A anti-B is anti-(B anti-A), and reverse enhancement. *J. Immunol.* **137**, 61-68.

Hoffmann, G.W., T.A. Kion, R.B. Forsyth, K.G. Soga, and A. Cooper-Willis. (1988). The N-dimensional network. In *Theoretical Immunology, Part 2*, A. S. Perelson, (ed.), pp. 291-319, Addison-Wesley, Redwood City CA.

Hoffmann, G.W. (1988). On I-J, a network centre pole and AIDS. In *The Semiotics of Cellular Communication in the Immune System,* E. Sercarz, F. Celada, N.A. Mitchison and T. Tada (eds.), pp. 257-271, Springer-Verlag, New York.

Hoffmann, G.W. and F. Tufaro. (1989). Serological distance coefficients. Immunol. Letters, in press.

Hughes, R.A.C. (1974). Protection of rats from experimental allergic encephaphalomyelitis with antiserum to guinea pig spinal cord. *Immunology* **26,** 703-711.

Hsia, S., D.M. Doran, R.K. Shockley, P.C. Galle, C.L. Lutcher, and L.D. Hodge. (1984). Unregulated production of virus and/or sperm specific antibodies as a cause of AIDS. *Lancet,* June 2.

Imagawa, D.T., M.H. Lee, S.M. Wolinsky, K. Sano, F. Morales, S. Kwok, J.J. Sninsky, P.G. Nishanian, J. Giorgi, J.L. Fahey, J. Dudley, B.R. Visscher and R. Detels. Human immunodeficiency virus type 1 infection in homosexual men who remain seronegative for prolonged periods. *The New England Journal of Medicine.* **320,** 1458-1462.

Jerne, N.K. (1974). Towards a network theory of the immune system. *Ann. Immunol. (Inst. Pasteur)* **125C,** 373-389.

Kingman, S. (1988). Virus develops even with antibodies absent. *New Scientist,* 26 May.

Kion, T.A. and G.W. Hoffmann. (1989). MHC-mimicking antibodies in MRL-*lpr/lpr* mice. Manuscript in preparation.

Kopelman, R.G. and S. Zolla-Pazner. (1988). Association of human immunodeficiency virus infection and autoimmune phenomena. *Am. J. Med.* **84,** 82.

Martinez A.C., M.A.R. Marcos, A. de la Hera, C. Marquez, J.M. Alonso, M.L. Toribio, and A. Coutinho. (1988). Immunological consequences of HIV infection: advantage of being low responder casts doubts on vaccine development. *Lancet,* Feb. 27.

Meuer, S.C., J.C. Hogdon, R.E. Hussey, J.F. Protentis, S.F. Schlossman and E.L. Rheinherz. (1983). Antigen-like effects of monoclonal antibodies directed at receptors on human T cell clones. *J. Exp. Med.* **158,** 988.

Nakao, A. and Roboz-Einstein, E. (1965). Chemical and immunochemical studies with a dialyzable encephalitogenic compound from the bovine spinal cord. *Ann. N.Y. Acad. Sci.* **122,** 171.

Paterson, P.Y. and Harwin, S.M. (1963). Suppression of allergic encephalomyelitis in rats by means of antibrain serum *J. Exp. Med.,* **117,** 755.

Perelson, A.S. (1988). (ed.) *Theoretical Immunology, Part 2* Addison-Wesley, Redwood City CA.

Richter, P.H. (1975). A network theory of the immune response. *Eur. J. Immunol.* **5**, 350-354.

Safford, J.W. Jr. and S. Tokuda. (1971). Antibody-mediated suppression of the immune response: effect on the development of immunologic memory. *J. Immunol.* **107**, 1213-1225.

Shearer, G.M. (1986a). AIDS: An autoimmune pathologic model for the destruction of a subset of helper T lymphocytes. *Mount Sinai J. Med.* **53**, 609-615.

Shearer, G.M. (1986b). Allogeneic leukocytes as a possible factor in induction of AIDS in homosexual men. *N. Engl. J. Med.* **308**, 223-224.

Siliciano, R.F., T.J. Hemesath, J.C. Pratt, R.Z. Dintzis, H.M. Dintzis, O. Acuto, H.S. Shin and E.L. Reinherz (1986). Direct evidence for the existance of nominal antigen binding sites on T cell surface Ti αβ heterodimers of MHC restricted T cell clones. *Cell* **47**, 161-171.

Spouge, J.L. (1986). Increasing stability with complexity in a system composed of unstable subsystems. *J. Math. Analysis and Applications* **118**, 502-518.

Staerz, U.D., H-G. Rammensee, J.D. Benedetto and M.J. Bevan. (1985). Characterization of a murine monoclonal antibody specific for an allotypic determinant on T cell antigen receptor. *J. Immunol.* **134**, 3994-4000.

Stricker, R.B., T.M. McHugh, D.J. Moody, W.J.W. Morrow, D.P. Stites, M.A. Shuman, and J.A. Levy. (1987). An AIDS-related cytotoxic autoantibody with a specific antigen on stimulated $CD4^+$ T cells. *Nature* **327**, 710-713.

Tarkowski, A., Holmdahl, R., Rubin, K., Klareskog, L.A., Nilsson, L.A. and Gunnarsson, K. (1986). *Clin. exp. Immunol.* **63**, 441-449.

Thomas, D.W. and M.J. Solvay (1986). Direct stimulation of T lymphocytes by antigen-conjugated beads. *J. Immunol.* **137**, 419-421.

Uhr, J.W. and Baumann, J.B. 1961. Antibody formation. I. The suppression of antibody formation by passively administered antibody. *J. exp. Med.* **120**, 987.

Uhr J. W. and G. Möller (1968). Regulatory effect of antibody on the immune response. *Adv. Immunol.* **8**, 81-127.

Vulpé, M. (1959). *'Allergic' Encephalomyelitis* (M. W. Kies and E.C. Alvcord, Eds.), p. 457. Thomas, Illinois.

Walden, P., Z.A. Nagy and J. Klein (1986). Major histocompatability complex-restricted and unrestricted activation of helper T cell lines by liposome-bound antigens. *J. Mol. Cell. Immunol.* **2**, 191.

Ziegler, J.L. and D.P. Stites. (1986). Hypothesis: AIDS is an autoimmune disease directed at the immune system and triggered by a lymphotropic retrovirus. *Clin. Immunol. and Immunopath.* **41**, 305-313.

Zon, L.I. and Groopman, J.E. (1988). Hematologic manifestations of the human immune deficiency virus (HIV). *Seminars in Hematology* **25**, 208-218.

Lecture Notes in Biomathematics

Vol. 58: C. A. Macken, A. S. Perelson, Branching Processes Applied to Cell Surface Aggregation Phenomena. VIII, 122 pages. 1985.

Vol. 59: I. Nåsell, Hybrid Models of Tropical Infections. VI, 206 pages. 1985.

Vol. 60: Population Genetics in Forestry. Proceedings, 1984. Edited by H.-R. Gregorius. VI, 287 pages 1985.

Vol. 61: Resource Management. Proceedings, 1984. Edited by M. Mangel. V, 138 pages 1985.

Vol. 62: B. J. West, An Essay on the Importance of Being Nonlinear. VIII, 204 pages. 1985.

Vol. 63: Carme Torras i Genís, Temporal-Pattern Learning in Neural Models. VII, 227 pages, 1985.

Vol. 64: Peripheral Auditory Mechanisms. Proceedings, 1985. Edited by J.B. Allen, J.L. Hall, A. Hubbard, S. Neely and A. Tubis. VII, 400 pages. 1986.

Vol. 65: Immunology and Epidemiology. Proceedings, 1985. Edited by G.W. Hoffmann and T. Hraba. VIII, 242 pages. 1986.

Vol. 66: Nonlinear Oscillations in Biology and Chemistry. Proceedings, 1985. Edited by H.G. Othmer. VI, 289 pages. 1986.

Vol. 67: P.H. Todd, Intrinsic Geometry of Biological Surface Growth. IV, 128 pages. 1986.

Vol. 68: The Dynamics of Physiologically Structured Populations. Edited by J.A.J. Metz and O. Diekmann. XII, 511 pages. 1986.

Vol. 69: S.H. Strogatz, The Mathematical Structure of the Human Sleep-Wake Cycle. VIII, 239 pages. 1986.

Vol. 70: Stochastic Methods in Biology. Proceedings, 1985. Edited by M. Kimura, G. Kallianpur and T. Hida. VI, 229 pages. 1987.

Vol. 71: Mathematical Topics in Population Biology, Morphogenesis and Neurosciences. Proceedings, 1985. Edited by E. Teramoto and M. Yamaguti. IX, 348 pages. 1987.

Vol. 72: Modeling and Management of Resources under Uncertainty. Proceedings, 1985. Edited by T.L. Vincent, Y. Cohen, W.J. Grantham, G.P. Kirkwood, and J.M. Skowronski. VIII, 318 pages. 1987.

Vol. 73: Y. Cohen (Ed.), Applications of Control Theory in Ecology. Proceedings, 1986. VII, 101 pages. 1987.

Vol. 74: A.Y. Yakovlev, A.V. Zorin, Computer Simulation in Cell Radiobiology. VI, 133 pages. 1988.

Vol. 75: H. Knolle, Cell Kinetic Modelling and the Chemotherapy of Cancer. VIII, 157 pages. 1988.

Vol. 76: C.A. Macken, A.S. Perelson, Stem Cell Proliferation and Differentiation. VIII, 113 pages. 1988.

Vol. 77: A. Hastings (Ed.), Community Ecology. Proceedings, 1986. VII, 131 pages. 1988.

Vol. 78: J.J. Linderman, D.A. Lauffenburger, Receptor/Ligand Sorting Along the Endocytic Pathway. VI, 164 pages. 1989.

Vol. 79: P. Prusinkiewicz, J. Hanan, Lindenmayer Systems, Fractals, and Plants. V, 120 pages. 1989.

Vol. 80: D. House, Depth Perception in Frogs and Toads. VII, 135 pages. 1989.

Vol. 81: C. Castillo-Chavez, S.A. Levin, C.A. Shoemaker (Eds.), Mathematical Approaches to Problems in Resource Management and Epidemiology. Proceedings, 1987. VII, 327 pages.

Vol. 82: A. Yu. Yakovlev, N.M. Yanev, Transient Processes in Cell Proliferation Kinetics. VI, 214 pages. 1989.

Vol. 83: C. Castillo-Chavez (Ed.), Mathematical and Statistical Approaches to AIDS Epidemiology. IX, 405 pages. 1989.

www.ingramcontent.com/pod-product-compliance
Ingram Content Group UK Ltd.
Pitfield, Milton Keynes, MK11 3LW, UK
UKHW051449290926
15471UKWH00008B/1100
* 9 7 8 3 6 4 2 9 3 4 5 5 1 *